Principles and Practice of Regional Anaesthesia

For Churchill Livingstone

Publisher: Geoffrey Nuttall
Project Editor: Lowri Daniels
Copy Editor: Rich Cutler
Indexer: June Morrison
Production Controller: Neil Dickson
Sales Promotion Executive: Caroline Boyd

Principles and Practice of Regional Anaesthesia

Edited by

J. A. W. Wildsmith MD FRCAnaes
Consultant Anaesthetist, Royal Infirmary, Edinburgh and Part-time Senior Lecturer, University of Edinburgh

Edward N. Armitage MB BS DObstRCOG FRCAnaes
Consultant Anaesthetist, Brighton General Hospital and Royal Alexandra Hospital for Sick Children, Brighton

Foreword by
D. B. Scott MD FRCP (Edin) FFARCS
Consultant Anaesthetist, Edinburgh

Illustrated by
Patrick Elliott, *Medical Artist, Royal Hallamshire Hospital, Sheffield*

Photographs by
Ken Crowe, *Publicity Manager, Portex Ltd, Hythe, Kent*

SECOND EDITION

CHURCHILL LIVINGSTONE
EDINBURGH LONDON MADRID MELBOURNE NEW YORK AND TOKYO 1993

CHURCHILL LIVINGSTONE
Medical Division of Longman Group UK Limited

Distributed in the United States of America by Churchill
Livingstone Inc., 650 Avenue of the Americas, New York,
N.Y. 10011, and by associated companies, branches and
representatives throughout the world.

First edition 1987
Second edition 1993

ISBN 0-443-04475-9

British Library Cataloguing in Publication Data
A catalogue record for this book is available from the British
Library.

Library of Congress Cataloging in Publication Data
Principles and practice of regional anaesthesia/edited by J.A.W.
Wildsmith, Edward N. Armitage; foreword by D.B. Scott;
illustrated by Patrick Elliott; photographs by Ken Crowe.
— 2nd ed.   p.   cm.
Includes bibliographical references and index.
ISBN 0-443-04475-9
1. Conduction anesthesia.   I. Wildsmith, J. A. W.
II. Armitage, Edward N.
[DNLM: 1. Anesthesia, Conduction. WO 300 P957]
RD84.P75 1993
617.9′64—dc20
DNLM/DLC
for Library of Congress   92-49107
                                               CIP

The
publisher's
policy is to use
**paper manufactured
from sustainable forests**

Produced by Longman Singapore Publishers Pte. Ltd.
Printed in Singapore

Contents

Contributors

E. N. Armitage MB BS DObstRCOG FRCAnaes
Consultant Anaesthetist, Brighton General
Hospital and Royal Alexandra Hospital for Sick
Children, Brighton, UK

G. R. Arthur MSc PhD
Associate Professor of Anesthesia, Harvard
Medical School, Boston; Associate
Pharmacologist, Anesthesia Research
Laboratory, Brigham and Women's Hospital,
Boston, Massachusetts, USA

D. T. Brown MB ChB FRCAnaes
Consultant Anaesthetist, Royal Infirmary,
Edinburgh; Part-time Senior Lecturer,
University of Edinburgh, Edinburgh, UK

L. E. S. Carrie MB ChB FRCAnaes
Consultant Anaesthetist, John Radcliffe
Maternity Hospital and Nuffield Department of
Anaesthetics, John Radcliffe Hospital, Oxford;
Clinical Lecturer, University of Oxford, Oxford,
UK

W. A. Chambers MD FRCAnaes
Consultant Anaesthetist, Royal Infirmary,
Aberdeen, UK

J. E. Charlton FRCAnaes
Consultant in Anaesthetics and Pain Relief,
Royal Victoria Infirmary, Newcastle upon
Tyne, UK

D. A. Desgrand MB BS FRCAnaes
Consultant Anaesthetist, Queen Alexandra
Hospital, Portsmouth, UK

T. J. Hughes FRCAnaes
Consultant Anaesthetist, Doncaster Royal
Infirmary, Doncaster, UK

D. M. Justins MB BS FRCAnaes
Director, Pain Management Centre, St Thomas'
Hospital, London, UK

A. Lee MB ChB FRCAnaes
Consultant Anaesthetist, Royal Infirmary,
Edinburgh; Honorary Senior Lecturer,
University of Edinburgh, Edinburgh, UK

D. G. Littlewood BSc MB ChB FRCAnaes
Consultant Anaesthetist, Royal Infirmary,
Edinburgh; Honorary Senior Lecturer,
University of Edinburgh, Edinburgh, UK

J. H. McClure BSc MB ChB FRCAnaes
Consultant Anaesthetist, Simpson Memorial
Maternity Pavilion, Edinburgh and Royal
Infirmary, Edinburgh; Honorary Senior Lecturer,
University of Edinburgh, Edinburgh, UK

W. A. Macrae MB ChB FRCAnaes
Consultant Anaesthetist, Ninewells Hospital,
Dundee, UK

L. V. H. Martin MB ChB FRCAnaes DA
DObstRCOG
Consultant Anaesthetist, Royal Infirmary,
Edinburgh; Honorary Senior Lecturer,
University of Edinburgh, Edinburgh, UK

R. S. Neill MD FFARCSI
Consultant Anaesthetist, Royal Infirmary,
Glasgow, UK

A. P. Rubin MB BChir FRCAnaes
Consultant Anaesthetist, Charing Cross
Hospital, London, UK

N. B. Scott MB ChB FFARCSI
Lecturer in Anaesthesia, University of Glasgow,
Glasgow, UK

G. T. Tucker BPharm PhD
Professor of Clinical Pharmacology, University
of Sheffield, Sheffield, UK

J. A. W. Wildsmith MD FRCAnaes
Consultant Anaesthetist, Royal Infirmary,
Edinburgh; Part-time Senior Lecturer,
University of Edinburgh, Edinburgh, UK

Foreword

Since its first appearance in 1987, *Principles and Practice of Regional Anaesthesia* has achieved very considerable and not unexpected popularity. Thus the second edition is most welcome. The need for high-quality educational books in anaesthesia is especially great in the case of regional anaesthesia. Training in general anaesthesia in the United Kingdom and the Irish Republic are second to none, and the high standards are jealously protected by the Royal College of Anaesthetists in London and the Faculty of Anaesthetists in Dublin. The teaching of regional anaesthesia, on the other hand, has largely been left to individual centres where it is employed clinically in a sufficient proportion of cases to allow trainees the necessary exposure to become proficient.

The wave of popularity for regional anaesthesia which began 20 years ago, and is now worldwide, has continued unabated since 1987. In many centres the demand for training far outstrips the availability.

This book, with its clear style and no-nonsense approach, is ideal for the practical anaesthetist wishing to increase both his knowledge and the safe acquisition of skills. It does not, however, achieve this at the expense of the scientific basis of the subject. Controversial subjects are not shirked, and add to the pleasure and interest of the reader. It is now some 50 pages longer and has three new contributors, Nick Scott, Alastair Lee and Doug Justins.

We look forward to many new editions in the future.

D. B. S.

Preface

Over 100 years after the discovery of the local anaesthetic effects of cocaine there is wide variation in the extent to which regional anaesthesia is practised and taught in the United Kingdom. We hope that this book will give an indication of the scope and potential place of regional anaesthesia in British practice, as well as providing instruction in its use. The word *anaesthesia* is employed advisedly, because most patients wish to be totally unaware of surgery. *Analgesia* has been reserved for the provision of pain control in the postoperative period. The adjectives *local* and *regional* have been used interchangeably.

The successful use of regional anaesthesia requires a thorough knowledge of anatomy and skill in the appropriate technique of needle insertion, but there is much more to the subject. The anaesthetist must be able to determine which patients will and will not benefit. To do this successfully he must understand the effects of the techniques and the ways in which they differ from those of general anaesthesia. He must then choose from the several techniques and drugs available the most suitable for the particular patient and surgical procedure. Finally he must understand and cater for the needs of the patient during and after the operation itself.

The aim of this book is to help the specialist anaesthetist who is unfamiliar with the use of regional anaesthesia. The book is divided into two parts. The first outlines the general principles for safe, effective practice and the second describes anatomy and technique. Some aspects are considered in both sections. The main reason for this is to allow each chapter to stand on its own, but we have tried to avoid extensive repetition.

We have confined ourselves to those methods which our authors find useful in British practice and we have made no attempt to describe every known block. Few anaesthetists can expect to master the whole range of regional techniques to a level at which they can instruct others and we are grateful to our authors for contributing material on subjects in which they have special expertise. In an attempt to produce a uniform appearance and a cohesive style all the illustrations were prepared by the same artist or photographer and every script has been subjected to editorial changes.

No text can provide all the necessary information in such a practical subject – clinical training and experience are essential. Neither can anatomy be learnt entirely from a book, for there is no substitute for a visit to the dissecting or autopsy room, or for asking a surgical colleague to demonstrate structures exposed during surgery. We believe that regional anaesthesia has much to offer our patients, but it requires just as much attention to detail as general anaesthesia. Regional anaesthesia is *not* an excuse for taking short cuts in patient care – it is a very satisfying way of making patient care better.

J.A.W.W.
E.N.A.

Acknowledgements to the First Edition

We are very grateful to Glaxo Ltd., who contributed most generously towards the production costs of the book, and to Kenneth Crowe of Portex Ltd., who volunteered to take the photographs. We were very fortunate to secure the services of Patrick Elliott, medical artist at the Royal Hallamshire Hospital, Sheffield. It is a pleasure to acknowledge the contribution of our publishers. Fiona Foley first suggested the book and supported its early development; Peter Richardson helped see it to maturity.

Many others have helped us. Elspeth Taylor (secretary to the Department of Anaesthetics, University of Edinburgh), Iris Talloch (secretary to John Mills, South-East Thames Regional Librarian, who allowed us the use of a word processor) and Margaret Armstrong helped with script preparation. Mary Keyes, Sister-in-charge of Theatres, Royal Sussex County Hospital kindly gave us access to a theatre for clinical photography; Denise Laraway, Mary Hillis, Hannah and Helen Armitage acted as models; Dr Jane Turrill drew the clinical landmarks; and both Tony Morris, senior operating department assistant, and Jim Ruddle, instrument technician, gave invaluable help at the sessions.

Last, but far from least, we must thank our wives and families for their support and their tolerance of the many long editorial sessions that were necessary.

J.A.W.W.
E.N.A.

Acknowledgements to the Second Edition

The first edition of this book was very well received and we are grateful to all those who commented favourably upon it. We are also grateful to those who suggested improvements and we have taken every such suggestion into account when preparing this new edition. In that task we are delighted to have had the continued services of Patrick Elliot as Illustrator and Kenneth Crowe of Portex Limited as Photographer. It is impossible to exaggerate the value of their contribution to this book.

We again thank our authors for their manuscripts and for their acceptance and tolerance of our editorial intervention. Jill Halliday (Secretary to the Department of Anaesthetics, Royal Infirmary of Edinburgh) has provided secretarial services and Dr Alastair Nimmo (Research Fellow in the Department of Anaesthetics, Royal Infirmary of Edinburgh) assisted with the transfer of text from one word-processor to another. We also thank those patients and operating theatre staff at Charing Cross Hospital, London, and the Royal Sussex County Hospital, Brighton, for making possible the clinical photographs. Finally, we gratefully acknowledge the contribution of our publishers. Peter Richardson, Simon Fathers and Clare Wood-Allum have all been a great support to us.

J.A.W.W.
E.N.A.

1. The history and development of local anaesthesia

J. A. W. Wildsmith

The first steps

The possible production of local anaesthesia by this or by other means, is certainly an object well worthy of study and attainment. Surgeons everywhere seem more and more acknowledging the facility, certainty, and safety with which the state of general anaesthesia can be produced at will before operating, as well as the moral and professional necessity of saving their patients from all requisite pain. But if we could by any means induce a local anaesthesia, without that temporary absence of consciousness, which is found in the state of general anaesthesia, many would regard it as a still greater improvement in this branch of practice. If a man, for instance, could have his hand so obtunded that he could see, but not feel, the performance of amputation upon his own fingers, the practice of anaesthesia in surgery would, in all likelihood, advance and progress even still more rapidly than it has done.

This striking appreciation of the benefits of local anaesthesia was published in 1848, decades before local anaesthesia became a practical possibility. The paper from which it is taken was by James Young Simpson (Fig. 1.1) and in it he also described his own (unsuccessful) experiments with the topical application of various liquids and vapours (Simpson 1848). As it was published less than 2 years after Oliver Wendell Holmes had suggested the word 'anaesthesia' to William Morton, it probably represents the first use of the term 'local anaesthesia'. However, Simpson was aware that his were far from being the first attempts to produce peripheral insensibility, for he refers to some ancient methods (which he considered

'apocryphal') and to Moore's method of nerve compression (Fig. 1.2). Some success had been achieved with the latter towards the end of the 18th century and there are even earlier reports of its use.

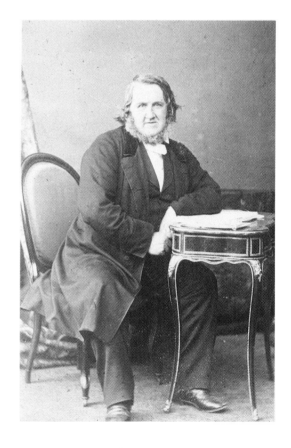

Fig. 1.1 James Young Simpson. Photograph courtesy of the Royal Medical Society.

1

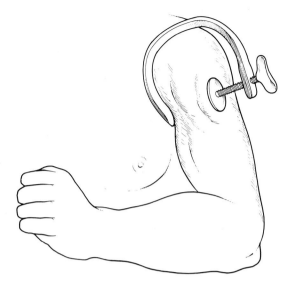

Fig. 1.2   James Moore's method of nerve compression.

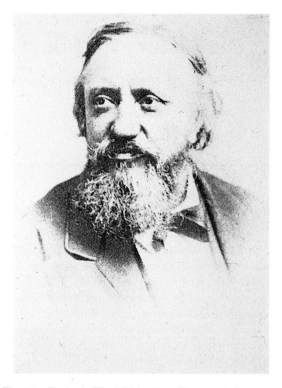

Fig. 1.3   Benjamin Ward Richardson. Photograph from Disciples of Aesculapius.

Another eminent Victorian who became interested in the possibility of producing local anaesthesia, and who appreciated its potential advantages over general anaesthesia, was Benjamin Ward Richardson (Fig. 1.3). He experimented with electricity before turning his attention to the use of cold. As with nerve compression, there are reports of the numbing effect of cold which go back to antiquity, the best known being by Napoleon's surgeon, Baron Larrey. Richardson's interest in this method (Richardson 1858) culminated in his introduction of the ether spray (Fig. 1.4), which worked by

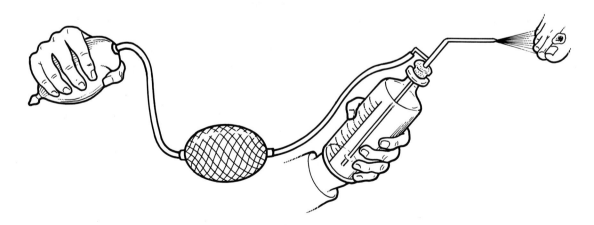

Fig. 1.4   Richardson's ether spray.

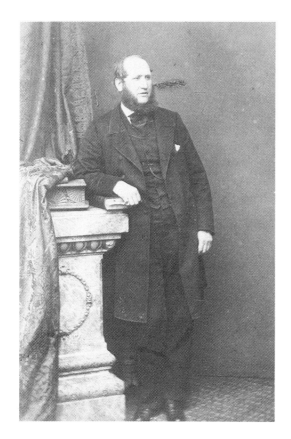

Fig. 1.5 Alexander Wood. Photograph courtesy of the Royal Medical Society.

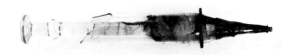

Fig. 1.6 Syringe devised by Wood. Photograph courtesy of the Royal College of Surgeons of Edinburgh.

Wood was nevertheless the first to think of the possibility of producing nerve blockade by drug injection and he has been called the 'father-in-law' of local anaesthesia – all he lacked was an agent which worked.

The introduction of cocaine

The sequence of events leading to the introduction of cocaine, the alkaloid derived from the leaves of *Erythroxylon coca*, into clinical practice began shortly after Wood's experiments with local morphine injection. Sporadic reports of the systemic effects of chewing the leaves had reached Europe from the time of the Spanish conquest, but it was not until 1857 that Montegazza gave the first detailed description of these actions. Prior to that, Gaedke had extracted some reddish crystals, but it was Niemann in 1860 who produced pure white crystals which he named cocaine. Niemann noted that these crystals produced numbness of the tongue, an observation subsequently confirmed by several other workers. Alexander Hughes Bennett was the first to demonstrate in animals that *injection* of cocaine produces sensory block, but, as with the work of others, the significance of his observation was not appreciated (Wildsmith 1983).

During this time cocaine came to be looked upon as a universal panacea and was even used to treat morphine addiction. A report of this latter use attracted the attention of Sigmund Freud, who reviewed the literature and started a programme of research, for which he enlisted the assistance of his friend Carl Koller (Fig. 1.7). Koller, like Freud, was a young graduate of the Vienna medical school who spent a portion of his time in Stricker's research laboratories. He wished to become an

evaporation and was the only practical method of local anaesthesia until the local action of cocaine was fully appreciated. Ethyl chloride supplanted ether as the cooling agent after 1880.

The development of the hypodermic syringe and needle was an important prerequisite for the use of cocaine for anything but topical application. They both evolved over many years and their introduction cannot be ascribed to any one person, but Alexander Wood (Fig. 1.5), a contemporary of Simpson, was, in 1853, the first to combine these items for hypodermic medication (Fig. 1.6). Wood was a physician interested in the treatment of neuralgia and he reasoned that morphine might be more effective if it was injected close to the nerve supplying the affected area (Wood 1855). The effect of his morphine was of course central, but

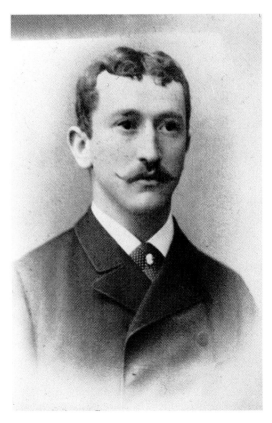

Fig. 1.7   Carl Koller. Photograph courtesy of Mrs Hortense Koller Becker.

ophthalmologist and, having heard from his teacher – Ferdinand Arlt – of the disadvantages of general anaesthesia for eye surgery, had applied a variety of agents to the conjunctiva without success (Wildsmith 1984). Koller was aware of the reports of cocaine's ability to produce local insensibility, but even he did not appreciate their significance at first. It was only a chance comment from a colleague that made him realize that he had in his possession the local anaesthetic agent for which he had been searching (Becker 1963). Experiments, firstly with animals, then on himself and colleagues, led on to clinical trial during the summer of 1884. A preliminary communication was read (by a former colleague – Joseph Brettaur – since Koller could not afford the trip) at the Heidelberg meeting of the German Ophthalmological Society on 15 September 1884 and from there the news spread with amazing speed.

Immediate developments

The full account of his own work (Koller 1884) appeared shortly after and many others reported their experience before the end of the year. Although there is evidence (Faulconer & Keys 1965) that William Burke may have absolute priority for the first nerve block, which was performed before the end of November 1884, credit is usually given to William Halsted and Richard Hall of New York. Before the end of 1885 they had blocked virtually every peripheral somatic nerve, including the brachial plexus, and had demonstrated the effectiveness of such methods (Boulton 1984).

Central neural blockade may be considered to have been introduced almost as soon. We will never know for certain whether the New York neurologist Leonard Corning produced epidural or subarachnoid block in 1885, but there is no doubt that at that early stage he deliberately injected cocaine between the posterior spinous processes of both a dog and a patient and produced block of the lower half of the body. Although he suggested that it might be used in surgery no further development of the method took place until nearly the end of the century. In 1891 Quincke in Kiel, Germany, had shown lumbar puncture to be a practical procedure and it was in the same centre in 1898 that August Bier performed the first spinal blocks for surgery. However, Bier abandoned the technique before he had gained much experience with it and it was Tuffier, working independently in Paris, who was responsible for popularizing the method in Europe. In the USA Tait, Caglieri and Matas were the early pioneers.

Pharmacological advances

The major factor in Bier's decision to abandon spinal anaesthesia was the toxicity of cocaine. It was also difficult to sterilize, brief in duration and had exacted a terrible price from pioneers like Halsted and Hall, who became addicted to it as a result of experimenting on themselves. Because of these factors the early use of cocaine was largely

limited to topical application. Later Schleich in
Germany and Reclus in France developed safe
dose regimes for, and popularized, infiltration
anaesthesia. Braun increased its duration and
reduced toxicity, first by the use of a tourniquet
and later by adding adrenaline to the solution.

Widespread use of local methods had to await
the introduction of safer drugs. Niemann in his
pioneer work had hydrolysed benzoic acid from
cocaine and it was the search for other benzoic
acid esters that produced new local anaesthetics.
Amylocaine (Stovaine) was introduced in 1903
and was popular for spinal anaesthesia until it was
shown to be irritant, but it was the development of
procaine by Einhorn in 1904 that was the really
significant advance. Its low toxicity, lack of
addictive properties and relative stability ensured
its popularity for the techniques already in use and
made feasible the development of new techniques
for which larger doses of drug were required.

Procaine is still far from ideal for it hydrolyses
when heated in solution, does not have a particularly long duration of action and may induce
allergic reactions. Many other drugs were tried,
but in the first 50 years after Koller's introduction
of cocaine the only ones to become established
were amethocaine and cinchocaine. Both are
potent and toxic, but were well suited to spinal
anaesthesia for which they have become the
standard agents.

The 1930s saw the start of the next major
advance. Working in Stockholm on the structure
of the alkaloid gramine, Erdtman – an organic
chemist believing in the importance of the senses
in analysis – tasted one of the substances that had
been produced as a precursor of gramine. The
significance of the ensuing numbness was appreciated immediately and the search for a clinically
useful derivative was started by Erdtman and
continued by Nils Lofgren, who synthesized
lignocaine in 1943. Perhaps almost as important as
the synthesis of lignocaine was Lofgren's system-
atic study of a whole range of compounds
(Lofgren 1948), so laying the foundations for all
subsequent studies of local anaesthetic drugs.
From these studies have come derivatives of
lignocaine such as mepivacaine, prilocaine, bupivacaine and etidocaine.

While the introduction of these agents has
considerably widened the scope of local anaesthesia they are essentially variations on a theme. Since
the development of lignocaine the most important
work has been in the field of membrane physiology. Many workers have contributed to this, the
most notable being Hodgkin and Huxley. Use of
apparatus such as the voltage clamp has produced
major advances in our knowledge of the mechanism of nerve conduction and its block by drugs at
the molecular level. This has yet to lead to the
development of new drugs, but a number of
alternative approaches continue to be investigated
(Kendig & Courtney 1991).

Concurrent studies of the pharmacokinetics of
local anaesthetic drugs have made a more practical
contribution to our knowledge for they have
indicated the most appropriate doses and agents
for the various techniques. They have thus played
an important part in basing clinical local anaesthesia on sound scientific principles.

Developments in technique

As has been mentioned, most local techniques had
been described by 1900, even if they were not
widely used. In 1906 Sellheim introduced paravertebral and intercostal block and 2 years later Bier,
taking advantage of the low toxicity of procaine,
developed his technique for intravenous regional
anaesthesia. Another important development at
about this time was Barker's description of the way
in which the curves of the lumbar spine and gravity
affect the spread of intrathecally injected solutions.

Epidural block is very much a product of the
20th century. The sacral approach, described
independently by Sicard and Cathelin in 1901, was
used by Stoeckel for analgesia during vaginal
delivery in 1909. The lumbar approach is considered to have been first described by Pages in Spain
in 1921, but he died soon afterwards and the
technique was 'rediscovered' and popularized by
Dogliotti in Italy a decade later. He used the loss
of resistance technique. The lumbar approach was
first used in labour in 1938 by Graffagnino and
Seyler. Massey Dawkins performed the first
epidural in Britain in 1942.

Most other subsequent advances in technique may be looked upon as being refinements or rediscoveries of techniques that had been described previously. This is not to deny the importance of these latter authors because they did a great deal to improve and popularize the practice of local anaesthesia. One important technical development that does deserve mention is the introduction of continuous methods of local anaesthesia. Continuous spinal anaesthesia was introduced by Lemmon in the USA in 1940. He left the spinal needle in situ (projecting through a gap in the operating table) and connected it to a length of rubber tubing through which repeated injections of procaine were made. In 1945 Tuohy described his needle for the insertion of a catheter into the subarachnoid space. This was adapted by Curbelo in 1949 to produce continuous lumbar block, although the first continuous epidural blocks are attributed to Hingson and Edwards, who used the caudal approach in 1942.

The popularity and use of local anaesthesia

Ever since Koller's original work, the popularity of local anaesthesia has waxed and waned, like that of many other medical developments. The announcement of his work produced a massive wave of enthusiasm, which was tempered as the problems of cocaine became appreciated. The first resurgence of interest came with the introduction of safer drugs at the beginning of the century, and the second as a result of the efforts of Labat, Lundy, Maxson, Odom and Pitkin in the USA in the years between the two World Wars.

In Britain, general anaesthesia has traditionally been administered by a qualified doctor (though not always by a specialist who practised anaesthesia exclusively). Since the conduct of general anaesthesia has been his entire responsibility, standards have usually been high. In contrast, local and regional techniques, if they were used at all, were performed by the surgeon, whose interest and attention were divided between anaesthetic and operation. Local anaesthesia was not seen to best advantage under such circumstances. However, when the examination for the Diploma in Anaesthesia was instituted in 1935, the curriculum

included local anaesthesia. This, together with the establishment of anaesthesia as an independent speciality within the National Health Service in 1948, did much to encourage local techniques.

Unfortunately the years between 1950 and 1955 saw a sharp decrease in the use of local, particularly spinal, anaesthesia in Britain. The many advances in general anaesthesia then taking place were partly responsible since they encouraged the belief that a local technique was unnecessary. More important though was the fear of severe neurological damage. The report entitled 'The grave spinal cord paralyses caused by spinal anesthesia' written in 1950 in New York by a British-trained neurologist, Foster Kennedy (Kennedy et al 1950), was followed by the Woolley and Roe case (Cope 1954, Hutter 1990), and the use of local anaesthesia all but died out. That it did not do so entirely was due to anaesthetists such as Macintosh, Gillies, Massey Dawkins and Lee who were prepared to advocate, use and teach local techniques. Subsequently, many reports (Lee and Atkinson 1978) appeared describing very large numbers of cases without neurological sequelae, and local anaesthesia became re-established in British practice during the 1980s.

There were more positive influences. The advantages of lignocaine and its derivatives – potent, predictable, heat-resistant and virtually free of allergic side-effects – should not be underestimated. The introduction of bupivacaine was particularly important because its long duration of action allows repeated injection with relatively little risk of cumulative toxicity. This was a major factor in the increased use of continuous epidural techniques in labour. Local techniques are very appropriate for the obstetric patient because they are effective and exert minimal effects on the child. Anaesthetists observing these benefits were encouraged to teach these methods and to try them in other branches of practice.

As anaesthetists gradually became aware that general anaesthesia cannot provide the ideal answer to every anaesthetic problem they turned increasingly to local methods. Even in very major surgery local anaesthetic techniques are of value in providing block of afferent stimuli and reducing the pain and stress suffered by the patient. This concept is far from new. As early as 1902 Harvey Cushing was advocating the combination of local with general anaesthesia to reduce 'shock', a concept that was developed by Crile into 'Anociassociation'. The term 'balanced anaesthesia' is very common today, but it implies the triad of sleep produced by inhalational means, profound analgesia with opioid drugs and muscle relaxation by neuromuscular block. In fact, when Lundy first used the term in 1926 he intended that the second and third parts of the triad would be produced by local anaesthetic injection.

There have been other advances which, although more difficult to quantify, have directly or indirectly helped the cause of local anaesthesia. For example, developments in the field of medical plastics have resulted in safe and reliable syringes, catheters and filters; and the anaesthetist can select from a wide variety of sedative and anxiolytic drugs which, carefully used, can greatly improve the patient's acceptance of a nerve block. Of great importance has been the understanding of the effects and treatment of sympathetic block. Ephedrine became available in 1924 and was first used to treat hypotension during spinal anaesthesia in 1927, but readily available intravenous fluids and equipment for their administration are more recent developments.

It is not inappropriate to conclude by mentioning the organizations which seek to promote the use of local anaesthetic techniques. The American Society of Regional Anesthesia was formed in 1975 and became firmly established and its younger European counterpart has grown rapidly. The fundamental aim of both is to ensure that properly managed local anaesthesia is an essential part of the armamentarium of the specialist anaesthetist.

FURTHER READING

Atkinson R S, Rushman G B, Lee J A 1982 A synopsis of anaesthesia, 8th edn. Wright-PSG, Bristol
Ellis E S 1946 Ancient anodynes: primitive anaesthesia and allied conditions. Heinemann, London

Keys T E 1963 The history of surgical anesthesia, 2nd edn. Dover, New York
Liljestrand G 1971 The historical development of local anesthesia. International encyclopedia of pharmacology and therapeutics, vol 1, pp 1–38. Pergamon Press, Oxford

REFERENCES

Becker H K 1963 Carl Koller and cocaine. Psychoanalytic Quarterly 32: 309–373
Boulton T B 1984 Classical file. Survey of Anesthesiology 28: 150–152
Cope R W 1954 The Woolley and Roe case. Anaesthesia 9: 249–270
Faulconer A, Keys T E 1965 Foundations of anesthesiology, vol II, pp 769–845. Charles C Thomas, Springfield
Hutter C D D 1990 The Woolley and Roe case. A reassessment. Anaesthesia 45: 859–864
Kendig J J, Courtney K R 1991 Editorial: New modes of nerve block. Anesthesiology 74: 207–208
Kennedy F G, Effron A S, Perry G 1950 The grave spinal cord paralyses caused by spinal anesthesia. Surgery, Gynecology and Obstetrics 91: 385–398
Koller C 1884 On the use of cocaine for producing anaesthesia of the eye. Lancet ii: 990–992
Lee J A, Atkinson R S 1978 Sir Robert Macintosh's lumbar puncture and spinal analgesia: intradural and extradural, 4th edn. pp179–181. Churchill Livingstone, Edinburgh.
Lofgren N 1948 Studies on local anesthetics: xylocaine, a new synthetic drug. Morin Press, Worcester (reprinted)
Richardson B W 1858 On local anaesthesia and electricity. Medical Times and Gazette i: 262–263
Simpson J Y 1848 Local anaesthesia, notes on its production by chloroform etc in the lower animals, and in man. Lancet ii: 39–42
Wildsmith J A W 1983 Three Edinburgh men. Regional Anesthesia 8: 1–5
Wildsmith J A W 1984 Carl Koller (1857–1944) and the introduction of cocaine into anesthetic practice. Regional Anesthesia 9: 161–164
Wood A 1855 New method of treating neuralgia by the direct application of opiates to the painful points. Edinburgh Medical Journal 82: 265–281

2. The features of regional anaesthesia

N. B. Scott   D. T. Brown

Local and regional anaesthesia have much to offer patients, surgeons and anaesthetists. The simplicity of administration of topical, infiltration and minor nerve block anaesthesia has ensured, and will continue to ensure, their popularity for casualty work, dentistry and minor surgery. General anaesthesia in these situations is usually unnecessary and in any case there are insufficient anaesthetists to provide it for all patients. Regional anaesthesia preserves consciousness and the patient's protective reflexes, and is widely used for more major surgery where there is a shortage of anaesthetists. Single handed, practitioners can perform a local block, observe its effects and then operate in relative safety. They are often working in situations where there is not the money to purchase supplies of expensive drugs and maintain modern general anaesthetic equipment. The lower cost of regional anaesthesia can be a considerable advantage in such circumstances.

Regional block has also been advocated as a means of avoiding the morbidity and mortality associated with general anaesthesia. It has been argued (Rosen 1981) that this would not necessarily reduce the number of anaesthesia-related deaths since unskilled use of spinals and epidurals might be at least as dangerous. This might be so, but misses the real point that, for a patient treated by an anaesthetist with the same degree of competence at both general and regional anaesthesia, the latter should be safer. Failure to intubate the trachea and aspiration of gastric content are far more difficult to manage than hypotension of sympathetic origin, no matter how skilled the anaesthetist.

General anaesthesia tends to be preferred where there are the staff and facilities to provide it safely, but even when it is practised to a high standard it is increasingly apparent that there are other reasons for using local blocks. Many of the minor sequelae and complications of general anaesthesia can be minimized or avoided altogether. The conditions required for a particular operation may be provided simply and without polypharmacy. There is an increasing body of evidence to show that the physiological 'stress' to which the patient is exposed during and immediately after surgery is considerably decreased by local anaesthesia. Few clinicians appreciate that neither general anaesthesia nor the opioids significantly reduce the endocrine response to surgery and trauma, while effective regional anaesthesia ablates it (Scott 1991). As a result the morbidity, and perhaps even the mortality, of anaesthesia and surgery have been reduced by the use of local blocks even for major operations (see below).

This is not to deny that there are potential drawbacks to the wider use of local blocks by the specialist anaesthetist. One very practical objection is that they will significantly prolong the operation list. This may be true for the occasional and inexpert user because the block may take longer to perform than the induction of general anaesthesia, and it is particularly true if the theatre staff are unused to the routine of such procedures. These delays may be quite justifiable in the interests of a particular patient, but soon become unacceptable if lists are repeatedly interrupted. However, proficiency, speed and success rate increase when blocks are practised regularly and time may actually be saved at the end of the procedure because there is little to do but move a conscious pain-free patient back to bed. If consecutive patients are to have local blocks it is possible, given the right circumstances, to save time by performing the second block while the first operation is being finished. Appropriate assistance and careful planning are the essential requirements.

The major complications of regional anaesthesia are related to systemic toxicity, either from the injected drug, which may contain a vasoconstrictor, or from the effects of the block itself. Drug toxicity is usually due to accidental intravascular injection or, more rarely, to the administration of an overdose. Both mishaps are avoidable. Careful technique and the correct choice of drug, concentration and volume should virtually eliminate them as causes of complications. Arterial hypotension due to sympathetic paralysis is the commonest 'systemic' effect of central blocks. Choice of an appropriate technique should minimize unwanted spread of local anaesthetic solution to the upper thoracic dermatomes, but if this should occur, or if it is necessary for a particular case, clear guidelines for management are available (Ch. 5).

Hypotension is a good example of a feature of regional anaesthesia which is usually considered undesirable, but which can be an advantage in certain circumstances. Conversely, preservation of consciousness – commonly considered an advantage – may be unacceptable to the nervous patient undergoing anything more than the most minor procedure. Similarly, each feature of regional anaesthesia has its good and bad aspects. When choosing an anaesthetic for a particular patient and operation, the anaesthetist should be able to assess the advantages and disadvantages of all techniques – local and general – and decide which is the most appropriate.

For many patients and situations, local anaesthesia is the only appropriate technique. During highly specialized surgery it may have little if any place, although the instances in which this is true are becoming fewer. In between these extremes there are many patients for whom a correctly chosen and well-managed local anaesthetic technique has much to offer, especially if the anaesthetist is prepared to combine it with sedation or light general anaesthesia. The aim of this chapter is to suggest why, where, how and when local anaesthesia may be of benefit by discussing its main features.

Simplicity of administration

The simplicity of local anaesthesia for the non-specialist anaesthetist undertaking relatively minor surgery has been referred to. For the specialist, dealing with more major surgery, regional anaesthesia may also simplify the procedure. A single intrathecal injection of one drug will produce excellent conditions for many procedures – complete anaesthesia, muscle relaxation and a reduction in the amount of bleeding. The patient's life is not dependent on the proper functioning and constant monitoring of complex general anaesthetic equipment. Because such equipment is unnecessary and the drugs employed are relatively inexpensive, the costs are lower. Simplicity of administration also means that the practitioner with a good knowledge of anatomy can easily become proficient in these methods.

The ease of administration, particularly of infiltration and topical anaesthesia, does produce problems. Minimal training or complacency may result in a lack of awareness of, or an inability to treat, complications. Drug overdose producing systemic toxicity, cardiorespiratory arrest from poorly managed high spinal or epidural block and pneumothorax after supraclavicular brachial plexus block are all potentially fatal complications. It is important to be aware that the combination of sympathetic block with even a minor degree of blood loss or dehydration will cause more hypotension than will general anaesthesia in the same circumstances. Thus, knowledge of the pharmacology of the drugs, of the complications of the techniques to be used, and training in appropriate methods of resuscitation are essential.

Preservation of consciousness

By its nature, uncomplicated regional anaesthesia will preserve consciousness, a desirable end it itself for the occasional patient who is terrified of being made unconscious. However, it is the secondary effects of unconsciousness that are important for the majority of patients. For example, the obstetric patient receiving regional analgesia is aware of her surroundings and the birth of her child, is able to maintain and protect her own airway and can cooperate with her attendant staff. There is also minimal fetal depression. These factors add up to a major argument for the use of local techniques.

The ability of the conscious patient to maintain and protect the airway and to cooperate are also of great value in dental practice, a field where airway obstruction during general anaesthesia is an ever-present risk. Minor orthopaedic trauma is often dealt with under general anaesthesia although it is recognized that gastric emptying is delayed in such patients. Many of these injuries are peripheral and eminently suitable for local techniques.

In some circumstances general anaesthesia may be preferred even though the risk of pulmonary aspiration is high, as for example in emergency surgery for gastrointestinal obstruction. The general condition of these patients tends to be poor because of the effects of the obstruction – particularly dehydration leading to hypovolaemia – and the presence of intercurrent disease. If a spinal or an epidural is to be used, a block to the mid-thoracic region is required. Controlled fluid administration with central venous pressure monitoring and therapy with inotropes and vasopressors will probably be necessary to prevent the hypovolaemia causing serious hypotension. Each of these treatments has its own complications which will increase the overall morbidity of the procedure.

A conscious, cooperative patient is an advantage in other situations. Surgery for varicose veins on the back of the legs or for pilonidal sinus requires the patient to be prone. If a local technique is used the patient can help to position him- or herself, indicate that the position is comfortable and confirm that respiration is unimpeded. A spinal anaesthetic can be used very effectively, although it is important to use a solution that will not spread to the thoracic dermatomes because treatment of a high block in a prone patient is difficult. Finally, the conscious or lightly sedated patient may be able to warn of the subjective effects of complications

at an early stage. The diabetic may recognize and report the initial symptoms of hypoglycaemia and, during transurethral surgery, patient distress may arouse suspicion that bladder irrigation fluid has entered the circulation.

Most of the problems of regional anaesthesia due to preservation of consciousness relate to patients' anxiety about being aware during the performance of the block and the surgical procedure. The majority of British patients expect to be asleep and it is at least arguable that, although many European and North American patients expect to be awake during their operations, they might prefer to be asleep. To undergo major surgery under regional anaesthesia alone is an unpleasant experience and occasionally an anxious patient will faint. This *can* occur in the supine patient and it may be mistaken for other causes of hypotension. In addition, a whole operating list of conscious patients can place an added strain on all members of the theatre team. Finally, because most operating tables are uncomfortable, the conscious patient may become restless.

Explanation and reassurance can help, but the more nervous the patient and the longer the surgery, the greater is the need for some kind of sedation. Oral premedication is rarely contraindicated, and intravenous or inhalational sedation can both be used to produce amnesia while preserving the benefits of consciousness. However, some patients may be so frightened that they will not tolerate surgery with anything but complete loss of consciousness and then of course these particular benefits may be lost.

Analgesia

The most outstanding advantage of even *single-shot* local anaesthetic techniques is the excellent analgesia (without central depression) produced. For the patient this means a period of complete postoperative analgesia during which the administration of oral or parenteral analgesics can be timed to become effective before the block wears off. This results in a gradual, rather than a sudden, awareness of pain and reduces the requirement for subsequent analgesic therapy with a consequent reduction in the side-effects of both opioids and non-steroidal anti-inflammatory drugs (NSAIDs). For instance, the use of caudal block for haemor- rhoidectomy results not only in much greater patient comfort, but in an earlier return of bowel function because of reduced opioid requirements (Berstock 1979).

Catheter techniques may be used to prolong analgesia for as long as is necessary. Continuous epidurals make the postoperative period consider- ably less unpleasant and will allow the patient to cooperate fully during nursing procedures, chest physiotherapy and mobilization. Gastric emptying is much closer to normal when epidural block is used for postoperative analgesia than it is if systemic opioids are used (Nimmo et al 1978). As a result oral intake and medication can be commenced earlier than is possible after opioid analgesia.

The analgesia produced by local blocks may also simplify certain general anaesthetics as well as providing greater comfort for the patient. This is best seen in surgery for certain minor but ex- tremely painful operations such as nail-bed ablation, distal orthopaedic procedures (e.g. Mitchell's osteotomy) or Lord's anal dilatation. Opioids are contraindicated in ambulant patients because of their sedative and emetic effects. A local technique will provide very useful postoperative analgesia, even if the block is, in itself, insufficient for the surgery. A lighter plane of general anaes- thesia can then be used, so recovery time is shorter and the patient can mobilize sooner.

Side-effects and sequelae

In addition to its effect on postoperative pain, regional anaesthesia may also reduce the incidence of other less major sequelae of anaesthesia and surgery, although freedom from wound pain may make the patient more aware of other sources of discomfort such as a venepuncture site and a nasogastric tube. Few controlled studies have been performed of the relative incidence of these sequelae, but Table 2.1 shows data from two reasonably comparable groups of patients having surgery with either spinal or general anaesthesia. All but one of the symptoms occurred less frequently after spinal anaesthesia, the exception

Table 2.1   Total incidence (%) of minor postoperative complications after spinal and general anaesthesia (from Dempster 1984). The incidence of complications graded by the patient as severe is also shown.

Side-effect	Spinal		General anaesthesia	
	Total	Severe	Total	Severe
Nausea	9	0	40	6
Vomiting	15	2	43	6
Headache	34	6	23	6
Sore throat	2	0	30	0
Muscle pains	4	0	9	0
Backache	28	2	32	6
Urinary difficulty	6	0	30	0

being headache, although the proportion of pa- tients who graded this as 'severe' was the same in each group.

Other published work (Lanz et al 1982) has suggested that the differences in minor sequelae might not be quite so clearly in favour of regional anaesthesia, but in that study the patient was responsible for the selection of the type of anaesthesia. Patients who have suffered severe nausea and vomiting after previous general anaes- thetics are particularly appreciative of regional techniques which minimize the requirement for opioids. However, no method can prevent certain patients from reacting to the psychological stress of surgery by becoming nauseated and even vomiting, particularly if they are given little in the way of perioperative sedation.

In addition, there are some disadvantages to the extension of the effects of these techniques into the postoperative period. Some patients find pro- longed lack of feeling, especially in the legs, unpleasant and urinary retention may occur, notably if large volumes of intravenous fluids have been used to maintain blood pressure. A high standard of medical and nursing care will minimize these complications and in the obstetric unit the staff/patient ratio is high enough for this to be provided. In the general ward the routine use of continuous epidurals requires careful appraisal of the staffing available. Finally, there will always be concern about the major sequelae of continuous blocks such as haematoma and abscess formation.

In a recent review (Scott & Hibbard 1990) of 505 000 obstetric epidurals there were two cases of epidural haematoma and one abscess, with two of the patients suffering permanent sequelae.

Sympathetic block

Until recently sympathetic block was widely considered to be a disadvantage of regional anaesthesia, but there is increasing evidence that it is beneficial. Because of the improved outcome in cardiac surgical patients receiving β-adrenoceptor blocking agents, Roizen (1988) has advocated that they should be used routinely in the surgical patient. Virtually all regional anaesthetic techniques produce sympathetic, as well as somatic, block so that many of the same effects are produced. The influence of these will depend not only on the site and level of the block, but also on the dose of local anaesthetic, the dose of vasoconstrictor (if used), the presence of intercurrent disease and the pre-existing state of the circulation. The detailed effects of sympathetic block produced by epidural injection have been reviewed (Bowler et al 1985), and the balance between sympathetic and parasympathetic nerve activity is particularly important so a sound knowledge of the autonomic control of the circulation is needed (Mason 1965).

Cardiovascular effects. In supine, healthy volunteers block up to, and including, the upper thoracic segments may have remarkably little effect on arterial pressure. Cardiac output and limb and organ blood flow are maintained, or even increased. Studies in normovolaemic patients without pain tend to confirm this except that hypotension is more likely to be seen as the block extends above T_5, when the sympathetic innervation to the heart is interrupted. Peripheral flow is usually increased in spite of the hypotension.

When a block is performed in a patient in pain, cardiac output and arterial pressure decrease, but this is usually only to 'normal' levels because pain causes an increase in sympathetic activity. Sympathetic block may result in cardiovascular collapse in the sitting or hypovolaemic patient because the circulation has been maintained by the increased sympathetic activity. The patient with severe valvular heart disease may be less able to compensate for peripheral vasodilation, because cardiac output may be relatively 'fixed'. Sympathetic block may also cause an unexpected degree of hypotension in the anxious patient, because the accompanying parasympathetic overactivity is then unopposed, and the patient simply faints.

The effects of an epidural block may be different from those of a spinal of similar extent. Very high systemic concentrations of local anaesthetic may be produced by the former and may contribute to circulatory depression, but it is usually considered that epidural block is less likely to cause hypotension. This may be because an epidural block usually spreads more slowly than a spinal so that there is more time for auto-compensation to occur. However, hypotension may be more marked when a local anaesthetic solution containing adrenaline is used for an epidural (Kennedy et al 1966) because the dose absorbed is only sufficient to produce β-adrenergic effects. A comparison of the cardiovascular effects of epidurals and spinals was carried out by Ward and colleagues (1965).

Moderate hypotension improves the surgical field and decreases blood loss by a combination of arterial *and* venous hypotension (Modig 1988). Even in the cardiac patient, a moderate degree of hypotension will improve performance because it is accompanied by reductions in preload, afterload and heart rate (Merin 1981). Thoracic epidural techniques have also been shown to improve endocardial blood flow (Klassen et al 1980). Sympathetic block produces an increase in lower limb blood (and arterial graft) flow and this may be partly responsible for the reduction in thromboembolic disease reported after regional anaesthesia (Thorburn et al 1980). This antithrombotic effect may also be related to a direct pharmacological action of the local anaesthetic drug on blood coagulability and fibrinolysis (Modig et al 1983a, b).

Respiratory effects. Sympathetically mediated reflexes result in substantial inhibition of normal breathing patterns for many days after surgery (Guenter 1984). This may partially explain the beneficial effect that high spinal or epidural block has on postoperative respiratory function (Spence & Smith 1971). However, these techniques also block the sympathetic supply to the lungs and airways. In theory this may precipitate severe bronchospasm in the asthmatic patient because of unopposed parasympathetic activity. Therefore the anaesthetist must be aware of the need to avoid this complication and to treat it promptly if it occurs. It should be remembered that severe bronchospasm may develop during general anaesthesia. By removing the need for airway instrumentation and by blocking afferent stimuli (both potent causes of reflex bronchospasm) regional anaesthesia can prevent this complication.

Gastrointestinal effects. Because of unopposed parasympathetic activity, sympathetic block leads to an increase in gastrointestinal motility and relaxation of many sphincters, although oesophageal sphincter tone is preserved (Thoren et al 1988). Incontinence is a theoretical consequence, but occurs no more often than during general anaesthesia. Bowel rupture may be more likely if there is an obstruction and this is another reason why spinal and epidural blocks should be used with great caution, if at all, in such cases. However, in elective bowel surgery regional anaesthesia has very definite benefits (for a review see Aitkenhead 1984). The sympathetic block may increase colonic blood flow (Johansson et al 1988), and use of a regional technique to provide muscle relaxation avoids the need to administer neostigmine, which may increase the incidence of anastomotic breakdown. However, if neostigmine *is* used to reverse neuromuscular block in a patient who also has a central nerve block, bowel motility is increased unless atropine is given well in advance.

If the block is continued into the postoperative period, distension and anastomotic leakage secondary to opioid-induced ileus may be minimized.

The neuroendocrine response

Physiological measurements have indicated that the metabolic and hormonal changes which have been noted when surgery is performed under general anaesthesia are reduced when regional techniques are employed, and that this reduction in 'stress' may increase the patient's well-being in the postoperative period. General anaesthesia does not in itself seem to be detrimental to patients and

the evidence suggests that it is the trauma of surgery that is responsible for most of the observed changes.

These changes include an increased rate of catabolism, a negative nitrogen balance and salt and water retention. Plasma levels of cortisol, glucose, catecholamines and antidiuretic hormone increase soon after the start of surgery (Gordon et al 1973) and the increases are maintained well into the postoperative period. In clean, uncontaminated surgery the response is generated by noxious stimuli being transmitted from the operative site to the central nervous system. The part played by somatic and sympathetic afferent, and by sympathetic efferent, impulses to the pancreas and adrenal medulla in the generation of the response has long been appreciated. More recently, it has been recognized that humoral factors such as the interleukins and tumour necrosis factor are also involved. General anaesthesia may do little more than reduce the response intraoperatively (Roizen et al 1981).

Complete block can be achieved more easily for many types of surgery with local anaesthetic techniques. The reduction in response has been shown most convincingly during and after lower abdominal surgery and the effect is more marked if the regional block extends form T_4 to S_5 (Engquist et al 1977). During upper abdominal surgery, epidural block, even when combined with vagal nerve block, may be insufficient to prevent some rise in the plasma levels of stress-related hormones (Traynor et al 1982).

The immune response. Changes in immunocompetence parallel the endocrine response which follows major surgery and have been implicated in the formation of tumour metastases and postoperative sepsis (Lennard et al 1985). The changes involve non-specific, humoral and cellular elements, are proportional to the degree of 'trauma', are unaffected by general anaesthesia and may be exacerbated by opioids (for a review see Scott 1991). Depression of lymphocyte transformation, which is one indication of immune suppression after major surgery, has been shown to be reduced by regional anaesthesia (Cullen & van Belle 1975). As with the hormonal and metabolic changes, there is still relatively little objective evidence to indicate whether the patient benefits from such inhibition. Even if the patient does benefit (and there are those who doubt it) it must be remembered that a very extensive block is required when major surgery is performed and that it must be continued well into the postoperative period, otherwise the subsequent changes will be the same as if no block had been used.

Muscle relaxation

Local techniques produce motor as well as sensory block. During surgery the resulting muscle relaxation has the advantage of being confined to the operative field (unlike that due to neuromuscular blocking drugs) so the patient can continue to breathe spontaneously. Spinal and epidural block may result in impairment of the nerve supply to some respiratory muscles, but unless a very high block is produced this is of little consequence. Blocks to the level normally required for abdominal surgery produce only a slight decrease in expiratory reserve volume and expulsive ability (for a review see Bowler et al 1985).

These latter effects may become important in patients with respiratory disease. In general, though, the effect of the block in preventing pain and the consequent reduction in the requirement for opioid drugs more than compensates for any decrease in muscle power. The latter will in any case be minimized by careful choice of concentration of local anaesthetic.

Weakness of the legs may be relatively prolonged after spinal anaesthesia, because the highest concentration of local anaesthetic in the cerebrospinal fluid occurs around the lumbar and sacral nerve roots. Provided patients are warned in advance that motor block is likely, they should not become very concerned about it. However, some patients who develop profound motor block during an infusion may prefer an alternative, albeit less effective, analgesic technique which preserves mobility.

Effect on morbidity and mortality

Given the beneficial effects of regional anaesthesia in controlling pain, suppressing adverse cardiovas-

cular reflexes, reducing pulmonary dysfunction and minimizing the factors contributing to thromboembolic disease, it is reasonable to expect a consequent decrease in the incidence of some of the major complications of surgery. In an attempt to show whether the clear physiological benefits translate into a demonstrable effect on outcome, a large number of workers have studied a variety of its aspects. This work has been reviewed in detail (Scott & Kehlet 1988) and is summarized below.

Cardiac morbidity. A number of studies, mostly in relatively healthy patients, have shown a statistically insignificant reduction in the incidence of ischaemic electrocardiographic changes with regional anaesthesia compared to general anaesthesia. More positive results have been obtained in higher-risk patients. Firstly, Reiz and colleagues (1982) found the epidural block resulted in significantly better intraoperative stability than general anaesthesia in patients undergoing major vascular surgery within 3 months of a myocardial infarction. Postoperative reinfarction (1 in 23 versus 5 in 22) and death from myocardial infarction (1 in 23 versus 3 in 22) were also less. Secondly, Yeager and colleagues (1987) found that the incidence of cardiovascular failure after major surgery in high-risk patients was reduced.

Pulmonary morbidity. Regional anaesthesia has long been known to reduce the degree of both pulmonary dysfunction (Spence & Smith 1971) and hypoxia after surgery (McKenzie et al 1980). These effects are presumably produced by the reduced incidence of atelectasis shown in a number of studies (see Scott 1991). However, the significance of atelectasis as such is questionable, the important postoperative complication being infection. More recently, though, three studies have shown that this can be reduced (Cushieri et al 1985, Cook et al 1986, Yeager et al 1987).

Gastrointestinal morbidity. The effects of regional anaesthesia, or perhaps of the reduction in use of drugs such as neostigmine and morphine, on the minor sequelae of surgery were considered above. The same factors might be expected to influence more major complications, and the duration of ileus after both hysterectomy (Ahn et al 1986) and colonic surgery (Thoren et al 1988) has been shown to be reduced. There is some retrospective evidence that regional anaesthesia may even decrease the incidence of breakdown of bowel anastomoses (Aitkenhead et al 1978), although a follow-up prospective study did not confirm this (Worsley et al 1988).

Blood loss. Although spinal anaesthesia was one of the earlier techniques of induced hypotension, the relationship between blood pressure and blood loss is far from clear. Notably, it has been shown that artificial maintenance of blood pressure does not increase blood loss (Thorburn 1985) and other studies have suggested that the main effect of the blocks is to diminish venous oozing (Modig 1988). Controlled studies suggest that a fairly consistent decrease in bleeding with regional anaesthesia occurs, but that the effect is only statistically significant in surgery to the lower half of the body (Scott 1991).

Thromboembolism. A large number of studies have now shown that regional anaesthesia has a significant impact on the incidence of thromboembolic complications of surgery to the lower half of the body. Fewer studies have been performed in patients undergoing surgery to the upper half of the body and have tended to show that regional anaesthesia makes little difference. However, one study did find that epidural block was as effective as low-dose heparin (Scheinin et al 1987).

Convalescence. By controlling pain, regional anaesthesia has a profound effect on well-being and ease of mobilization in the early postoperative period. As a result, Yeager and colleagues (1987) were able to show a marked reduction in the duration of intensive care after major surgery in high-risk patients. The use of regional anaesthesia may also influence events later in the postoperative period and even decrease the length of hospital stay, although statistically significant data to support this view have yet to be published.

An overview. In 1988 Scott & Kehlet reviewed the then current data from controlled clinical studies comparing the morbidity of surgery performed under regional or general anaesthesia. They found good statistical support for the use of regional anaesthesia for procedures below the umbilicus, but the choice between regional and general anaesthesia did not seem to have a clear influence on the outcome of surgery above that level. The study performed by Yeager and colleagues (1987) has since provided statistically significant evidence in favour of regional anaesthesia in more extensive surgery and more recent work is confirming this (Tuman et al 1991).

There are a number of reasons why it is more difficult to demonstrate objectively the benefits of regional anaesthesia in more extensive surgery. It is more difficult to block completely the neuroendocrine response to such procedures and this requires a very extensive block with the potential risks which that entails. Because of concerns about these risks, many previous workers may not have provided a block which was extensive or profound enough, or may not have continued it for long enough. It is, nonetheless, worth noting that *no study* has found regional anaesthesia to cause *more* morbidity than general anaesthesia.

However, it must be recognized that regional procedures are associated with the risk of certain complications which would not occur if 'traditional' methods of anaesthesia and analgesia were used. It may be argued that these complications are very often the results of a failure of proper care, but this only serves to emphasize that clinicians must learn how to manage regional anaesthesia properly if the potential benefits is to accrue to the patient (Wildsmith 1990).

Benefits to the anaesthetist

A most important benefit to the specialty as a whole is the way in which local techniques have enabled anaesthetists to extend their practice beyond the operating theatre. The provision of epidural services in the labour wards and the staffing of chronic pain clinics are two good examples, and the wider use of these methods in the management of acute pain is an area of great current interest.

The anaesthetist who is prepared to learn and practise regional anaesthesia has a larger armamentarium with which to deal with the many clinical problems presented to him or her. Finally, regional anaesthesia causes neither atmospheric pollution nor adverse effects on the liver after repeated administration. Those who use these methods successfully obtain considerable satisfaction, not only from the technical skill required, but also from the benefits that accrue to their patients.

There is no more warming sight than the cheerful wave of a patient leaving theatre wide awake, but free from pain.

FURTHER READING

Hall G M 1985 The anaesthetic modification of the endocrine and metabolic response to surgery. Annals of the Royal College of Surgeons of England 67: 25–29

Kehlet H 1984 The effect of regional anaesthesia on the stress response to surgery and postoperative morbidity. In:

Scott D B, McClure J H, Wildsmith J A W (eds) Regional anaesthesia: 1884–1984, pp159–162. I C M, Sodertalje

Scott N B, Kehlet H 1988 Regional anaesthesia and surgical morbidity: British Journal of Surgery 75: 299–304

REFERENCES

Ahn H, Lindhagen J, Bronge A, Ygge H 1986 The effect of postoperative epidural local anaesthetics on gastro-intestinal motility. Proceedings of 5th Annual Meeting of the European Society of Regional Anaesthesia, Malmo (abstract)

Aitkenhead A R 1984 Anaesthesia and bowel surgery. British Journal of Anaesthesia 56: 95–101

Aitkenhead A R, Wishart H Y, Peebles-Brown D A 1978 High spinal nerve block for large bowel anastomosis: a retrospective study. British Journal of Anaesthesia 50: 177–183

Berstock D A 1979 Haemorrhoidectomy without tears. Annals of the Royal College of Surgeons of England 61: 51–54

Bowler G M R, Wildsmith J A W, Scott D B 1985 Epidural administration of anesthetics. Clinics in Critical Care Medicine: Acute Pain Management 8: 187–235

Cook P T, Davis M J, Cronin K D, Moran P 1986 A prospective randomised trial comparing spinal anaesthesia using hyperbaric cinchocaine with general anaesthesia for lower limb vascular surgery. Journal of Anaesthesia and Intensive Care 14: 373–380

Cullen B F, van Belle G 1975 Lymphocyte transformation and changes in leukocyte count: effects of anesthesia and operation. Anesthesiology 43: 563–569

Cushieri R J, Morran C G, Howie J C, McArdle C S 1985 Postoperative pain and pulmonary complications: comparison of three analgesic regimes. British Journal of Surgery 72: 495–498

Dempster S 1984 The sequelae of spinal analgesia as opposed to general anaesthesia. Undergraduate prize essay. Association of Anaesthetists of Great Britain and Ireland.

Engquist A, Brandt M R, Fernandes A, Kehlet H 1977 The blocking effect of epidural anaesthesia on the adrenocortical responses to surgery. Acta Anaesthesiologica Scandinavica 21: 330–335

Gordon N H, Scott D B, Percy-Robb I W 1973 Modification of plasma cortiocosteroid concentrations during and after surgery by epidural blockade. British Medical Journal i: 581–583

Guenter C A 1984 Toward prevention of postoperative pulmonary complications. American Review of Respiratory Disease 130: 4–5

Johansson K, Ahn H, Lindhagen J, Tryselius U 1988 Effect of epidural anaesthesia on intestinal blood flow. British Journal of Surgery 75: 73–76

Kennedy W F, Bonica J J, Ward R J, Tolas A G, Martin W E, Grinstein A 1966 Cardiorespiratory effects of epinephrine when used in regional anesthesia. Acta Anaesthesiologica Scandinavica Supplement XXIII: 320–333

Klassen G A, Bramwell R S, Bromage P R, Zborowska-Sluis D 1980 Effect of acute sympathectomy by epidural anesthesia on the canine coronary circulation. Anesthesiology 52: 8–15

Lanz E, Theiss D, Emmerich E A, Emmerich M 1982 Regional versus general anaesthesia: attitudes and experiences of patients. Regional Anaesthesia 7: S163–S171

Lennard T W, Shenton B K, Bortotta et al 1985 The influence of surgical operation on components of the immune system. British Journal of Surgery 72: 771–776

McKenzie P J, Wishart H Y, Dewar K M S, Gray I, Smith G 1980 Comparison of the effects of spinal anaesthesia and general anaesthesia on postoperative oxygenation and perioperative mortality. British Journal of Anaesthesia 52: 49–53

Mason D T 1965 The autonomic nervous system and regulation of cardiovascular performance. Anesthesiology 29: 670–680

Merin R G 1981 Local and regional anesthetic techniques for the patient with ischemic heart disease. Cleveland Clinic Quarterly 48: 72–74

Modig J 1988 Beneficial effects on blood loss in total hip replacement when performed under lumbar epidural anaesthesia versus general anaesthesia: an exploratory study. Acta Chirurgica Scandinavica Supplement 550: 95–103

Modig J, Borg T, Bagge L, Saldeen T 1983a Role of extradural and of general anaesthesia in fibrinolysis and coagulation after total hip replacement. British Journal of Anaesthesia 55: 625–629

Modig J, Borg T, Karlstrom G, Maripuu E, Sahlstedt B 1983b Thromboembolism after total hip replacement: role of epidural and general anesthesia. Anesthesia and Analgesia 62: 174–180

Nimmo W S, Littlewood D G, Scott D B, Prescott L F 1978 Gastric emptying following hysterectomy with extradural analgesia. British Journal of Anaesthesia 50: 559–561

Reiz S, Balfors E, Sorensen M B et al 1982 Coronary hemodynamic effects of general anesthesia and surgery. Modification by epidural analgesia in patients with ischemic heart disease. Regional Anesthesia 7: S8

Roizen M F 1988 Should we all have a sympathectomy at birth? Or at least preoperatively? Anesthesiology 68: 482–484

Roizen M F, Horrigan R W, Frazer B M 1981 Anesthetic doses blocking adrenergic (stress) and cardiovascular responses to incision – MAC BAR. Anesthesiology 54: 390–398

Rosen M 1981 Editorial comment. Anaesthesia 36: 36–37

Scheinin B, Asantila R, Orko R 1987 The effect of bupivacaine and morphine on pain and bowel function after colonic surgery. Acta Anaesthesiologica Scandinavica 31: 161–164

Scott D B, Hibbard B M 1990 Serious non-fatal complications associated with extradural block in obstetric practice. British Journal of Anaesthesia 64: 537–541

Scott N B 1991 The effects of pain and its treatment. In: McClure J H, Wildsmith J A W (eds) Mechanisms and management of conduction blockade for postoperative analgesia. Edward Arnold, London

Spence A A, Smith G 1971 Postoperative analgesia and lung function: a comparison of morphine with extradural block. British Journal of Anaesthesia 43: 144–148

Thorburn J 1985 Subarachnoid blockade and total hip replacement: effect of ephedrine on intraoperative blood loss. British Journal of Anaesthesia 57: 290–293

Thorburn J, Louden J R, Vallance R 1980 Spinal and general anaesthesia in total hip replacement: frequency of deep vein thrombosis. British Journal of Anaesthesia 52: 1117–1121

Thoren T, Carlsson E, Sandmark S, Watwil M 1988 Effects of thoracic epidural analgesia with morphine or bupivacaine on lower oesophageal sphincter pressure: an experimental study in man. Acta Anaesthesiologica Scandinavica 32: 391–394

Traynor C, Paterson J L, Ward I D, Morgan M, Hall G M 1982 Effects of extradural analgesia and vagal blockade on the metabolic and endocrine response to upper abdominal surgery. British Journal of Anaesthesia 54: 319–323

Tuman K J, McCarthy R J, March R, Ivankovich A D 1991 Epidural anesthesia/analgesia improves outcome after major vascular surgery: a hypothesis reconfirmed. Anesthesia and Analgesia 72: S302

Ward R J, Bonica J J, Freund F G, Akamatsu T J, Danziger F, Engelson S 1965 Epidural and subarachnoid anesthesia: cardiovascular and respiratory effects. Journal of the American Medical Association 191: 275–278

Wildsmith J A W 1990 Regional anaesthesia must be properly managed. Anaesthesia 45: 984

Worsley M H, Wishart H Y, Peebles-Brown D A, Aitkenhead A R 1988 High spinal nerve block for large bowel anastomosis. A prospective study. British Journal of Anaesthesia 60: 36–40

Yeager M P, Glass D D, Neff R K, Brinck-Johnsen T 1987 Epidural anesthesia and analgesia in high-risk surgical patients. Anesthesiology 66: 729–736

3. Pain pathways

J. H. McClure

Pain is the conscious interpretation of a noxious stimulus. This stimulus is transmitted along peripheral nerves to the central nervous system (CNS) where responses are initiated to protect the organism from harm. Noxious stimuli also initiate reflex sequences which are not perceived consciously. Both conscious and reflex responses may be modified at various relay stations along the route of transmission. Previous experience, mood and the general state of arousal all play major roles in the modification of these responses. Impulses generated by noxious stimuli do not travel along simple pathways. Various routes through the CNS are available and the signal may be modified by 'facilitation' and 'inhibition' at the junctions (synapses) between individual nerve cells (neurones).

THE PAIN PATHWAY

Peripheral nerves (Fig. 3.1) are made up of motor, sensory and autonomic nerve fibres (axons) ar-ranged in bundles (fasciculi). The fibres vary considerably in size and these differences may be related to differences in function. In general, large diameter fibres conduct faster than smaller ones. This is due to the presence around larger fibres of a sheath of myelin, which acts as an insulating layer and increases the rate of transmission. If a mixed peripheral nerve is stimulated electrically it is possible to record with extracellular electrodes a compound action potential (Fig. 3.2) with 'peaks' which correspond to the arrival of signals in the different types of fibre. Detailed analysis of compound action potentials allows peripheral nerve fibres to be classified according to their rates of conduction, and for this classification to be related to the various modalities of nerve function (Table 3.1).

In mammals Aδ and C fibres are thought to be involved in the transmission of pain impulses through peripheral nerves. The impulses are initiated by receptors at the nerve endings which translate noxious stimuli into changes in mem-

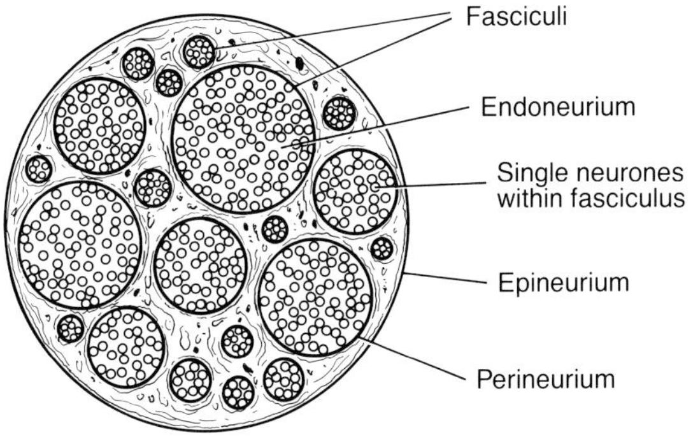

Fasciculi

Endoneurium

Single neurones within fasciculus

Epineurium

Perineurium

Fig. 3.1 Transverse section through a peripheral nerve.

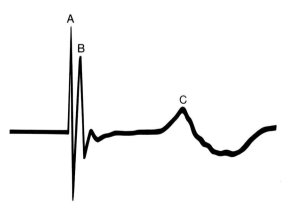

Fig. 3.2 Compound action potential of a peripheral nerve.

Table 3.1   Classification of mammalian nerve fibre types (Ganong 1987)

Fibre type	Diameter (μm)	Conduction speed (m s^{-1})	Function
Aα	12–20	70–120	Proprioception, somatic motor
β	5–12	30–70	Touch, pressure
γ	3–6	15–30	Motor to muscle spindle
δ	2–5	12–30	*Pain*, temperature, touch
B	<3	3–15	Preganglionic autonomic
C	0.3–1.3	0.5–2.3	*Pain*, reflexes, postganglionic sympathetic

brane excitability. In the case of pain these changes in excitability may be mediated by prostaglandins and other substances released when tissues are damaged. If the stimulus is adequate the membrane will depolarize and initiate an action potential. The frequency with which these action potentials are generated depends on the intensity of the original stimulus.

The axons in the peripheral nerve are extensions of the cell bodies of the first-order sensory neurones. The cell body is located in the ganglion of the posterior root of the segmental nerve (Fig. 3.3) and it also has a centrally projecting axon which synapses with the second order nerve in the dorsal horn of the spinal cord. These synapses are located in Rexed's laminae I, II, IV and V (Fig. 3.4), which are also known as the marginal layer, the substantia gelatinosa and the nucleus proprius.

The second-order neurones cross the spinal cord and ascend in the anterolateral spinothalamic tract. These neurones pass to the posteroventral nucleus of the thalamus and synapse with the third-order neurones which radiate to the post-

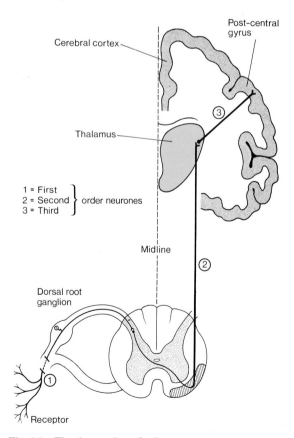

Fig. 3.3   The three orders of pain neurone.

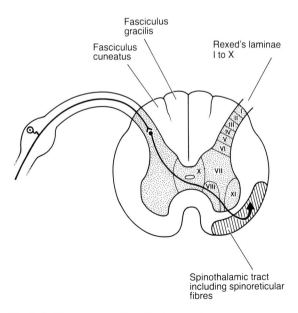

Fig. 3.4   Transverse section of spinal cord.

central gyrus of the cerebral hemisphere (Fig. 3.3). This essentially simplistic outline of the main pathway serves as a framework for more detailed knowledge. There is good neurophysiological evidence that other pathways exist. For instance, spinoreticular fibres from Rexed's laminae VII and VIII are thought to transmit pain to the region of the hypothalamus (Lipton et al 1978).

Peripheral transmission

The nervous impulses that lead to the sensation of pain are generated by receptors which are situated on free nerve endings and respond to harmful stimuli – nociceptors. Their features vary according to the nerve fibre type with which they are associated.

Aδ nociceptors are unimodal and respond to heat or mechanical stimuli such as pinching and pin-prick. Impulses are transmitted rapidly and lead to a sensation of sharp, localized pain.

C nociceptors are polymodal and respond to mechanical, thermal and chemical stimuli, including substances released by tissue damage such as bradykinin, potassium, histamine and substance P. The sensation they generate is of a diffuse, burning pain.

Both types of nociceptor are widely distributed in the dermis and have terminations which penetrate the epidermis. They are also found in deeper structures in the musculoskeletal system. Nociceptors have been described in the viscera and are connected to unmyelinated C fibres that run with the efferent autonomic nerves to those viscera. Visceral pain is produced by ischaemia, extreme muscle contraction, and traction upon or distension of a hollow viscus, and is poorly localized.

The sensitivity of both types of receptor can be increased by repeated stimulation, which lowers the threshold for excitation so that the receptors respond to previously innocuous stimuli. This increased sensitivity is mediated by prostaglandins released at the same time as the agents that stimulate nociceptors directly. Axon reflexes may further increase and maintain the release of all these mediators of the inflammatory response. The local vasodilatation and increased capillary permeability initiate the process of repair, and the accompanying sensitization of nociceptors (as evidenced by the hyperalgesia of surgical wounds) protects the injured area.

The pain transmitted by Aδ fibres is opioid-resistant, but that transmitted by C fibres may be modified by both opioid and non-steroidal anti-inflammatory drugs (NSAIDs). Local anaesthetics block transmission in both types of nerve fibre and they also influence the inflammatory response by suppressing sensitization of nociceptors. This can reduce wound hyperalgesia, so that infiltration of the abdominal wall before surgery can reduce postoperative pain after herniorrhaphy for a time greatly exceeding the nerve-blocking action of the drug (Tverskoy et al 1990).

Central modulation

The primary afferent fibres from the nociceptors terminate in the dorsal horn of the spinal cord, the first point at which integration of the signal can occur. This is the site of significant processing of the afferent input. The *gate control theory* was first put forward by Melzack & Wall (1965) to explain this central modulation which at times can block the transmission of a massive influx of 'painful' stimuli, but at other times can allow apparently benign stimuli to be interpreted as pain.

The release of neurotransmitter by the primary neurone is inhibited by endogenous opioids (known as enkephalins) produced by short intermediary or control neurones (Fig. 3.5). The activity of the control neurone is, in turn, influenced by a wide range of inputs from the same and other levels in the nervous system. For example, stimulation of the brain stem in awake animals can cause inhibition of transmission and produce a state in which severe noxious stimuli evoke no response (Willis 1982). However, other descending impulses may enhance the activity of sensory neurones sufficiently to generate a positive spino-bulbo-spinal feedback loop (Cervero & Wolstencroft 1984).

A number of transmitter substances are involved (Fig. 3.5) and provide a physiological basis for the spinal analgesic action of a number of different types of drug. Exogenous opioids are known to act on the same receptors as the enkephalins and it is possible that derivatives of the benzodiazepines and the α_2-adrenergic agonists will be developed for spinal use in the future. Clinically useful antagonists to the neurotransmitters released by the primary pain neurones are not yet available, but an understanding of their physiology is important to the control of acute pain.

The primary pain neurone releases both amino acid (glutamate) and peptide (substance P) transmitters. Glutamate acts as a 'classic' transmitter and produces short-lived depolarizations of the postsynaptic membrane. The release of substance P is slower in onset and longer in duration, so that in situations of high neuronal activity its action is cumulative. Its main effect, mediated through a range of actions, is to increase the sensitivity of the secondary neurone so that identical stimuli produce successively larger responses – the phenomenon of *wind-up* (Woolf 1989). If such stimulation is prolonged, virtually permanent increases in sensitivity can be induced. This ability of the CNS to adjust its level of sensitivity in response to changes in sensory input is known as *plasticity* and produces a physiological basis for the development of some chronic pain states (Dubner 1991, Woolf 1991).

The therapeutic implication is clear. By preventing the arrival of impulses from nociceptors during

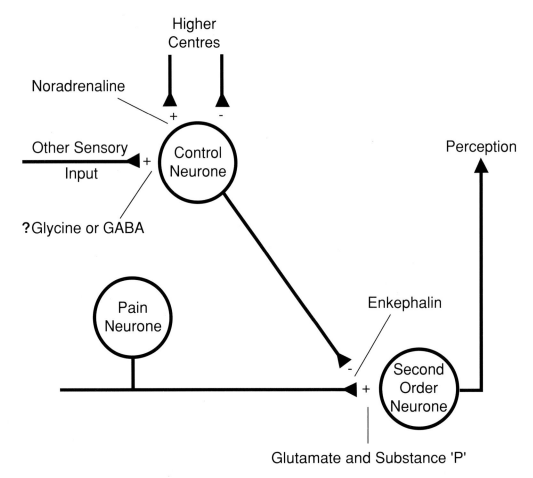

Fig. 3.5 Gate theory of pain. Release of enkephalin by the control neurone inhibits transmitter release. Exogenous opioids have the same effect. Benzodiazepines and adrenergic agonist drugs may produce spinal analgesia at the spinal level by increasing the activity of the control neurone as depicted here, or perhaps more directly.

Table 3.2 Effects of opioid receptor stimulation in man

Receptor	Effects
μ	Supraspinal analgesia Euphoria Respiratory depression Dependence
κ	Spinal analgesia Sedation
σ	Dysphoria Hallucinations Mydriasis

surgery, a peripheral or central nerve block will prevent both this and the positive-feedback phenomenon mentioned above. Similarly, a small dose of opioid given *before* a noxious stimulus can suppress the spinal cord hyperexcitability which develops during injury. Much larger doses are required to achieve a similar effect once that hyperexcitability has developed (Wall 1988).

Opioid receptors have been identified at various sites in the CNS. They are concentrated in the substantia gelatinosa and the marginal zone of the dorsal horn in the spinal cord, the hypothalamus, the limbic system, the peri-aqueductal grey matter of the IVth ventricle and the reticular activating system in the brain stem (Pert and Snyder 1973, Pert and Yaksh 1974, Snyder 1977). Since these receptors are present, it is assumed that enkephalins are released there and that all these areas are involved in the modulation of pain transmission, although the receptors are *not* all the same. At least five have been described (μ, κ, σ, δ and ε), but only the first three (Table 3.2) are thought to be important in the central nervous system of man (Wood 1990).

Peripheral nerve distribution

The distribution of the peripheral nerves is related to man's embryological development. Every embryological segment is supplied by a pair of nerves, each of which has a ventral (motor) and a dorsal (sensory) root (Fig. 3.3). The area of skin supplied by the branches of each pair of nerves is known as a dermatome (Fig. 3.6 – see Fig. 11.1 for a 'typical' segmental nerve). The development of

the limb buds, with their subsequent rotation, causes some distortion and there is also considerable overlap between adjacent nerves. The segmental pattern may be tracked from the periphery through the spinal cord and the hypothalamus to the sensory homunculus in the postcentral gyrus of the cerebral cortex.

An adequate block of cutaneous sensation will not guarantee full anaesthesia of the underlying structures. In the limbs this is because the distribution of the segmental nerves to the deep structures is not the same as it is to the superficial tissues. In the trunk it is because the viscera are not supplied directly by the segmental nerves, but by autonomic nerves distributed through various ganglia and plexuses.

Pain originating in the thoracic and abdominal viscera is transmitted by sympathetic afferent fibres through the sympathetic chain to the segmental nerves T_1–L_2, and by parasympathetic vagal fibres. Other parasympathetic fibres transmit deep pain from structures in the pelvis (spinal parasympathetic outflow, S_2–S_3) and the head and neck (cranial nerves III, VII and IX). Referred pain, such as shoulder tip pain secondary to diaphragmatic irritation, indicates the common embryonic origin of the nerve supply to the two structures involved. The clinical problems associated with this difference in innervation between deep and superficial structures are considered in the relevant practical chapters.

The site of block

The pain pathway may be interrupted at many points along its course. Morphine and other opioids have a partial effect on the synaptic transmission of pain only. Local anaesthetics have the advantage of producing a complete but reversible block of all types of first order neurone. They may thus be used at many points along the pain pathway, but when choosing the point of block the deep and superficial innervation of the operative field must be considered carefully.

The standard methods (Fig. 3.7) of local anaesthetic administration are as follows:

Topical. Local anaesthetics may be applied directly to the mucous membranes of the nose,

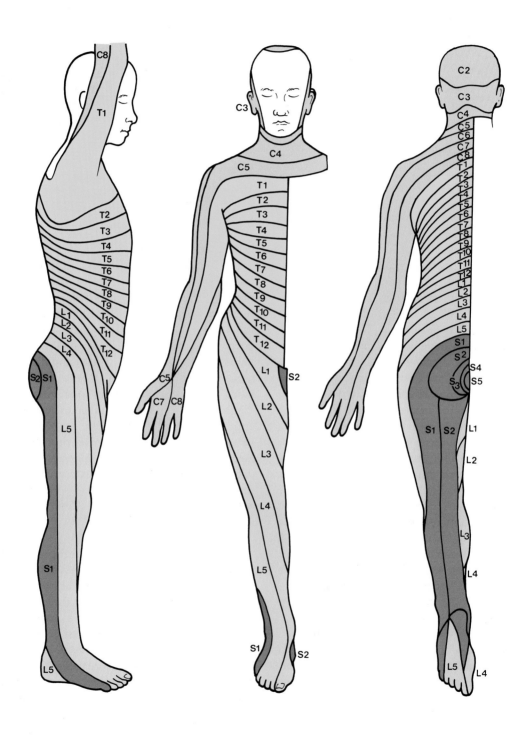

Fig. 3.6   Cutaneous dermatomes.

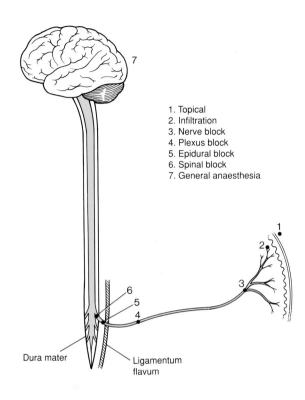

1. Topical
2. Infiltration
3. Nerve block
4. Plexus block
5. Epidural block
6. Spinal block
7. General anaesthesia

Dura mater

Ligamentum flavum

Fig. 3.7 Possible sites for local anaesthetic application.

points by reference to anatomical landmarks, by eliciting paraesthesiae or by electrical stimulation. The lumbosacral plexus is not so easily identified and the sciatic nerve is deeply placed in the buttock and upper leg. Paravertebral somatic block involves injecting local anaesthetic close to the vertebral column where the segmental nerves emerge from the intervertebral foramina. This technique has been virtually superseded by epidural block, which anaesthetizes several nerves with a single injection.

Epidural block. Ease of identification of the epidural space and unimpeded spread of the local anaesthetic solution make this a most useful technique. Continuous block can be produced with catheter techniques.

Spinal (subarachnoid) block. This is a simpler technique than epidural block since identification of cerebrospinal fluid (CSF) is an unambiguous end point. It is usually performed in the lumbar region to avoid needle damage to the spinal cord.

General anaesthesia. Local anaesthetic drugs stabilize *all* excitable membranes and procaine infusions have been used to produce general anaesthesia. The technique is rarely used now.

Selection and timing of nerve block

If a local anaesthetic technique is to be used, it is obvious that the one chosen should produce an adequate distribution and quality of block for the duration of surgery. Of the several techniques that might be suitable, the one least likely to give rise to complications in the particular patient should be used. As a general rule this means using the most distal method, but the risks of systemic toxicity, hypotension, needle trauma, etc., must all be borne in mind. The anaesthetist must also consider any intercurrent disease in the patient, the facilities available (especially the availability of particular drugs, equipment and the quality of after-care), and, not least, his or her own level of training and experience.

Since peripheral and central nerve blocks decrease both the amount of postoperative pain and the requirements for other analgesic drugs (McQuay et al 1988, Cousins 1989, Tverskoy et

mouth, throat and urethra, and also to the external surfaces of the eye. Standard preparations will penetrate these surfaces, but until recently intact skin presented a relatively impermeable barrier. The development of a eutectic mixture of lignocaine and prilocaine (the eutectic mixture of local anaesthetics – EMLA) in a cream formulation has overcome this difficulty, although prolonged application (up to 1 hour) is necessary (Lundh 1984).

Infiltration. The extent of infiltration will depend on the area of anaesthesia required. Large volumes of dilute local anaesthetic solution are commonly used.

Peripheral nerve block. Many small peripheral nerves are readily accessible and easily blocked, given a reasonable knowledge of the relations of the nerve trunks and their distribution.

Proximal nerve block. Accessibility is the essential prerequisite for a proximal nerve block. The brachial plexus is easily located at a number of al 1990) the block may be used simply as an analgesic 'supplement' to a general anaesthetic. If this is the case, a decision has to be made about timing. Convenience may dictate that it will be performed at the end of the operation, but the physiological considerations outlined above indicate that the optimum time is *before* surgery commences.

Subarachnoid and epidural opioids

Since the discovery of opioid receptors in the spinal cord (La Motte et al 1976), a wide variety of opioid drugs has been injected into the vertebral canal with the aim of producing profound analgesia. The epidural route was first used in man in 1979 for the treatment of intractable pain (Behar et al 1979), but the initial enthusiasm for the technique and its possibilities was tempered by reports of side-effects, the most serious being respiratory depression (Scott and McClure 1979, Davies et al 1980). This has been observed at widely varying intervals after both subarachnoid and epidural administration of most of the commonly used drugs (Morgan 1989).

Opioids vary in lipophilicity, and drugs like morphine, which has a relatively low lipid solubility, remain in the CSF long after injection and so may diffuse rostrally to affect the respiratory centre. Theoretically, it is more appropriate to use a lipid-soluble drug which will bind strongly to the spinal cord and not remain in the CSF in significant concentration (Morgan 1989). However, significant respiratory depression has been reported (Brockway et al 1990) even after epidural fentanyl, which is short-acting as well as lipid-soluble. In the light of present knowledge, continuous monitoring of respiration and constant nursing supervision is recommended. In some situations this may be needed for up to 24 hours after drug administration.

The respiratory depression occurring after epidural fentanyl noted above was in a patient given a *bolus* dose in combination with bupivacaine. Current research is directed towards the view that continuous infusion of relatively low doses may be safer, particularly if they are given in combination with local anaesthetics. Combinations are certainly more effective (Lee et al 1988) and the synergistic effects of the two classes of drug may allow dose reductions to levels below those which cause complications. In addition, diamorphine is more effective as a supplement to epidural bupivacaine when it too is given epidurally rather than systemically (Lee et al 1991), but this does not mean that the therapeutic ratio of the method is greater. Therefore, much more research is needed before the routine use of these methods can be advocated. The possibility that an enkephalin-like drug might be developed with pure spinal analgesic properties and no psychotropic, gastrointestinal or respiratory effects is a most attractive prospect.

FURTHER READING

McClure J H, Wildsmith J A W (eds) 1991 Conduction blockade for postoperative analgesia. Edward Arnold, London

Wildsmith J A W (ed) 1989 Postgraduate educational issue: symposium on aspects of pain. British Journal of Anaesthesia 63: 135–226

REFERENCES

Behar M, Magora F, Olshwang D, Davidson J T 1979 Epidural morphine in treatment of pain. Lancet i: 527–528

Brockway M S, Noble D W, Sharwood-Smith G H, McClure J H 1990 Profound respiratory depression after extradural fentanyl. British Journal of Anaesthesia 64: 243–245

Cervero F, Wolstencroft J H 1984 A positive feedback loop between spinal cord nociceptive pathways and antinociceptive areas of the cat's brain stem. Pain 20: 125–128

Cousins M J 1989 Acute pain and the injury response: immediate and prolonged effects. Regional Anesthesia 14: 162–179

Davies G K, Tolhurst-Cleaver C L, James T L 1980 Respiratory depression after intrathecal opiates. Anaesthesia 35: 1080–1083

Dubner R 1991 Neuronal plasticity and pain following peripheral tissue inflammation or nerve injury. In: Bond M R, Charlton J E, Woolf C J (eds) Proceedings of the VIth World Congress on Pain, pp 263–276. Elsevier, Amsterdam

Ganong W F 1987 Review of medical physiology, 13th edn. p 45. Appleton and Lange, Norwalk, Connecticut, USA

La Motte C, Pert C B, Snyder S H 1976 Opiate receptor changes after dorsal root section. Brain Research 112: 407–412

Lee A, Simpson D, Whitfield A, Scott D B 1988 Postoperative analgesia by continuous extradural infusion of bupivacaine and diamorphine. British Journal of Anaesthesia 60: 845–850

Lee A, McKeown D, Brockway M, Bannister J, Wildsmith J A W 1991 Comparison of extradural and intravenous diamorphine as a supplement to extradural bupivacaine. Anaesthesia 46: 447–450

Lipton S, Miles J B, Williams N, Barke-Jones N 1978 Pituitary injection of alcohol for widespread cancer pain. Pain 5: 73–82

Lundh R 1984 Topical anaesthesia from Koller to the present. In: Scott D B, McClure J H, Wildsmith J A W (eds) Regional Anaesthesia 1884–1984, pp 72–73. ICM, Sodertalje

McQuay H J, Caroll D, Moore R A 1988 Postoperative orthopaedic pain – the effect of opiate premedication and local anaesthetic blocks. Pain 33: 291–296

Melzack R, Wall P D 1965 Pain mechanisms, a new theory. Science 179: 1011–1014

Morgan M 1989 The rational use of intrathecal and extradural opioids. British Journal of Anaesthesia 63: 165–188

Pert C B, Snyder S H 1973 Opiate receptor: demonstration in nervous tissue. Science 179: 1011–1014

Pert C B, Yaksh T L 1974 Sites of morphine-induced analgesia in the primate brain: relation to pain pathways. Brain Research 80: 135–140

Scott D B, McClure J H 1979 Selective epidural analgesia. Lancet i: 1410

Snyder S H 1977 Opiate receptors in the brain. New England Journal of Medicine 296: 266–270

Tverskoy M, Cozacov C, Ayache M, Bradley E L, Kissin I 1990 Postoperative pain after inguinal herniorrhaphy with different types of anesthesia. Anesthesia and Analgesia 70: 29–35

Wall P D 1988 The prevention of postoperative pain. Pain 33: 289–290

Willis W D 1982 Control of nociceptive transmission in the spinal cord. Progress in Sensory Physiology 3: 1–155

Wood M 1990 Opioid agonists and antagonists. In: Wood M, Wood A J J (eds) Drugs and anesthesia, pp 129–178. Williams and Wilkins, Baltimore

Woolf C J 1989 Recent advances in the pathophysiology of acute pain. British Journal of Anaesthesia 63: 139–146.

Woolf C J 1991 Central mechanisms of acute pain. In: Bond M R, Charlton J E, Woolf C J (eds) Proceedings of the VIth World Congress on Pain, pp 25–34. Elsevier, Amsterdam

4. Pharmacology of local anaesthetic drugs

G. R. Arthur   J. A. W. Wildsmith   G. T. Tucker

A local anaesthetic is a drug which reversibly blocks the transmission of peripheral nerve impulses. Many classes of drug have a local anaesthetic action (e.g. β blockers and antihistamines), but all those known and used as local anaesthetics can trace their origin back to cocaine (see Ch. 1). These agents conform to a common structural arrangement consisting of a benzene ring attached to an amine group by an intermediate chain, which includes either an ester or an amide linkage (Fig. 4.1).

Local anaesthetics work by blocking membrane depolarization, a non-specific process common to other excitable tissues (such as brain and heart) besides peripheral nerve. Since local anaesthetics are injected near their sites of action, only peripheral nerves should be exposed to concentrations high enough to produce a significant effect. However, if sufficient drug reaches other organs via the circulation their function will also be affected.

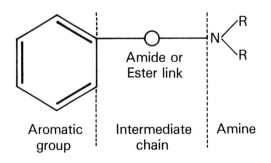

Fig. 4.1   General formula for local anaesthetic drugs.

MODE OF ACTION

Neural transmission (Fig. 4.2)

During the resting phase the interior of a peripheral nerve axon has a potential difference of about −70 mV relative to the outside. When the nerve is stimulated there is a rapid increase in the membrane potential to about +20 mV, followed by an immediate return to the resting level. This whole depolarization/repolarization sequence lasts 1–2 ms and produces the familiar action potential associated with the passage of a nerve impulse.

The resting potential exists because there are more anions than cations within the cell. In concentration terms this difference is small, but it is the net result of the several forces that affect the distribution of ions across the membrane. The Donnan effect, the sodium/potassium pump and the semipermeable nature of the membrane all combine to produce marked differences in intracellular and extracellular ion concentrations. In the present context the most important ions are sodium and potassium. The high extracellular sodium concentration is maintained because at rest the membrane is impermeable to sodium. However, it is relatively permeable to potassium ions, which diffuse out of the cell until the negative intracellular electrochemical potential created by their loss balances the concentration gradient.

Depolarization of the fibre is the result of a sudden increase in membrane permeability to sodium, which can then diffuse down both concentration and electrochemical gradients. Sodium ions enter as a result of changes in the configuration of large protein molecules present in the cell membrane. Nerve stimula-

29

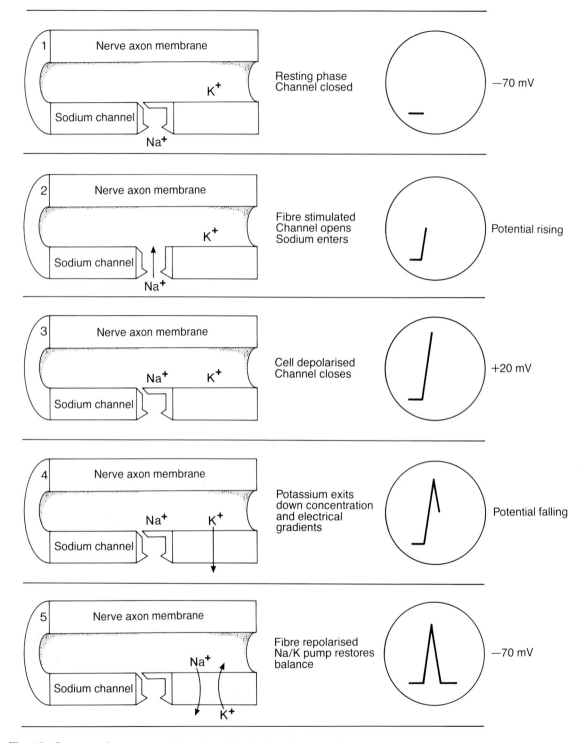

Fig. 4.2   Sequence of events at a sodium channel during impulse transmission.

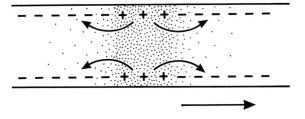

Fig. 4.3 Local current flow from depolarized section of nerve axon. In spite of the bidirectional current flow the impulse is only transmitted orthodromically because sodium channels are inactivated for a finite period of time after opening and closing.

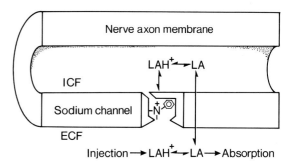

Fig. 4.4 Effect of local anaesthetic on a sodium channel.

tion causes 'channels' in these proteins to open and it is through these channels that sodium ions enter the axoplasm. Entry of the positively charged sodium ions raises the membrane potential to about +20 mV, at which point the electrochemical and concentration gradients for sodium balance one another and the channels close. Both concentration and electrochemical gradients then favour movement of potassium out through the membrane until the resting potential is restored. Like sodium, potassium passes through specific channels, some of which are permanently open and others of which open only during repolarization. Only a small proportion of the total number of ions present take part in this exchange and the sodium/potassium pump rapidly restores their distribution during the resting phase.

At sensory nerve endings the initial opening of sodium channels is produced by an appropriate physiological stimulus, which may be chemically mediated in some cases. The impulse is transmitted along the axon because a local current (Fig. 4.3) flows between the depolarized segment of nerve (which has a positive charge) and the next segment (which has a negative charge). The voltage change associated with this current opens the sodium channels in the next section, so that the action potential is propagated along the nerve.

Effect of local anaesthetic drugs (Fig. 4.4)

Local anaesthetics are usually injected as acid solutions of the hydrochloride salt (pH <5). In this form the amine group is ionized and the drug

becomes soluble in water and therefore suitable for injection. After injection, tissue buffering raises the pH and a percentage of the drug dissociates to become free base, the amount depending on the pK_a of the individual drug. Being lipid-soluble, the free base is able to penetrate both the nerve's coverings and the lipid cell membrane to reach the interior of the axon where a portion reionizes. The reionized portion then enters the sodium channels and may be thought of as simply 'plugging' them so that sodium ions cannot enter the cell. As a result, action potentials are neither generated nor propagated – conduction block has occurred. Because it is the ionized form of the drug that is active and reionization has to take place intracellularly, individual drug pK_a has little effect on the rate of onset of block, although it *may* affect diffusion through nerve coverings. As well as diffusing into the nerves at the site of injection, the drug will also enter the capillaries and be removed by the circulation. Eventually tissue concentration will fall below that in the nerves and the drug will diffuse out, thus allowing restoration of normal function.

SYSTEMIC TOXICITY

Local anaesthetics have exactly the same membrane-stabilizing effect on the cells of the heart and brain as they have on peripheral nerve fibres. Because these drugs are injected at their sites of intended action, the concentrations found in the systemic circulation are usually below those that produce overt toxic effects. The most severe reactions result from accidental intravascular injection, but they may follow repeated administration during prolonged pain control, or simple over-dosage.

Clinical features

The early features of systemic toxicity are all subjective. Patients may note numbness of the tongue or circumoral structures (due to a direct effect of drug in an area with a high blood supply), light-headedness or tinnitus and they may become acutely anxious. Objective features include slurring of speech, muscle twitching and drowsiness. In the most severe cases consciousness is lost, convulsions occur and the patient will almost certainly become apnoeic. Without immediate resuscitation, hypoxia and acidosis will develop rapidly, due not only to the apnoea, but also to the high oxygen consumption of the muscles of a convulsing patient.

The cardiovascular system is much less sensitive to the effects of local anaesthetic drugs than the central nervous system and circulatory collapse during a toxic reaction is most likely to be due to hypoxia and acidosis (which will increase the proportion of ionized, active drug present intracellularly). The local anaesthetic drugs do have a primary depressant action on the myocardium which is proportional to their local anaesthetic potency, but the effect is of little significance at the systemic concentrations produced during uneventful regional anaesthesia or in the therapy of arrhythmias (Covino & Vassallo 1976). Low concentrations of most of the drugs tend to produce slight vasoconstriction, but vasodilation occurs at higher concentrations.

These peripheral and myocardial effects are modified by central actions which result in an increase in sympathetic nerve activity (Bonica 1971). The intravenous injection of 1–2 mg kg^{-1} of lignocaine may thus produce measurable increases in blood pressure, heart rate and cardiac output. However, the epidural injection of about 400 mg of plain lignocaine will produce the expected decrease in these parameters (even though similar systemic concentrations of drug are produced) because the sympathetic nerves are blocked.

It is important to realize that the rapid intravenous injection of a large dose of a local anaesthetic will almost certainly produce frank convulsions or cardiorespiratory collapse without any of the more minor manifestations of systemic toxicity being apparent.

Factors affecting toxicity

Central nervous system toxicity is related to the amount of drug in the blood being supplied to the brain. This will depend on the dose administered, the rate of absorption, the site of injection, the pattern of distribution to other tissues and the rate of metabolism and excretion (Fig. 4.5).

Dosage

It has become common for 'safe' dose recommendations for local anaesthetics to be related to the patient's weight. Such recommendations have no valid basis. For instance, the epidural administration of a fixed dose of lignocaine to patients with a considerable range in weight produced no correlation with maximum plasma lignocaine concentration (Scott & Cousins 1980). The anaesthetist should be aware of the factors which affect systemic concentrations of local anaesthetics and relate these to the *particular block, patient and*

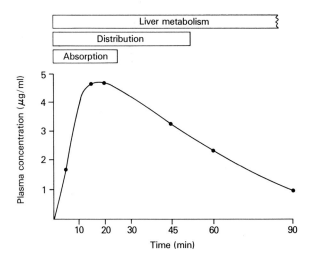

Fig. 4.5 Factors affecting plasma concentrations of a local anaesthetic after injection.

drug with which he is concerned. Local anaesthetic drug requirements may be smaller in the pregnant patient and obviously extremes in size are important. It should be said that dosage information for young children is very limited.

The volume and concentration of a solution used for any procedure have little direct effect on resultant systemic concentrations. It is the mass of drug injected that is important, i.e. 20 ml of 2% lignocaine will produce the same systemic effect as 40 ml of 1% lignocaine.

Absorption

Absorption from the site of injection depends on the blood flow – the higher the blood flow the more rapid will be the rise in, and the greater will be the peak, systemic drug concentration. The rate of absorption is greatest after intercostal block, followed by epidural, brachial plexus and lower limb blocks. Absorption is slowest after subcutaneous infiltration, but high concentrations may follow topical application to the upper respiratory and gastrointestinal tracts. Absorption may be reduced by the addition of a vasoconstrictor to the injected solution. In most cases this will allow the safe dose to be increased by 50–100%, but use of a vasoconstrictor may not always be appropriate.

Intravenous regional anaesthesia (Bier's block) is a special case. Premature tourniquet release will result in the rapid entry of a large dose of local anaesthetic into the circulation. When the tourniquet has been applied for 20 minutes, however, much of drug has diffused into the tissues of the limb. Tourniquet release then results in slower increases in systemic concentrations than after brachial plexus block.

The overall state of the circulation will also affect the systemic concentrations achieved. For example, 400 mg of drug injected intravenously over 1 minute into a patient with a cardiac output of 4 litres min^{-1} will result (theoretically) in a peak concentration of 100 $\mu g\ ml^{-1}$. Any alteration in cardiac output or rate of injection will produce a proportionate alteration in concentration.

Distribution (Fig. 4.6)

Distribution throughout the body buffers the rise in systemic concentration. Before blood containing

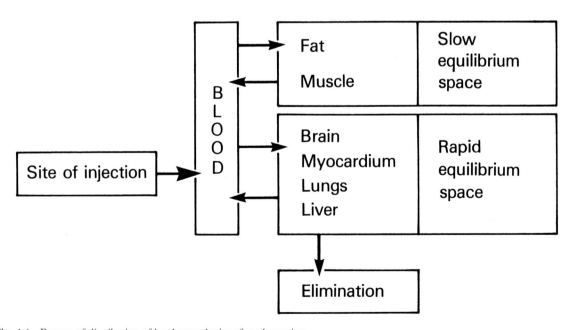

Fig. 4.6   Pattern of distribution of local anaesthetics after absorption.

local anaesthetic reaches the systemic circulation it will pass through the right side of the heart, where it will have no effect, and through the lungs, which are capable of temporarily sequestering, and possibly metabolizing, large amounts of local anaesthetic. The percentage that is so distributed decreases as the dose increases, so the buffering capacity of the lungs will be less able to prevent a toxic reaction should an intravenous injection be made rapidly. After passage through the lungs local anaesthetics are distributed preferentially to those organs with a high blood supply and high affinity such as brain, heart, liver and spleen. Fat and muscle, having low blood supplies, equilibrate slowly, but the high affinity of fat for these drugs means that large amounts may be absorbed there temporarily, prior to release back to the circulation before metabolism.

Metabolism

Generally the *ester* drugs are metabolized by plasma cholinesterase so rapidly that it is very difficult to measure their concentrations in blood after a regional block. Because of this rapid metabolism systemic toxicity is very rare. Theoretically an abnormal cholinesterase level could result in an increased risk of toxicity (cf. suxamethonium) but it has been shown that enzyme activity must be reduced dramatically to impair significantly the rate of hydrolysis of the ester drugs.

The *amide* local anaesthetics are metabolized in the liver and it is probable that prilocaine may undergo some extrahepatic metabolism as well. Hepatocellular damage has to be severe before the rate of breakdown is affected, but because some amides (*not* bupivacaine) have relatively high hepatic extraction ratios their rate of metabolism is more dependent on hepatic blood flow. This has practical relevance to the use of lignocaine as an anti-arrhythmic agent in cardiogenic shock, where liver blood flow will be reduced.

The metabolic pathways for all the amides are similar to that of lignocaine (Fig. 4.7). Initially lignocaine is dealkylated and then hydrolysed before or after a second dealkylation. Hydroxylation of the ring structure also occurs. Its

metabolites are less toxic than the parent compound, but inability to excrete these products may contribute to lignocaine toxicity in renal failure. Negligible amounts of both ester and amide drugs are eliminated as the parent compound.

Protein binding

Like many other drugs, local anaesthetics bind to plasma proteins to some degree, the two proteins involved being α_1-acid glycoprotein and albumin.

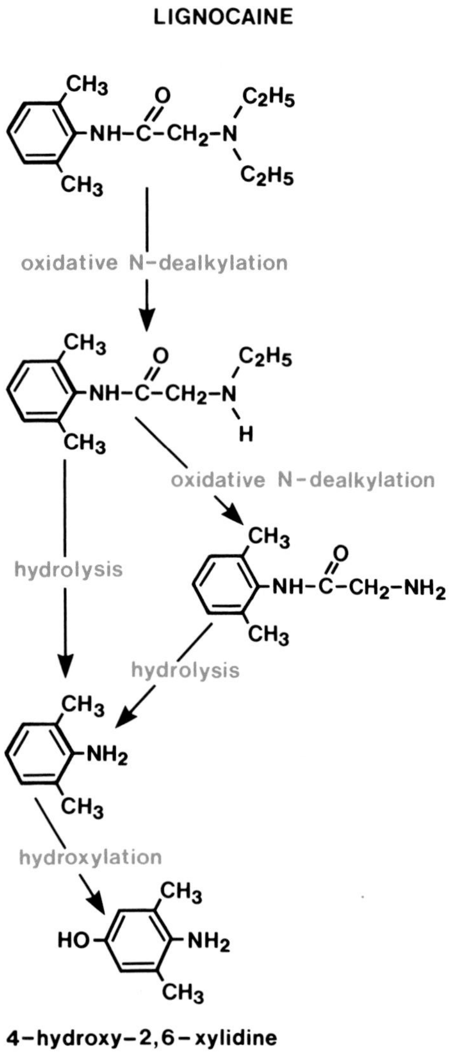

Fig. 4.7 Metabolic pathway for lignocaine.

Table 4.1 Approximate percentages of amide local anaesthetics that are protein-bound at two different serum concentrations

	Serum concentration (μg ml^{-1}):	
	1	50
Bupivacaine	95	60
Etidocaine	95	60
Ropivacaine	94	63
Lignocaine	70	35
Mepivacaine	75	30
Prilocaine	40	30

The former binds the drugs avidly, but has a limited capacity for them, whereas albumin has a low affinity and a large capacity. As a result, the greater proportion of a low concentration is bound, but once the binding sites on α_1-acid glycoprotein are occupied the proportion that is bound decreases as the concentration increases (Table 4.1).

The measurement of protein binding was originally undertaken to provide a physicochemical property which related to duration of action in the laboratory assessment of new compounds. It is often assumed that drugs with greater affinity for protein are less toxic because only a small part of the total amount present in plasma is 'available' to diffuse into the tissues and produce toxic effects. However, figures for protein binding are obtained *in vitro* under equilibrium conditions and probably bear little relationship to the very dynamic situation existing during the phase of rapid drug absorption. In addition the assumption that these figures relate to toxicity is illogical because the bound fraction is in simple equilibrium with that which is free in plasma. Thus, drug from either fraction in plasma is available to diffuse down a concentration gradient into the tissues. The ready availability of bound drug is illustrated by the fact that the percentage hepatic extraction of amide local anaesthetics considerably exceeds the free fraction in blood.

It is noteworthy that prilocaine, the least protein-bound of all the amides, is the least toxic. In animals, at least, the concentration of prilocaine

must be much greater than that of lignocaine to produce the equivalent convulsive activity (Englesson et al 1965). It may be that its low binding to plasma protein is paralleled by lower binding to nerve cell protein, and that it thus produces a lesser effect.

Figures for protein binding are not related to acute toxicity.

Placental transfer

Local anaesthetic present in maternal blood will equilibrate through the placental membrane with the fetus just like any other organ. Fetal plasma contains less α_1-acid glycoprotein than maternal plasma and as a result concentrations are usually lower in fetal than in maternal plasma. However, at equilibrium the concentration of 'free' drug will be the same in both circulations. There is evidence that tissue drug concentrations are much closer in mother and fetus than comparison of maternal and fetal plasma concentrations would imply (Morishima et al 1983).

Even if tissue concentrations of local anaesthetics are much the same in the fetus as in the mother it is important to stress that the effects of these drugs are, in the vast majority of cases, of minimal significance particularly when compared with those of conventional methods of analgesia and anaesthesia. Immaturity of some neonatal enzyme systems may mean that the drugs are metabolized more slowly. This will be of little importance unless delivery takes place just after a high peak concentration in the mother. Neonatal concentrations may then remain elevated for some time. Toxicity may manifest itself more in the child than in the mother in one situation – the acidotic fetus. Acidosis will result in a greater proportion of any intracellular drug being in the active ionized form so its effect will be more pronounced. Latent toxicity may become overt in that situation.

Prevention and treatment of toxicity

The single most important factor in the prevention of toxicity is the avoidance of accidental intra-

venous injection. Careful aspiration tests are vital
and should be repeated each time the needle is
moved, but a negative test is not an absolute
guarantee of extravascular placement, especially
when catheter techniques are used. The initial
injection of 2–3 ml of solution containing adrenaline (1:200 000) has been advocated – an
increase in heart rate during the next 1–2 minutes
indicating an intravascular injection. However, the
heart rate may vary considerably while a block is
being established (particularly during labour) and
adrenaline is not the safest of drugs. In addition,
no test dose can guarantee against subsequent
migration of the catheter or needle into a vein.

An alternative to the test dose is to repeat the
aspiration test after each 5 ml of solution and to
inject slowly while watching the patient carefully
for early signs of toxicity. A very distinct pause
in injection should be allowed after the first 5 ml
increment to allow such features to appear. In the
elderly a period of at least a minute should elapse
in case a slow circulation time delays the onset of
symptoms such as tinnitus or circumoral numbness. Finally, particular care should be taken with
head and neck blocks because the injection of
only a small dose of drug into a carotid or
vertebral artery will produce a major cerebral
reaction.

Systemic toxicity from absorption of a correctly
placed but excessive dose of drug is very rare and
may be avoided by taking into account the known
behaviour of the individual drug when injected at
the particular site. Each chapter in the second
section of this book indicates the appropriate
drugs and doses for the various blocks considered. The pharmacokinetic basis behind these
figures lends little support for the principle of the
'maximum recommended dose', whether this is
related to patient weight or not. Scott (1989) has
argued cogently the case against adherence to
such a maximum because it can result in the use
of an inadequate amount of drug for the procedure. A better concept is to keep in mind the
'median' dose required for a specific block and
to modify this *up or down* in the light of the
patient's physique and state of health.

The treatment of toxic reactions is discussed in
Chapter 5.

OTHER SIDE-EFFECTS

Local anaesthetics are relatively free from other
side-effects. Complications of specific drugs will
be discussed later, but four general features are
worth mentioning here.

Allergic reactions

Allergy to the esters is relatively common, particularly with procaine, since *p*-aminobenzoic acid is
produced when this agent is hydrolysed. Most
reactions are dermal in personnel handling the
drugs, but fatal anaphyllaxis has been recorded.
Allergy to the amides is extremely rare and most
'reactions' are due to systemic toxicity, or the
effects of added vasoconstrictors or are due to
manifestations of anxiety such as fainting. The
occasional truly allergic reaction is usually due to
a preservative in the solution rather than to the
actual drug, but true drug allergy has been
reported (Brown et al 1981). The investigation of
allergic reactions is considered in Chapter 5.

Drug interactions

Interactions with other drugs are possible, but
rarely give rise to clinical problems. All local
anaesthetics have a weak neuromuscular blocking
action. It is theoretically possible that this might
result in potentiation of the relaxants or cause
problems in myasthenic patients, but there is no
clear evidence to indicate that this happens.
Therapy with anticholinesterases for myasthenia,
or the concomitant administration of other drugs
hydrolysed by plasma cholinesterase, could slow
the metabolism of ester drugs. The amide local
anaesthetics are potent inhibitors of plasma cholinesterase (Zsigmond et al 1978) and the
administration of an ester to a patient who has
recently received an amide might have unexpectedly toxic effects. Lignocaine and the other agents
may be displaced from plasma protein-binding
sites by a variety of other drugs (McNamara et al
1981) but this is of minimal clinical significance.

The benzodiazepines mask the early signs of
systemic toxicity and may be used for that effect.

Large doses given as premedication may even prevent convulsions, but cardiorespiratory collapse could then be the first sign of a toxic reaction. The dose of any anticonvulsant used to treat toxicity must be adjusted with care since it may exacerbate cardiorespiratory depression. The depressant action of drugs used in the treatment of cardiovascular disease might combine with the systemic effect of a local anaesthetic to precipitate cardiac failure.

Tissue toxicity

The local anaesthetic drugs in clinical use rarely produce nerve damage. Any neuropathy developing after surgery is more likely to be due to other factors such as faulty patient positioning or trauma from the needle, the catheter or the operative procedure itself. However, a few years ago there were several reports in the American literature of neurological damage after the use of chloroprocaine. It would seem that this was caused by sodium bisulphite added to the solution as an antioxidant (for a review see Covino 1984). In the epidural space the nerve sheath probably protects the nerve from the effects of this preservative, but when accidental intrathecal injection occurs – a feature common to most of the reported cases – the bisulphite has free access to the nerve tissue.

This emphasizes the particular care which must be taken with intrathecal injection. The recent renewed interest in continuous spinal anaesthesia has resulted in the publication of several reports of the cauda equina syndrome (Rigler et al 1991). The common factor here seems to have been the repeated injection of hypertonic solutions of local anaesthetic (usually with dextrose) in an attempt to extend an initially restricted block. The solution would seem to have accumulated in the sacral region and resulted in osmotic injury to the unsheathed nerve roots. Isotonic solutions may be preferable.

Antiplatelet activity

One side-effect of local anaesthetic drugs may be looked upon as a benefit rather than a complication. Regional techniques can result in a reduction in the risk of the thromboembolic complications of surgery (Ch. 2). One of the mechanisms of this is a direct pharmacological effect, decreasing both platelet aggregation and blood viscosity (Borg and Modig 1985, Henny et al 1986). The relative importance of this and the indirect effect on lower limb blood flow have yet to be established.

PHARMACOLOGY OF INDIVIDUAL DRUGS

The available local anaesthetic drugs vary somewhat in their stability, potency, duration and toxicity. Differences in these features may be related to variations in physicochemical properties, and these in turn to the underlying chemical structures.

Local anaesthetic drug chemistry

As was indicated above (Fig. 4.1), local anaesthetic molecules have a three-part structure which includes either an ester or amide bond at the centre. The main differences between these two classes – route of metabolism and allergenicity – have been discussed. The esters tend also to hydrolyse spontaneously in storage and should only be heat-sterilized once. The amides are far more stable in solution, unless mixed with dextrose for spinal anaesthesia, in which case they too should only be heat-sterilized once.

The aromatic portion of the molecule is the more lipophilic and the amine portion hydrophilic, but addition of an alkyl radical to any part of the basic 'skeleton' tends both to increase lipid solubility and decrease water solubility. The base forms of the drugs that are sufficiently potent for clinical use are of low water solubility and that is why they are usually prepared as the more water-soluble hydrochloride salt.

Quite small changes in chemical structure produce profound changes in physicochemical properties and in clinical profile. For instance, substitution of a butyl group for the methyl group on the piperidine ring of mepivacaine produces bupivacaine, which is more potent, longer-acting and more toxic on a weight-for-weight basis.

Table 4.2 The features of individual local anaesthetic drugs – **esters**

Proper name/ formula	% equivalent concentration[a]	Relative duration[a]	Toxicity	pK_a	Partition coefficient	%protein bound	Main use by anaesthetists in the UK
COCAINE	1	$\frac{1}{2}$	Very high	8.7	?	?	Nil
BENZOCAINE	NA	2	Low	NA	132	?	Topical
PROCAINE	2	$\frac{3}{4}$	Low	8.9	3.1	5.8	Nil
CHLOROPROCAINE	1	$\frac{3}{4}$	Low	9.1	17	?	Not available
AMETHOCAINE	$\frac{1}{4}$	2	High	8.4	541	76	Topical

Potency is related to lipid solubility, because this determines the agent's ability to penetrate lipid cell membranes. *Rate of onset* may also be affected by lipid solubility, but pK_a, by influencing the proportion of drug in the non-ionized form, is at least as important. The lower the pK_a, the faster the onset. *Duration of action* increases with lipid solubility, but also relates to the affinity for binding to protein. Sodium channels are formed from large protein molecules and presumably the longer-acting drugs bind to them for longer. Alterations in structure also affect the rate, and the nature of the products, of metabolism.

In addition to their influence on potency, rate of onset and duration of action, the physicochemical properties of an agent also determine the order in which different types of peripheral nerve fibre are blocked (Wildsmith et al 1989). It is often observed clinically that pain sensation is blocked before the other more discriminatory sensations and motor function. Yet laboratory work has indicated that, at axonal level, the A fibres which transmit motor and most sensory impulses are more sensitive to the action of local anaesthetics than the C fibres thought to carry pain sensation (Gissen et al 1980). This is because lipid diffusion barriers, such as the myelin sheaths and other Schwann cell structures, surround A fibres to a greater extent than C fibres. These diffusion barriers will delay the access of most drugs to the A fibre axon. It is only when an agent of extremely high lipid solubility and low pK_a is used that the

Table 4.2 (cont.) The features of individual local anaesthetic drugs – **amides**

Proper name/ formula	% equivalent concentration[a]	Relative duration[a]	Toxicity	pK_a	Partition coefficient	% protein bound	Main use by anaesthetists in the UK
LIGNOCAINE	1	1	Medium	7.8	110	64	Infiltration Nerve block Epidural
MEPIVACAINE	1	1	Medium	7.7	42	77	Not available
PRILOCAINE	1	$1\frac{1}{2}$	Low	7.7	50	55	Infiltration Nerve block IVRA
CINCHOCAINE	$\frac{1}{4}$	2	High	7.9	?	?	Not available
ROPIVACAINE	$\frac{1}{4}$	2–4	Medium	8.1	230	94	Not yet marketed
BUPIVACAINE	$\frac{1}{4}$	2–4	Medium	8.1	560	95	Extradural Spinal Nerve block
ETIDOCAINE	$\frac{1}{2}$	2–4	Medium	7.9	1853	94	Not available

[a]Lignocaine = 1; NA, not applicable (not used in solution); ?, information not available. NB: published figures vary. See Strichartz and colleagues (1990) for more details.

greater sensitivity of the A fibre is apparent clinically. One of the striking features of the relatively new drug etidocaine is its ability to produce motor block out of proportion to the degree of analgesia – an indication of its ability to penetrate lipid membranes.

One other inherent drug property which might modity its clinical profile is its direct effect on blood vessels. Most local anaesthetics produce some degree of vasodilatation, but exceptions are cocaine and ropivacaine, which are vasoconstrictors, and prilocaine, which appears to have no effect.

Clinical factors affecting drug profile

Before making direct comparisons between the various local anaesthetic drugs, it is important to emphasize that several clinical factors affect rate of onset, potency, duration of action and toxicity. Onset time will be decreased, and duration increased, by the use of a larger dose. The dose may be increased by increasing volume or concentration, but given the same total dose, a large volume of a dilute solution will produce a better block than a small volume of a concentrated one.

There are marked differences in onset time between the different types of block. Onset is almost immediate after infiltration and is progressively longer for spinal, peripheral nerve, epidural and brachial plexus blocks. This order correlates with variations in diffusion barriers, both around and within the nerve trunks, at the different sites. In the cerebrospinal fluid the nerve rootlets are bare, but they acquire a sheath after piercing the dura mater. Further coverings are acquired as the nerves leave the intervertebral foramina, but these become progressively thinner as the nerves spread distally and become smaller. The dose of drug required for the different blocks and the likely duration of action also increase in much the same order as onset time.

Individual drug features

Because of the above factors, comparisons between different agents should be made only using data collected for the same block. It is at least

Table 4.3 Pharmacokinetic data for parenterally administered local anaesthetic drugs in man, specified with respect to arterial blood drug concentrations, except for prilocaine and cocaine data which are specified with respect to peripheral venous plasma drug concentrations

Drug	$t_{\frac{1}{2},z}$ (min)	CL (1 min^{-1})	V_{ss} (l)	E_H (%)
Cocaine	42–90	0.71–3.08	118^a	?
Procaine	<1	?	?	?
Chloroprocaine	<0.5	?	?	?
Amethocaine	?	?	?	?
Lignocaine	96	0.95	91	65
Mepivacaine	114	0.78	84	52
Prilocaine	93	2.84	261	?
Cinchocaine	?	?	?	?
Ropivacaine	111	0.73	59	49
Bupivacaine	162	0.58	73	38
Etidocaine	162	1.11	133	74

NB: published figures vary. $t_{\frac{1}{2},z}$ half-life of elimination; CL, rate of plasma clearance; V_{ss}, volume of distribution; E_H, hepatic extraction.
^{a} V_z for cocaine.

questionable whether there are any significant differences in onset time between agents if *equipotent* concentrations are used. However, there are real differences in potency, duration and toxicity. Much of our understanding of the safe clinical use of local anaesthetics has come from studies of their pharmacokinetics (Tucker 1984). Such information was the basis of the discussion earlier in this chapter of the factors that govern systemic toxicity. The features of the individual drugs are discussed below and some of the more quantitative data are shown in Tables 4.2 and 4.3.

The esters

Cocaine. Because of its systemic toxicity, central nervous stimulant and addictive properties and tendency to produce allergic reactions, cocaine has little if any place in modern anaesthesia. It is still used in ear, nose and throat practice for its vasoconstrictor action, but is becoming very difficult to obtain legitimately at a reasonable price.

In animals the main site of metabolism is thought to be the liver, but there is evidence that plasma esterases are more important in man (Van Dyke et al 1976).

Benzocaine. This ester does not contain the amine group common to all the other clinically useful agents. As a result it does not ionize and this has two implications. Firstly, it will not form water-soluble salts so it can only be used topically. Secondly, its mode of action must differ from that outlined above for the other local anaesthetics. It is thought that benzocaine diffuses into the cell membrane (but not the cytoplasm) and either causes the membrane to expand in a way similar to that postulated for general anaesthetics, or enters the sodium channel directly from the lipid phase of the membrane. It is possible that the other local anaesthetics may, in part, exert their action by these mechanisms.

Benzocaine is hydrolysed very rapidly to *p*-aminobenzoic acid so is of low toxicity, but may produce allergic reactions. It is very effective when used topically.

Procaine and chloroprocaine. The short shelf life, brief duration of action, incidence of allergic reactions and the introduction of better agents have all combined to limit the use of procaine. As its name suggests, chloroprocaine is structurally very similar. The simple addition of a chloride atom to the aromatic ring produces a drug that is hydrolysed even faster than procaine and is probably slightly more potent. Its metabolic product is 2-chloro-4-aminobenzoic acid which, from the lack of published reports, seems to be less likely to produce allergic reactions than *p*-aminobenzoic acid. The obvious advantages of this compound, which is used very widely in the USA, have been offset by reports of permanent neurological damage. Evidence is accumulating to suggest that this has been due to bisulphite included in the solution to prevent spontaneous hydrolysis (Covino 1984).

Amethocaine. This is the most potent and longest acting of the ester drugs in clinical use. It is hydrolysed by plasma cholinesterase, but relatively slowly, so it is quite toxic. In small doses it can be used safely and it is the standard drug for spinal anaesthesia in the USA, where it is known as tetracaine.

The amides

Lignocaine. Lignocaine is today the standard agent against which all other local anaesthetics are compared. All the general features of the amides outlined earlier apply to it and it has no unusual properties. It has been used safely for all types of local anaesthesia and is also a standard anti-arrhythmic agent.

Mepivacaine. Although chemically somewhat different from lignocaine, mepivacaine is very similar clinically. It seems to have no particular advantage or disadvantage although it may be slightly less toxic than lignocaine.

Prilocaine. Of all the amide drugs prilocaine has the lowest systemic toxicity. This is because it differs from lignocaine in several minor, but significant respects. It does not produce any vasodilatation, is sequestered or perhaps metabolized by the lungs (Akerman et al 1966a) in greater amounts, is distributed to the other tissues at a faster rate, and requires higher concentrations to produce convulsions. As a result the safe dose of this agent is twice that of lignocaine. Since it is equipotent with lignocaine and probably has a slightly longer duration of action, it is surprising that it is not more widely used.

The reason for its lack of popularity is related to the fact that there is only one methyl group on the aromatic ring. This means that the first stage of its metabolism is hydrolysis to *o*-toluidine, the hydroxylated products of which have the ability to reduce haemoglobin (Akerman et al 1966b). It is anxiety about producing methaemoglobinaemia that seems to restrict the use of prilocaine even though more than 600 mg must be used before the theoretical risk becomes real. This is far in excess of the amount that would be used for a single administration and *prilocaine is the agent of choice whenever the risk of systemic toxicity is high.*

It should not be used during labour, partly because 'top-up' injections may exceed the dose that will produce methaemoglobinaemia, but mainly because fetal haemoglobin is more sensitive to this transformation. It would seem wise to try and avoid using it in anaemic patients, although it is important to stress that when methaemoglobinaemia becomes clinically apparent as cyanosis, only 1.5 g 100 ml^{-1} haemoglobin is reduced and the intravenous injection of 1 mg kg^{-1} of methylene blue will rapidly reverse this.

Cinchocaine. Cinchocaine was developed in 1925, nearly two decades before lignocaine, and was the first local anaesthetic to have an amide linkage. However, it is otherwise dissimiliar in structure. It is very toxic and this limits its use to spinal anaesthesia.

Bupivacaine. The introduction of bupivacaine was an important event because it is a long-acting agent, the acute toxicity of which is, relative to potency, much the same as that of lignocaine. Its duration allows single-shot local blocks to be used for more prolonged surgery; more importantly this means that the risk of toxicity is less during catheter techniques because the intervals between injections are longer. The other advantage of bupivacaine for catheter techniques is that effective analgesia can be provided with less motor block than other agents.

Unfortunately, bupivacaine was implicated in a series of very severe toxic reactions, some of which were fatal. In many of these instances the supervision of the patient left much to be desired, but evidence accumulated to suggest that the agent may occasionally produce cardiotoxicity before neurotoxicity, with primary ventricular fibrillation being described in both man and animals (Covino 1984). A common feature of most of the reactions was that a very large dose had been administered directly into the circulation. In some of the cases excessive concentrations were used for intravenous regional anaesthesia – a procedure for which this agent is most unsuitable. Many of the other reactions were associated with the use of the 0.75% solution and it would seem that, should the needle or catheter be placed accidentally in a vein, this concentrated formulation allows the very rapid injection of a large dose into the circulation. Peak systemic concentrations are thus likely to be higher than if the same dose were injected as a more dilute solution.

Obviously, such serious reactions can be prevented if the drug is administered correctly. However, concern about the problem led to renewed interest in finding an alternative agent with a similiar clinical profile to bupivacaine, but less cardiotoxicity. At the time of writing ropivacaine is undergoing intense clinical investigation to see if it meets these criteria.

Ropivacaine Chemically, this agent is intermediate in structure between mepivacaine and bupivacaine (Table 4.2). Like all members of this series it contains an asymmetric carbon atom and exists as two optically active isomers. Ropivacaine is prepared as a solution of the (*S*) isomer alone, whereas the other drugs are presented as a racemic mixture of the two isomers. In terms of local anaesthetic performance the (*S*) isomer is possibly more potent and certainly longer-acting than the (*R*) isomer (Akerman et al 1988), but (for bupivacaine at least) it is the (*R*) isomer that is the more cardiotoxic (Vanhoutte et al 1991).

In man, the pharmacokinetic properties of ropivacaine compare well with bupivacaine (Lee et al 1989) and its cardiotoxicity is less (Scott et al 1989). Early clinical studies have suggested that it performs very similarly to bupivacaine (Reynolds 1991), but that it may produce an even greater degree of 'separation' of motor and sensory block (Brockway et al 1991). If these findings are confirmed, ropivacaine may be a useful addition to the range of local anaesthetic drugs.

Etidocaine. This is a long-acting derivative of lignocaine, which is unlikely to become as widely used as bupivacaine. It seems to have the ability to produce a more profound effect on motor nerves than sensory ones and this may be related to its very high lipid solubility and low pK_a.

ADDITIVES

In addition to the active agent, local anaesthetic solutions may contain several substances added to adjust factors such as pH, tonicity and baricity. Those in multidose bottles, but not those in ampoules, will also contain a preservative which can be the cause of allergic phenomena. Manufacturers usually recommend that solutions containing preservative should not be used for spinal and epidural injection. Other additions may be made to the solution for pharmacological rather than pharmaceutical reasons.

Vasoconstrictors

Addition of a vasoconstrictor will reduce the toxicity, prolong the duration and probably improve the quality of block resulting from the injection of a local anaesthetic. Commendable though each of these features is, vasoconstrictors are not used universally. They are totally contraindicated for ring blocks and intravenous regional anaesthesia since they may produce tissue ischaemia. The most commonly used agent, adrenaline, has its own systemic effects and should be used with particular care, if at all, in patients with cardiac disease. Concentrations greater than 1:200 000 should not be used and the total dose should be limited. Doses greater than 200 µg have been shown to cause cardiovascular disturbances during brachial plexus block (Kennedy et al 1966). Interactions with other sympathomimetic drugs, such as tricyclic antidepressants, may occur, especially when vasoconstrictors are used systemically to treat hypotension. Felypressin has less systemic effect, but it may be a coronary vasoconstrictor and is usually only available for dental use.

Finally, there is the question as to whether vasoconstrictors increase the risk of permanent neurological damage by making nerves ischaemic. Their widespread use in the USA suggests that this is not a matter for practical concern, but many anaesthetists feel that they should only be used if there is no alternative method of reducing toxicity or prolonging duration. As with chloroprocaine, it might be the preservative that has been responsible for nerve damage. Most solutions containing adrenaline also contain sodium metabisulphite as an antioxidant.

Other adjuvants

At various times solutions of local anaesthetics have been introduced containing substances which, it is claimed, may improve the block in some way. Some drugs have been prepared as the *carbonated* salt instead of the standard hydrochloride in an effort to speed the onset of block. Laboratory studies have consistently shown that this is effective due to a combination of direct axon depression by carbon dioxide, enhanced diffusion of the local anaesthetic and a decrease in intracellular pH favouring formation of the ionized form of the drug (Catchlove 1972). Clinical studies are less consistent in their results, but the evidence suggests that carbonated solutions produce a significant improvement in blocks of slower onset (McClure & Scott 1981).

The *alkalinization* of standard solutions of local anaesthetics by the addition of sodium bicarbonate has also been employed in an attempt to speed the onset of block. The theory is that an increase in the pH of the solution will increase the proportion of the drug in the non-ionized, membrane-permeant form and thus speed nerve penetration. The results of clinical studies have not been entirely consistent, and, even where a positive effect has been demonstrated, doubt has been expressed about its clinical usefulness (Swann et al 1991). There is always the risk that the pH change will cause the drug to precipitate before injection and the method has little to commend it.

A much older strategy for speeding onset is the addition of the tissue enzyme *hyaluronidase*. There is little objective evidence (Keeler et al 1992) to support its use except in ophthalmology (Nicoll et al 1986), where it continues to be popular.

Local anaesthetics have also been injected with *high molecular weight dextrans* to try to prolong their duration. Again the clinical results are inconclusive, but dextrans of very high molecular weight may be effective, especially in combination with adrenaline (Simpson et al 1982).

A number of substances have been added to local anaesthetic preparations to try and improve their rate of penetration through intact skin. Until recently these have not been very successful, but a recent development has been the *eutectic mixture of local anaesthetics* (EMLA). This is an oil-in-water emulsion of equal amounts of the base forms of lignocaine and prilocaine. When crystals of these bases are mixed together at room temperature they assume a 'liquid' form because this eutectic mixture has a lower melting point than either constituent. This allows the drugs to be prepared in a formulation suitable for topical application. The cream has to be applied to the skin for about an hour, but sufficient base does penetrate to allow relatively painless venepuncture. In some patients it may even allow the cutting of skin grafts.

The addition of *opioids* to local anaesthetics is being employed increasingly for central nerve block and has been considered in Chapter 3.

CHOICE OF LOCAL ANAESTHETIC AGENT

One of the most important decisions to be made when using a local technique is how much of which drug is to be injected. Firstly the solution has to be of adequate strength. For lignocaine (the relative potencies of the other agents are in Table 4.2) the concentrations which are adequate to produce analgesia for skin incision are:

Infiltration Intravenous regional	0.5%
Minor nerve block	1.0%
Brachial plexus Sciatic/femoral	1.0–1.5%
Epidural	1.5–2.0%
Spinal	2.0–5.0%

Greater concentrations than these may be used to produce more profound blocks of faster onset. The volume to be injected will depend on the particular technique. Once the required concentration and volume are known, an appropriate drug should be selected on the basis of the likely rate of absorption and expected duration of surgery at that site.

Some workers employ mixtures of drugs, usually in an attempt to overcome the somewhat slower onset of the longer-acting agents by adding a short-acting drug with a rapid onset. The evidence that this actually works is at best conflicting and it may be that pharmaceutical interactions between solutions are responsible for the failure of the technique to work (Covino 1986). In most situations it is simpler to insert a catheter and make sequential injections.

Further consideration of drug selection for particular blocks is therefore given in the appropriate chapter in the second section of this book. It is important to remember that availability of particular agents may be limited by commercial factors. However, it is often possible to arrange for a hospital pharmacy in Britian to import a supply of an otherwise unavailable drug from a country where it is on sale.

FURTHER READING

Butterworth J F, Strichartz G R 1990 Molecular mechanisms of local anesthesia: a review. Anesthesiology 72: 711–734

Smith G, Scott D B (eds) 1986 A symposium on local anaesthesia. British Journal of Anaesthesia 58: 691–746

REFERENCES

Akerman B, Astrom A, Ross S, Telc A 1966a Studies on the absorption, distribution and metabolism of labelled prilocaine and lidocaine in some animal species. Acta Pharmacologica et Toxicologica 24: 389–403

Akerman B, Peterson S A, Wistrand P 1966b Methemoglobin forming metabolites of prilocaine. Third International Pharmacological Congress (Abstracts), Sao Paolo, Brazil, p 237

Akerman B, Hellberg I-B, Trossvik C 1988 Primary evaluation of the local anaesthetic properties of the amino amide agent ropivacaine (LEA 103). Acta Anaesthesiologica Scandinavica 32: 571–578

Bonica J J 1971 Regional anesthesia: recent advances and current status, pp 69–70. Blackwell, Oxford

Borg T, Modig J 1985 Potential antithrombotic effects of local anaesthetics due to their inhibition of platelet function. Acta Anaesthesiologica Scandinavica 29: 739–742

Brockway M S, Bannister J, McClure J H, McKeown D, Wildsmith J A W 1991 Comparison of extradural ropivacaine and bupivacaine. British Journal of Anaesthesia 66: 31–37

Brown D T, Beamish D, Wildsmith J A W 1981 Allergic reaction to an amide local anaesthetic. British Journal of Anaesthesia 53: 435–437

Catchlove RFH 1972 The influence of CO_2 and pH on local anesthetic action. Journal of Pharmacology and Experimental Therapeutics 181: 298–309

Covino B G 1984 Current controversies in local anaesthetics. In: Scott D B, McClure J H, Wildsmith J A W (eds) Regional anaesthesia 1884–1984, pp 74–81. ICM, Sodertalje

Covino B G 1986 Pharmacology of local anaesthetic agents. British Journal of Anaesthesia 58: 701–716

Covino B G, Vassallo H G 1976 Local anesthetics: mechanisms of action and clinical use, pp 131–140. Grune and Stratton, New York

Englesson S, Paymaster N J, Hill T R 1965 Electrical seizure activity produced by Xylocaine and Citanest. Acta Anaesthesiologica Scandinavica Supplement XVI: 47–50

Gissen A J, Covino B G, Gregus J 1980 Differential sensitivity of mammalian nerves to local anesthetic drugs. Anesthesiology 53: 467–474

Henny C P, Odoom J A, ten Cate H et al 1986 Effects of extradural bupivacaine on the haemostatic system. British Journal of Anaesthesia 58: 301–305

Keeler J F, Simpson K H, Ellis F R, Kay S P 1992 Effect of addition of hyaluronidase to bupivacaine during axillary brachial plexus block. British Journal of Anaesthesia 68: 68–71

Kennedy W F, Bonica J J, Ward R J, Tolas A G, Martin W E, Grinstein A 1966 Cardiovascular effects of epinephrine when used in regional anesthesia. Acta Anaesthesiologica Scandinavica 23: 320–333

Lee A, Fagan D, Lamont M, Tucker G T, Halldin M, Scott D B 1989 Disposition kinetics of ropivacaine in humans. Anesthesia and Analgesia 69: 736–738

McClure J H, Scott D B 1981 Comparison of bupivacaine hydrochloride and carbonated bupivacaine in brachial plexus block by the interscalene technique. British Journal of Anaesthesia 53: 523–526

McNamara P J, Slaughter R L, Pieper J A, Wyman M G, Lalka D 1981 Factors influencing serum protein binding of lidocaine in humans. Anesthesia and Analgesia 60: 395–400

Morishima H O, Hiraoka H, Tsuji A et al 1983 Pharmacodynamics of lidocaine in the mature, nonasphyxiated fetal lamb. Anesthesiology A412

Nicoll J M V, Trueren B, Acharya P A, Ahlen K, James M 1986 Retrobulbar anesthesia: the role of hyaluronidase. Anesthesia and Analgesia 65: 1324–1328

Reynolds F 1991 Editorial: ropivacaine. Anaesthesia 46: 339–340

Rigler M L, Drasner K, Krejcie T C et al 1991 Cauda equina syndrome after continuous spinal anesthesia. Anesthesia and Analgesia 72: 275–281

Scott D B 1989 Editorial: "maximum recommended doses" of local anaesthetic drugs. British Journal of Anaesthesia 63: 373–374

Scott D B, Cousins M J 1980 Clinical pharmacology of local anesthetic drugs. In: Cousins M J, Bridenbaugh D (eds) Neural blockade in clinical anesthesia and management of pain, pp 86–127. Lippincott, Philadelphia

Scott D B, Lee A, Fagan D, Bowler G M R, Bloomfield P, Lundh R 1989 Acute toxicity of ropivacaine compared with that of bupivacaine. Anesthesia and Analgesia 69: 663–669

Simpson P J, Hughes D R, Long D H 1982 Prolonged local analgesia for inguinal herniorrhaphy with bupivacaine and dextran. Annals of the Royal College of Surgeons of England 64: 243–246

Strichartz G R, Sanchez V, Arthur G R, Chafetz R, Martin D 1990 Fundamental properties of local anesthetics. II. Measured octanol:buffer partition coefficients and pK_a values of clinically used drugs. Anesthesia and Analgesia 71: 158–170

Swann D G, Armstrong P J, Douglas E, Brockway M, Bowler G M R 1991 The alkalinisation of bupivacaine for intercostal nerve blockade. Anaesthesia 46: 174–176

Tucker G T 1984 Pharmacokinetics of local anaesthetic agents – possible role in toxicity. In: Scott D B, McClure J H, Wildsmith J A W (eds) Regional anaesthesia 1884–1984, pp 61–71. ICM, Sodertaljer

Vanhoutte F, Vereecke J, Verbeke N, Carmeliet E 1991 Stereoselective effects of the enantiomers of bupivacaine on the electrophysiological properties of the guinea pig papillary muscle. British Journal of Pharmacology 103: 1275–1281

Van Dyke C, Barash B G, Jatlow P, Byck R 1976 Cocaine: plasma concentrations after intranasal application in man. Science 191: 859–861

Wildsmith J A W, Brown D T, Paul D, Johnson S 1989 Structure–activity relationships in differential nerve blockade at high and low frequency stimulation. British Journal of Anaesthesia 63: 444–452

Zsigmond E K, Kothary S P, Flynn K B 1978 In vitro inhibitory effect of amide-type local analgesics on normal and atypical human plasma cholinesterases. Regional Anesthesia 3/4: 7–9

5. The management of regional anaesthesia

J. E. Charlton

A well-conducted regional anaesthetic technique is a thing of beauty, and gives satisfaction and comfort to patient, anaesthetist and surgeon alike. However, the warm glow that success engenders is merely the residue of a great deal of hard work. Preoperative, intraoperative and postoperative management of regional anaesthesia may differ considerably from that required for general anaesthesia and this chapter outlines the principles of patient management.

PREOPERATIVE CONSIDERATIONS

Preoperative management is as important as the performance of the block itself. Several different factors have to be considered, including the patient's general health, the nature, site and duration of the intended surgery, and the availability of appropriate equipment and facilities.

Factors influencing the choice of technique

Pre-existing disease

A full history and physical examination is usually available, but it is the responsibility of the anaesthetist to check that all necessary information has been obtained. If indicated, further consultation or laboratory data should be sought. There is a widespread belief that regional anaesthesia is safer that general anaesthesia, especially in patients with severe or widespread systemic disease. There is little objective evidence to support this, but regional anaesthesia appears to offer a substantial advantage in many clinical situations. However, it should not be used simply because some inconven-

ient contraindication to general anaesthesia has arisen.

Cardiovascular system. The choice of a regional anaesthetic technique for patients with ischaemic heart disease or a fixed output state is a matter of fine judgement. Both the agent employed, and the technique chosen, may have profound effects upon an already jeopardized circulation. However, provided adequate oxygenation is maintained and meticulous attention is paid to the management of hypotension, there is no reason why it should not be used.

Surgery upon patients with *ischaemic heart disease* carries a higher risk than usual and this is markedly increased if there is any episode of prolonged hypotension (Mauney et al 1970). In patients with previous myocardial infarction Steen and colleagues (1978) found a five-fold increase in reinfarction rate if the systolic pressure fell by 30% or more for 10 minutes or longer. Hypotension will reduce myocardial perfusion and may be a major factor in reinfarction. Any situation which leads to a relative increase in cardiac work and myocardial oxygen demand is to be avoided, and hypoxaemia, tachycardia, hyper- and hypotension or combinations of these will cause problems in the cardiac patient. Using a dog model with reduced coronary flow, Klassen and colleagues (1980) found that sympathetic block from an epidural caused a beneficial redistribution of coronary flow to the endocardium, probably due to alterations in the tone of transmural resistance vessels. Human studies have shown that high spinal anaesthesia caused a decrease in coronary blood flow paralleling the decrease in mean arterial pressure. However, the myocardial oxygen extraction coefficient was not increased, indicating that myocardial oxygenation remained adequate for the lower workload (Hackel et al 1956).

Indications of the relative safety of regional anaesthesia can be found in the study of Reiz and colleagues (1980), who gave thoracic epidural anaesthesia to four patients with known coronary artery disease. They found a decrease in coronary blood flow, coronary and systemic vascular resistance, heart rate and myocardial oxygen extraction. The extensive sympathetic block from T_1 to T_{12} led to a decrease in blood pressure and there was some evidence of myocardial ischaemia. However, if the sympathetic block is limited, high thoracic epidural anaesthesia may have beneficial effects upon the diseased myocardium. Blomberg and colleagues (1989) studied nine patients with advanced coronary artery disease and unstable angina. Epidural blockade of T_1–T_5 relieved the pain and improved myocardial oxygenation without jeopardizing coronary perfusion. A study by Kock and colleagues (1990) found that high thoracic epidural anaesthesia with a block of T_1–T_5 improved ischaemia-induced abnormalities of left ventricular function during a stress test in patients with ischaemic heart disease. Reiz (1989) has reviewed current understanding of the circulatory changes induced by epidural anaesthesia in cardiac patients.

It should be emphasized that the role of regional anaesthesia-induced sympathetic block in the management of the surgical patient with heart disease is unclear, but there are some breathtaking precedents to consider – Griffiths & Gillies (1948) introduced the concept of induced hypotension by using high or total spinal anaesthesia in patients with severe hypertensive cardiovascular disease!

Patients with *valvular heart disease* and those receiving β adrenoceptor blocking drugs have a reduced ability to respond to stress and cannot increase their cardiac output. The use of spinal or extradural block will result in a degree of sympathetic paralysis which may lead to a decrease in blood pressure. An unexpectedly high level of anaesthesia may also block the cardio-accelerator fibres and superimpose a fixed output state upon an already dangerous hypotension. Controlling the extent of sympathetic block will limit these prob-lems, as shown by the study of Kock and colleagues (1990), in which all the patients were under complete β block.

Given that a low cardiac output will result in reduced hepatic blood flow and a reduced ability to metabolize local anaesthetic drugs, there may be a resultant increase in the systemic effects of these agents.

Respiratory system. Patients with severe respiratory disease are among the most willing to have a regional anaesthetic for their operation. They are keenly aware of the limitations that their disease places upon their activity and how local anaesthesia may be of benefit to them. For peripheral or lower abdominal surgery neural block avoids the complications of general anaesthesia and neuromuscular blocking agents, and enables the patient to look after his own airway and respiration. With regard to upper abdominal or thoracic surgery a supplementary general anaesthetic is usually necessary. In addition, some degree of motor block will be present and may lead to a decrease in vital capacity, maximum breathing capacity and the ability to cough and clear secretions. This can cause problems for those patients with chronic obstructive airways disease who have poor pulmonary compliance and rely upon muscular activity in expiration. Unfortunately, there is no evidence that any form of preoperative respiratory function testing can predict which patients may become compromised. The major advantage of regional anaesthetic techniques in upper abdominal or thoracic surgery is in the provision of postoperative analgesia.

Nervous system. Pre-existing disease of the nervous system presents the anaesthetist with a most contentious problem. Bromage (1978) has reviewed possible causes of neurological damage during the performance of regional anaesthesia, especially near the spinal cord. These include direct trauma, haematoma, infection, vasoconstriction and accidental injection of a neurotoxin. It is almost inevitable that, if a patient's neurological condition degenerates after a regional anaesthetic, the block will be blamed to the exclusion of all other possible causes. However, Bromage has elegantly shown that many peripheral nerve lesions occurring after extradural analgesia are not directly related to the technique itself. Marinacci & Courville (1958) carried out electromyography on 482 patients with neurological complications after subarachnoid anaesthesia; only four cases were considered to be due to the block.

Nonetheless, there are plenty of reports of permanent neurological deterioration after regional anaesthesia in patients with pre-existing problems (Chaudhari et al 1978, Hirlekar 1980, Ballin 1981). In this context, the use of regional anaesthesia for back surgery must be carefully considered. With regard to established neurological disease there are protagonists of regional anaesthesia who believe that it exerts no influence upon the clinical course of a wide range of conditions (Crawford et al 1981). They cite multiple sclerosis, Guillain–Barré syndrome, residual poliomyelitis and muscular dystrophy, but give no indication of the agents used, methods of assessment or length of follow-up. There is at least one case report of sudden cardiovascular collapse following the use of spinal anaesthesia in a patient with Guillain–Barré syndrome (Perel et al 1977).

The spinal cord develops reflex activity about 1 month after transection. Mass autonomic reflexes can be provoked by visceral stimulation such as a full bladder. These reflex responses may include hypertension and bradycardia and may be life-threatening if the transection level is above T_5. Procedures such as cystoscopy are particularly likely to provoke these reflexes and spinal anaesthesia can be employed with great benefit with the sole intention of blocking the reflex pathways (Schonwald et al 1981), However, there has been at least one report of such a mass reflex developing in the presence of an apparently adequate block (Lambert et al 1982). Subarachnoid baclofen may further attenuate these mass autonomic reflexes (Muller et al 1990).

It would seem reasonable to employ regional anaesthesia in patients with established neurological disease *only* when a clear clinical advantage can be obtained and after a full discussion of the possible consequences. There should be careful documentation of the neurological deficit before and after the procedure.

Gastrointestinal system. Pre-existing liver disease or decreased hepatic blood flow may reduce the metabolism of local anaesthetic drugs and thus increase the possibility of toxicity. This problem may be minimized by reducing the dose.

Obesity. There may be technical problems with the performance of regional anaesthesia in the morbidly obese. Fisher and colleagues (1975) have suggested that difficulty in positioning, identifying landmarks and needle location all combine to make regional anaesthesia extremely difficult. Conversely, the benefits of combining light general anaesthesia with regional anaesthesia for upper abdominal surgery in the morbidly obese have been well documented by Buckley and colleagues (1983). Many of their patients also had cardiovascular and respiratory disease, and postoperative complications were less than in a similar group given general anaesthesia alone. However, the two groups and techniques employed were not matched or randomized and the findings should be assessed in that light.

Renal system. Bromage & Gertel (1972) alleged that patients with chronic renal failure are more susceptible than healthy patients to toxicity from local anaesthetic agents. These authors suggested that this might stem from a difference in drug binding due to the hypoproteinaemia associated with renal failure. They also noted that anaemia may cause a high output circulation and thus lead to rapid systemic absorption. On the other hand, the sympathetic block caused by regional anaesthesia may improve circulation and perfusion to the site of operation, whether this is the kidney itself, or a limb during the fashioning of an arteriovenous fistula.

Diabetes. Diabetic patients have an increased incidence of atherosclerosis and its attendant complications. They are particularly prone to episodes of painless myocardial ischaemia and the cardiovascular system should be the focus of unremitting vigilance. In addition, diabetes is associated with microangiopathy, peripheral neuropathy, autonomic dysfunction and infection. However, these problems are more than offset on the occasions when regional anaesthesia allows surgery to be performed with minimal disruption of the diabetic patient's carbohydrate intake and insulin regime.

Infection. Infection at or close to the site of injection is an absolute contraindication to the use of all local anaesthetic techniques. Not only may it cause spread of the infection, but the block is unlikely to be effective (Bieter 1936), because pH changes in infected tissue will impair its clinical effect. It may be possible to block a nerve distant from the focus of infection, but this is not always effective, as many dental patients can confirm.

Systemic infection may also be a contraindication to the use of spinal and epidural techniques. Epidural abscesses may occur spontaneously from sources of infection elsewhere, but clearly they are more likely to develop in a haematoma produced by an epidural needle or catheter. The belief that the caudal approach presents a greater risk of infection than any other is unfounded as long as antiseptic precautions are adequate (Abouleish et al 1980).

Muscle disease. Malignant hyperthermia is probably the best known example of a muscle disease with anaesthetic significance. Regional anaesthesia avoids the use of volatile agents and muscle relaxants, but may still be associated with increased temperature in susceptible individuals (Katz & Krich 1976, Wadhwa 1977). Amide agents such as lignocaine can release calcium from the sarcoplasmic reticulum and should be avoided. Esters are probably safer (Gronert 1980), but there has been one report of a reaction in a susceptible individual (Katz & Krich 1976).

Regional anaesthesia has been advocated for patients with muscular dystrophy and myasthenia gravis, and for the latter may be the technique of choice for peripheral or lower abdominal surgery.

Haematological disorders. It has been stated frequently that the presence of any coagulation disorder is an absolute contraindication to the performance of regional anaesthesia. This is probably true only when regional anaesthesia is carried out at a site where any haemorrhage cannot be controlled by direct pressure. Thus, epidural and spinal anaesthesia should not be used in patients with bleeding disorders (e.g. thrombocytopenia, haemophilia, leukaemia) or those on long-term anticoagulant therapy. This may not apply to the patient who receives heparin during the course of the surgical procedure, some time after the insertion of an epidural catheter.

Epidural haematomas occur spontaneously in normal patients (Cooper 1967, Markham et al 1967). They occur more commonly in the presence of anticoagulant therapy (Cousins 1972, Bamford 1978) and more commonly still after epidural anaesthesia (Gringrich 1968, Butler & Green 1970, Helperin & Cohen 1971, Janis 1972, Varkey & Brindle 1974). Spinal cord compression and paraplegia may develop and become irreversible if not diagnosed and treated promptly. The presence of the block makes diagnosis difficult.

A possible solution is to insert the epidural catheter prior to anticoagulation, and then monitor the activated clotting time (Rao & El-Etr 1981). Heparin requirements vary greatly and excessive dosage can be avoided by close monitoring. The catheter should be removed an hour before a heparin top-up is due. Circulating heparin levels will then be low and this will minimize the possibility of bleeding into the epidural space. However, one case report has shown that insertion of the catheter prior to anticoagulation does not eliminate the possibility of a haematoma (Gringrich 1968). It is difficult to justify the placement of epidural catheters after the commencement of anticoagulant therapy, although this has been reported with apparent safety in 1000 cases (Odoom & Sih 1983).

Subarachnoid haematomas are much rarer (Lund 1971). Nevertheless, it would seem sensible to avoid spinal anaesthesia in patients with bleeding disorders and in those who are fully anticoagulated. Intercostal block should also be avoided in the anticoagulated patient (Nielsen 1989).

Low-dose heparin therapy. Subcutaneous heparin has become extremely popular since a major international trial showed it to be effective for prophylaxis against deep venous thrombosis and pulmonary embolism (Kakkar et al 1975). There has been much debate as to whether regional anaesthetic techniques should be used in patients receiving this therapy (Sage 1990,

Wildsmith & McClure 1991). The difficulty in deciding upon an appropriate anaesthetic technique is compounded by the variable nature of the response to heparin. Limitations in the benefits of low-dose heparin therapy (e.g. the risk of haematoma and haemarthrosis after major orthopaedic surgery) have led to a decrease in its use.

It would seem reasonable to use any peripheral regional technique in the presence of low-dose heparin therapy. Performing blocks where direct pressure cannot control haemorrhage is more controversial, and in such patients many anaesthetists do not employ spinal or epidural techniques, despite reports of their safe use (Alleman et al 1983).

Aspirin. Concern has been expressed about the use of regional anaesthesia in patients receiving aspirin for its antiplatelet activity or in the prevention and treatment of pre-eclampsia, a condition where both platelet count and bleeding time may be abnormal. This presents a dilemma because epidural block is often indicated in the management of this condition (Ramanathan et al 1989). McDonald (1991) has reviewed the problem and suggests that treatment with aspirin should be stopped 7–10 days before delivery, and that a bleeding time of less than 10 minutes permits safe use of epidural block. However, withdrawing aspirin therapy may not be desirable obstetrically, the clinical measurement of bleeding time is not precise (Hindman & Koka 1986) and there is little information on what constitutes an acceptable figure (Wildsmith & McClure 1991).

The place of regional anaesthesia in the presence of minor disorders of coagulation remains in doubt. It would seem reasonable to use peripheral blocks where pressure can be maintained at the injection site and central block can be used if the partial thromboplastin time and the activated clotting time are within normal limits (Dehring & Ahrens 1990). It is prudent to maintain a high index of suspicion for potential problems and record any neurological deficit before and after the block.

Sickle cell disease. Regional anaesthetic techniques are the methods of choice in sickle cell disease (Howells et al 1972). The usual precautions should be taken with regard to perfusion,

maintenance of adequate oxygenation and use of tourniquets. On theoretical grounds, prilocaine should be avoided in these patients.

Allergy. Many patients claim to be 'allergic' to local anaesthetics, but the history usually reveals that a previous reaction was due to systemic toxicity, the effect of an added vasoconstrictor or a psychological reaction. Most patients have only been exposed to local anaesthesia in the dental chair where fear and anxiety are relatively common, adrenaline is used in high concentration and injections are made into vascular tissues. Allergy to local anaesthetics is rare (see Ch. 4), but each suspected case should be investigated, since failure to do so may force the anaesthetist to avoid regional anaesthesia unnecessarily.

Intradermal injection is the usual method of testing for local anaesthetic sensitivity, but false positive responses are relatively common (Fisher 1984). Full resuscitation facilities should be available and the initial injection should be 0.1 ml of solution. Complete investigation should include progressive injection of increasing doses of the local anaesthetic drug (Weiss et al 1989). Cross-sensitivity is common between the ester drugs, but not between the amides. Sensitivity to the preservative methylparaben should always be checked at the same time.

Drug therapy. Drug interactions with local anaesthetic agents are also relatively rare (see Ch. 4), but might influence the choice of technique, especially in the elderly – patients over 60 years of age form 12% of the British population, but account for 50% of prescriptions.

Psychological. Regional anaesthesia is not contraindicated by psychological illness, but its use must be assessed in the context of the patient's ability to understand and consent to the intended procedure. He must be able to cooperate fully and it may be that the nature of his illness makes this impossible. Moore (1976) states that hysteria and malingering are both relative contraindications to the use of regional anaesthesia.

The operation

Regional anaesthesia is not suitable for all operations. In some cases, the appropriate block may be technically difficult with a high failure rate, or the operation may be so extensive that more than one block is required, and the problem of drug toxicity may arise. In many other cases though, regional anaesthesia can provide effective postoperative analgesia even if sedative or general anaesthetic supplementation is required for the operation itself. One of the chief advantages of regional anaesthesia in obstetrics is that the mother can be fully conscious and unsedated at the time of delivery.

Site and nature of the operation. Obviously the chosen regional technique should provide anaesthesia over the area of the skin incision, but it must also be extensive enough to block stimuli arising from deeper structures manipulated during surgery. For example, a block limited to T_{11} and T_{12}, although adequate for an inguinal herniorrhaphy incision, will be inadequate when the surgeon handles the spermatic cord and hernial sac; and perineal anaesthesia alone will be inadequate for a vaginal hysterectomy. When a spinal or epidural block is used, particular care should be taken to ensure that it 'matches' the operation and is not too high or too low.

Even if it is technically possible to supply complete anaesthesia for all stages of an operation, it is not always desirable that the patient should be fully aware throughout. No patient should be aware of sawing during amputation, and at least a few seconds of unconsciousness are required for this and other such critical moments.

Duration. This will have a bearing on the selection of the regional technique. Catheter methods, which allow increments of local anaesthetic to be given during surgery, should be used for operations which are likely to outlast the effect of a single dose. Single injection techniques should be reserved for operations which are certain to be finished before a single dose has worn off, and which do not require local analgesia for postoperative pain control.

The duration of the operation may also influence the decision as to whether sedation or general anaesthesia should be offered. Operating tables are not designed for the comfort of the conscious, and

a long period lying on one can become an ordeal even for the most resilient and cooperative patient.

Anaesthetist and surgeon. The extent to which regional anaesthesia is deemed suitable in various cases depends on the attitude of both anaesthetist and surgeon. Not everyone has had the author's good fortune to work with a surgical colleague whose surgeon father performed over 90% of his operations under local anaesthesia which he administered himself (McEvedy 1946). The main source of surgical prejudice against regional anaesthesia is the fear that the smooth running of the operating list will be impaired. With careful planning this need not happen (see Ch. 2). The cooperation and enthusiasm of surgeons should be cultivated at all times, and it is common courtesy to inform them in advance when regional anaesthesia is planned. Another area of surgical concern is the possibility that the operation might be compromised by inadequate anaesthesia or muscle relaxation. The surgeon is entitled to expect the best possible operating conditions, and the anaesthetist requires skill, experience and patience to provide these consistently.

The atmosphere in the operating theatre should be relaxed and free of stress. There is wide variation among surgeons as to what constitutes an 'ideal' environment. Some enjoy the technical challenge and social contact provided by the conscious patient, whereas others value freedom of speech and prefer general anaesthesia. The views of the latter must be respected, but many senior surgeons feel that surgical trainees should, at some stage, gain experience in operating upon conscious patients. They point out that this refines surgical technique and tightens operating theatre discipline.

There is a similar variation in attitude towards regional anaesthesia among anaesthetists. Modern training regulations ensure that all trainee anaesthetists get some experience from an early stage, but not everyone is temperamentally suited to cope with the special challenges which regional anaesthesia presents. Such anaesthetists should aim to master one or two widely applicable blocks so that their repertoire is not restricted to general anaesthetic techniques, and their patients are not entirely denied the benefits of regional anaesthesia. At the other end of the scale, the enthusiast must make sure that his main concern is the patients' overall welfare, and not his own keenness to perform blocks.

Available facilities

Before proceeding further it is necessary to consider the equipment and drugs required for the safe and effective performance of the chosen technique.

Resuscitation. Intravenous access and fluids, a tipping trolley, an oxygen supply and resuscitation drugs and equipment *must* be available. The equipment must include an anaesthetic machine as a source of oxygen, a means of lung ventilation, a laryngoscope, oropharyngeal airways, cuffed endotracheal tubes, a stilette and continuous suction. Thiopentone, diazepam, suxamethonium, ephedrine and atropine should be immediately available.

Local anaesthetic drugs. The pharmacology of local anaesthetic drugs has been described in Chapter 4. Obviously the appropriate drug for the planned procedure must be available. *Every care should be taken to ensure that the intended local anaesthetic solution is injected. The consequences of accidental injection of antiseptics and other irritant solutions, such as potassium chloride, are catastrophic.*

Presentation of local anaesthetic drugs. The contents of single-use glass or plastic ampoules from a reputable drug company are guaranteed sterile and should be used for all central blocks. The ampoules themselves may be double wrapped and autoclaved for use within a sterile field. Multidose vials contain additional bacteriostatic agents and are not suitable for spinal and epidural work. It has been suggested that multidose vials should not be used for any regional anaesthetic technique (Henderson & Macrae 1983), because pathogens may have been introduced during previous use. These objections can be overcome by using a multidose vial once only and then removing the top with a bottle opener and discarding it. Generic local anaesthetics should be regarded with suspicion unless the exact contents are known.

All injections should be made through a micro-pore filter if a filter straw (FS 5000, Burron Medical) has not been used initially, since problems may arise from particulate matter from ampoules (Somerville & Gibson 1973) and from disposable regional anaesthetic trays (Seltzer et al 1977).

Commercially produced local anaesthetic solutions containing adrenaline have a lower pH than plain solutions and contain a preservative. These factors prevent oxidation of the adrenaline, but might be related to neurotoxicity. Addition of adrenaline to the plain solution just before use does not lower the pH significantly (Tucker 1983).

The preoperative visit

Explanation to the patient

It cannot be overemphasized that the preoperative preparation of the patient is one of the keys to success with regional anaesthesia. It establishes rapport with the patient, ensures his cooperation and makes technical performance of the block easier. Patients with pre-existing medical conditions, such as obstructive respiratory disease, are often anxious to have regional anaesthesia. Healthier patients can be offered a choice of regional anaesthesia, general anaesthesia or a mixture of both. Most patients prefer to be asleep and their wishes should always be taken into account. It may be necessary occasionally to 'sell' the advantages of regional anaesthesia, but there should be no attempt at coercion.

An adequate explanation of what the patient can expect should be given in terms which he can understand. It is a great help if the anaesthetist has experienced regional anaesthesia himself. Specific mention should be made of paraesthesiae if they are to be elicited. If the patient is to remain conscious during surgery, it is prudent to advise him that some sensation may be preserved, and that he might experience feelings of movement, warmth or cold; otherwise any stimulus may be interpreted as pain and this may result in unnecessary action being taken by the anaesthetist. It should be emphasized that any truly painful sensation will be attended to immediately.

It is good practice to point out the advantages

associated with the chosen technique – early recovery, lack of postoperative pain, reduced amount of nausea and vomiting, etc. – and to follow this with an explanation of what the patient will experience before, during and after the block. An assurance that he will not see the operation is often required and the patient should be warned that motor block may outlast the sensory block postoperatively.

Preparation of the patient

Patients for major blocks should be treated in the sáme way as patients receiving general anaesthesia and should be starved from midnight on the day of operation. Patients scheduled for peripheral nerve blocks can receive a light diet, e.g. tea and toast, up to 4 hours before the expected time of operation. It is permissible for patients to take their normal medicines with a sip of water at their usual time provided there are no contraindications. Wherever possible patients should empty the bladder preoperatively. If the bladder becomes overdistended during spinal or epidural anaesthesia the need for postoperative catheterization is significantly increased. A full bladder in a patient with a peripheral block can be both uncomfortable and disruptive.

Premedicant drugs

Some patients require no more premedication than a preoperative visit and adequate explanation of the intended procedure by the anaesthetist. However, for many patients premedication is desirable and its aim should be the relief of pain and anxiety.

Opioids. Pain relief may be necessary in patients with fractures or other painful conditions. This will enable transport to the operating theatre and positioning for the block to be undertaken with the minimum of distress. In these circumstances opioid analgesics are appropriate, although they possess many properties that are undesirable in patients having regional anaesthesia, including nausea, vomiting, respiratory depression, sedation and delayed gastric emptying. However, there is evidence that opioid premedication prior to regional anaesthesia reduces postoperative analgesic requirements (McQuay et al 1988). Grant and his colleagues (1981) have suggested intramuscular ketamine (0.5 mg kg^{-1}) as an alternative to opioids.

Benzodiazepines. Anxiolytic drugs such as diazepam, lorazepam and temazepam are useful premedicants for patients about to undergo surgery under regional anaesthesia. Oral diazepam (2.5–10 mg 2 hours before surgery) has become very popular, particularly because it has been suggested that it has the advantage of suppressing convulsant activity and thus adds a margin of safety against the effects of inadvertent overdose (de Jong & Heavner 1974). However, there are at least two major drawbacks to the use of diazepam in these circumstances. First, diazepam has an extremely long duration of action, particularly in the elderly. Second, the depression of the central nervous system (CNS) can be detrimental, in that it may allow cardiotoxic effects to develop without any premonitory CNS signs or symptoms. In addition, Gregg and colleagues (1988) have questioned the protective effect of diazepam premedication before regional anaesthesia with bupivacaine. Bupivacaine increases sympathetic activity by a central action (Gerard et al 1989) and this may counteract its myocardial depressant effect.

Lorazepam (1–2.5 mg 2 hours before surgery) has a slow onset and prolonged duration of action. Like diazepam it can be given orally or parenterally. Many anaesthetists prefer oral temazepam 10–30 mg 1 hour before surgery. It has a relatively short duration of action, is an effective anxiolytic and has few side-effects (Beechey et al 1981). It does not produce amnesia and, if this is required, one of the other benzodiazepines such as lorazepam should be used.

Other premedicant drugs. With the exception of trimeprazine in paediatric practice, phenothiazines are rarely used for premedication. There is no place for the butyrophenones such as droperidol. They may produce an apparently relaxed and cooperative patient who, in reality, is extremely apprehensive. Anticholinergic and antiemetic drugs are not usually required as premedicants before regional anaesthesia although they may be used in special circumstances.

Before long operations it is the author's practice to administer long-acting non-steroidal anti-inflammatory drugs (NSAIDs). These are useful in preventing the stiffness caused by prolonged immobility. Even where a light general anaesthetic has been administered this can cause discomfort. Oral piroxicam 20 mg the night before surgery, or diflunisal 500 mg 2–4 hours preoperatively can be helpful. Care is needed to ensure that NSAIDs are not given to patients with gastrointestinal, renal or coagulation problems.

When excessive secretions are likely to prove troublesome, anticholinergic drugs such as atropine or hyoscine may be useful. For most patients undergoing regional anaesthesia, the dryness they produce is an unnecessary discomfort. If an antivagal effect is needed, atropine is better given intravenously at the time.

Premedication in the elderly. Heavy premedication should be avoided. The benzodiazepines may cause profound sedation, confusion and restlessness. Many elderly patients present for fracture surgery, and premedication should then include an analgesic. An intramuscular antiemetic such as cyclizine 50 mg, prochlorperazine 6.25 mg or metoclopramide 10 mg may be useful if an opioid is to be used. Hyoscine should be avoided.

BLOCK PERFORMANCE

Patient handling

Care in handling begins with the transport of the patient from his bed to the induction room. Sufficient help should be available to ensure this is achieved with minimal discomfort, especially if the condition requiring surgery is painful. The block may be performed with the patient on either the tipping theatre trolley or the operating table. The author prefers to use the theatre trolley as this offers more space for positioning the patient and is slightly more comfortable. In addition, the theatre table may be in use. All equipment for the block – including any special requirements, such as a stool if the block is to be carried out in the sitting position – should be ready before the patient arrives.

Adequate trained help must be available and more than one person may be necessary, especially when the block is being performed out of the patient's sight. One assistant can provide equipment and drugs as required and the other can reassure and observe the patient while the block is being performed. The induction room should be well lit and at a reasonable temperature. Pillows and foam rubber pads should be available to ensure patient comfort. The optimum design for a local anaesthetic induction room has been described by Rosenblatt & Shal (1984).

Pulse and blood pressure should be recorded and intravenous access should be secured before the patient is positioned. Intravenous fluids and additional oxygen may be given if indicated for the particular block, patient or operation. While this is being done, it is wise to remind the patient what he will experience during the performance of the block.

If general anaesthesia is to be used in association with spinal or epidural anaesthesia, the block may be performed before or after induction. The choice will depend on the anaesthetist's personal preference, training requirements and experience, and on the needs of the particular patient. In cases where general anaesthesia is induced first, the patient's condition should be stable before the block is performed. For peripheral blocks, the patient's subjective feelings are important if the blocks are to be successful and if complications are to be avoided. Warning signs and symptoms may be missed in the unconscious patient. Most anaesthetists agree that heavy sedation should not be administered prior to the block as the patient may become uncontrollable.

The patient is positioned under the supervision of the anaesthetist. As an *aide-mémoire*, or for teaching purposes, the relevant anatomy may be marked with a skin pencil. It is useless to do this before the patient is properly positioned as anatomical relationships may change. The skin is prepared with an antiseptic solution, and in conscious patients a skin wheal is raised at the site of injection after a preliminary warning. This gives the patient an indication of what is to come, and the anaesthetist a chance to assess the patient's response.

Equipment

Trolleys

A mobile trolley with shelf space underneath for storage of sterile packs, drugs and other equipment represents the ultimate luxury. A Mayo table for the block pack is the bare minimum and there should be enough bench space nearby for additional items. The sterile field must be large enough for easy use, and for maintenance of sterility.

Commercially prepared packs are now widely available. There is variation in design and content, but a major advantage is that sterility is guaranteed by the manufacturer. Many anaesthetists prefer hospital-prepared packs as they permit a wider range of choice to suit personal requirements. They are most suitable for hospitals with a large turnover and a central sterile supply department which can guarantee sterility and the exclusion of extraneous material. Commercial packs may be more suitable for smaller hospitals and 'occasional' users.

If hospital packs are to be used, the most difficult problem is getting all concerned to agree on the contents. One answer is to prepare a basic pack with sufficient equipment for skin preparation and towelling, possibly with a limited number of carefully maintained, reusable, high-quality glass syringes and needles. Alternatively, equipment such as syringes, needles, filters and catheters can be added as needed. A separate tray with a different selection of items can be prepared for peripheral nerve block.

If local anaesthetic drugs are to be included in any of these trays, the hospital pharmacist should be consulted so that sterility, potency and freedom from contamination can be guaranteed.

Needles

The alternatives for particular procedures are discussed in the appropriate chapters in the second section of this book. The choice lies between disposable and reusable needles. The range of disposable needles available in Britain is relatively small, but sufficient variety is available to permit their exclusive use and they have the advantage of guaranteed sterility. Short-bevel needles (Fig. 5.1)

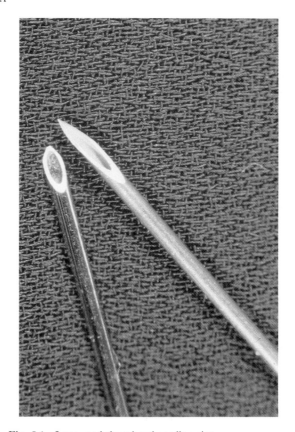

Fig. 5.1 Long- and short-bevel needle points.

have been shown to produce significantly less damage to nerves than hypodermic needles (Selander et al 1977), particularly if the bevel of the needle is parallel to the long axis of the nerve.

Disposable pencil-point needles (Regional Master Corporation) similar to the Whitacre spinal needle are also relatively atraumatic. They are Teflon coated and designed for use with a nerve stimulator. Intraneural injection is almost impossible because they have a side port (Galindo & Galindo 1980). They are available in three sizes (25 g 3.2 cm, 22 g 6.3 cm and 22 g 12.6 cm), although the smallest is not recommended because injection through it is very difficult. Disposable paediatric spinal needles are very useful for minor peripheral and cranial nerve blocks and trigger point injections. Translucent hubs allow the earlier recognition of intravascular placement during plexus or peripheral nerve block and anything which minimizes the possibility of an intravascular injection is to be encouraged.

Security beads on reusable needles are regarded as important since constant resterilization and use may weaken the junction between the hub and needle. With modern standards of manufacture this is unnecessary for a disposable needle if the guidelines listed below are followed: the needle should be discarded, not straightened, if it bends during the course of the block; the needle should be substantially withdrawn before changes in direction are made; if firm osseous contact occurs, the needle should be inspected and replaced if damaged.

Catheters

Disposable catheters should be biochemically inert, easy to sterilize, have a low coefficient of friction and a high tensile strength. They should be reasonably rigid, but should not kink easily and the tip should be atraumatic. Most modern catheters are marked at intervals and are radiopaque.

The Racz catheter (Arrow Intenational) has been developed for long-term use and consists of a spiral of wire with a straight length of similar wire acting as a permanent stilette. It is coated with a fluoropolymer (Racz et al 1982). When used as an epidural catheter care must be taken with its removal (Lingenfelter 1983). It is easiest to remove when the back is not flexed (Frankhouser 1983).

Epidural catheters are considered in Chapter 8.

Intravenous cannulae can be used for continuous caudal or plexus block. Ideally they should be radiopaque and made of Teflon. If the cannula has a metal hub and is filled with saline an alligator clip can be attached to allow nerve stimulation.

Syringes

Glass syringes with well-fitting glass or metal plungers are ideal, but the fit of the plunger in the barrel may vary between one syringe and another and even between different parts of the same syringe. The syringe should be assembled and tested before use and rejected if the plunger does not run smoothly. Aspiration of a little saline or local anaesthetic into the syringe and lubrication of the barrel is helpful in doubtful cases. Glove powder on the plunger can make the syringe stick, so the anaesthetist should not handle its ground-glass surface. Good-quality disposable plastic syringes, while lacking the finesse of smooth-running glass ones, have a more consistent feel and are the first choice of an increasing number of anaesthetists. They are certainly preferable to ill-fitting glass syringes. All syringes should have a standard Luer fitting, not a Luer-lock connection, because this requires more rotation to connect it and thus increases the likelihood of needle movement.

Peripheral nerve location

The first requirement for a successful nerve block is accurate knowledge of the anatomy. Because of anatomical variation and the fact that many nerves are deeply placed, objective evidence may be needed to show that the needle tip is close to the nerve. Elicitation of paresthesiae is the traditional solution to these problems, but more recently the nerve stimulator has been used. Both techniques have their advantages and disadvantages.

Paraesthesiae

Eliciting paraesthesiae can be unpleasant, if not painful, for the patient and may produce a sudden movement which may move the needle and cause neural damage (Selander et al 1979a). It does, however, ensure that the needle tip is very close to the nerve and makes the likelihood of a successful block greater. Paraesthesiae are subjective feelings and may be misinterpreted even by alert and cooperative patients, especially if there has been difficulty in finding the exact location of the nerve (Raj et al 1980). Success rates in performing blocks using paraesthesiae may be poor because of inappropriate responses from the patient, especially if he is apprehensive or unable to cooperate.

Nerve stimulator

The advantages of using a nerve stimulator are that:

1. There is no need to produce paraesthesiae, although they may occur.
2. Patient cooperation is unnecessary and the technique can be used in patients who are heavily sedated or anaesthetized.
3. It will give information on the optimal place to inject local anaesthetic, provided the stimulating unit gives some indication of current output.
4. Lack of a motor response indicates misplacement of the needle.

The disadvantages are that:

1. It is possible to stimulate the nerve when the needle tip is still some distance away. For instance, the brachial or lumbar plexus can be stimulated through the sheath if too high a current is used. This would result in an unsuccessful block.
2. It is not possible to stimulate sensory nerves in the same way as those with a motor component.
3. Some expense is incurred in the purchase and maintenance of the unit.

Further problems arise with the type of stimulating unit. Most of these are designed for testing neuromuscular transmission and give no indication of either voltage or current at the site of stimulation. Raj and colleagues (1980) have done much to popularize the use of these units for regional anaesthesia, but have pointed out that they suffer from a serious disadvantage in that they only control voltage, whereas it is current that causes a nerve to depolarize. Galindo (1982) has designed an instrument which delivers a constant current which is displayed visually (Nerve Finder, Regional Master Corporation). It is intended for use with the Teflon-coated side port needles described previously. Other stimulating units that give an indication of the current at the needle tip are the Neurostim LA (Hugo Sachs Elektronik) and the Model 750 peripheral nerve stimulator (Bard). The latter is a dual-purpose unit which can also be used for testing neuromuscular transmission. Both offer a range of stimulating currents up to 10 mA, which is far in excess of those required for accurate needle placement. Experience with these units suggests that the needle tip is close to the nerve when a current of less than 0.5 mA produces a response.

Insulated needles. There is some controversy as to whether an ordinary needle may be used with a nerve stimulator, or whether all but the tip should be insulated. Proponents of the insulated needle note that the current is precisely located at the tip (Bashein et al 1984), whereas any part of a non-insulated needle may stimulate the nerve. Supporters of non-insulated needles assert that these are effective because the *maximum* current density is localized to the tip (Montgomery et al 1973).

Some studies (Bashein et al 1984, Pither et al 1984) have considered whether the additional cost and reduced service life of insulated needles make their use worthwhile. It would seem that this more accurate, but relatively expensive, equipment can be justified for teaching, and for uncommon or unfamiliar blocks.

Aseptic technique

It is unnecessary to gown or wear sterile gloves for most regional anaesthetic procedures provided that strict no-touch technique is observed. At least one leading exponent of regional anaesthesia does not normally towel the area prior to a brachial plexus block (Winnie 1983), but it is probably wise to do so (and to wear sterile gloves) until expertise has been gained. Careful preparation and towelling should always be employed for central blocks, and a case can be made for gowning in techniques where catheters are being used as they are sometimes difficult to control. Starch-free gloves have the advantages that they give a better 'feel' to the skin and underlying tissues and avoid the risk of starch contamination.

The skin should be cleaned with an iodine-based bactericidal preparation, or chlorhexidine (Abouleish et al 1980). These solutions should be allowed to dry before the needle is inserted as they are then at their most effective and the risk of transferring a neurolytic solution to the needle is minimized. For this reason, care should be taken that preparation solutions do not drip on the equipment tray or the anaesthetist's gloves. Shaving may be necessary, but should not be performed in advance as the associated skin trauma predisposes to infection (Seropian & Reynolds 1971). Whether skin preparation actually provides any protection against infection is uncertain, but it does serve to keep the anaesthetist's hands and attention on a limited and relatively sterile area. The introduction of sterile, disposable equipment has probably done more to reduce the possibility of infection than skin preparation and towelling.

Needle insertion

All equipment should be checked and all solutions drawn up before the block is started. If possible these items should be kept out of the patient's sight at all times. When large or pencil point needles are being used, a small puncture should be made through the skin wheal to allow easier insertion. If this is not done, considerable force may be necessary, and the patient may become apprehensive and tense, and the needle may penetrate suddenly to a greater depth than intended.

Every attempt should be made to avoid touching the shaft of the needle. This may prove difficult where long and flexible needles are being used, and in these cases the shaft should be gripped as near to the hub as possible. The needle can be steadied by placing the back of the non-dominant hand against the patient whilst the thumb and index finger grasp the hub (see Fig. 8.10). This increases the control that can be exercised while the needle is steadily advanced by the dominant hand.

When altering the direction of the needle, the amount withdrawn is important. Withdrawing too little will result in virtually no change in the direction of the needle, no matter how much the hub is angled. This may cause it to follow a curved path with some risk of breakage. It is therefore better to withdraw the needle until it lies in pliable tissues and can be realigned without bending.

Intraneural injection. If paraesthesiae have been elicited, care must be taken that intraneural injection is not performed as this will cause considerable pain and may lead to permanent nerve damage (Lofstrom 1975, Selander et al 1979a). In order to prevent this, the needle should be withdrawn slightly (0.5–1 mm) once paraesthe-

siae have been elicited. Anything worse than minor discomfort during the early part of the injection indicates the need for further needle withdrawal.

Special considerations

Aids to success

A success rate of over 95% should be the aim in regional anaesthetic practice. A start can be made by careful case selection and rejection of patients with anatomical problems such as abnormal sacral landmarks. An unsuccessful or inadequate block is usually due to failure to place the local anaesthetic solution close enough to the nerve, but it may also be due to the use of an inadequate volume or mass of local anaesthetic solution. Tucker (1983), using evidence from studies of the systemic uptake of local anaesthetic drugs, has argued forcibly that the use of fixed maximum doses for these agents is inappropriate. The maximum doses quoted on data sheets in Britain represent very conservative safety margins for correctly administered nerve blocks (with the exception of intercostal and interpleural block). Adherence to these limits, without considering the site of injection, may contribute to high failure rates for the beginner and may inhibit even the experienced anaesthetist.

Plenty of time must be allowed for performance of the block and just as much time for it to work. The anaesthetist should never be rushed into abandoning a block – 'tincture of time' is often as effective as a supplement or a general anaesthetic. He should become competent at one technique before learning an additional one and should never miss an opportunity to study the anatomy of any nerve block.

The 'immobile needle'. Winnie (1969) has advocated the use of a length of small-bore, disposable intravenous extension tubing placed between the syringe and the needle (Fig. 5.2). This allows the anaesthetist to maintain the needle in the correct position without it being dislodged when the syringe is removed or replaced.

Testing the block

Observing the onset of a block after injection of the solution has two purposes. It indicates that the

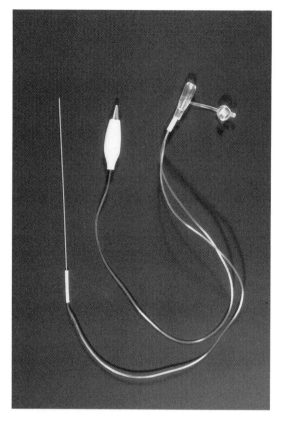

Fig. 5.2   An 'immobile' needle set. Note that this needle
has an insulated sheath and that there is an integral
attachment for a nerve stimulator.

distribution and quality of the block are adequate
for the proposed surgery and also warns if spread
has become excessive or if complications such as
hypotension are likely to develop. These are very
desirable aims, but formal testing has its drawbacks. It delays the start of surgery, possibly
engenders anxiety in the patient's mind about the
success of the procedure and may cause skin
trauma if repeated pinprick is used.

When the patient is in pain (i.e. in labour or with
a fracture) the onset of analgesia is a perfect
indication of block development. Surreptitious
gentle movement of a fractured limb will indicate
whether it is ready for manipulation. For elective
surgery informal assessment is more difficult, but
these are the patients more likely to be disturbed
by excessive testing. The best defence against
failure is to ensure that sufficient solution is

injected in the correct place, and for the anaesthetist's confident manner to communicate itself to
the patient. A latent period appropriate to the
block and drug in question should elapse before
signs of the developing block are sought. Useful
signs are vasodilatation in the area of the nerve or
plexus block, heaviness of the arm or legs and
some decrease in the blood pressure during spinal
or epidural block.

The ability to manage patients in this way only
comes with experience. The beginner should start
with simple blocks but, in his understandable
anxiety to test them, should use a blunt needle,
such as a safety pin, or a spirit-soaked swab. If in
doubt he should ask the surgeon to test the
operative site by squeezing the skin progressively
harder with a pair of forceps before the incision is
made.

Living with failure

Success in regional anaesthesia depends on many
different factors and may not always be achieved.
The only true failure is a failure to learn something
from the experience. The block may be slow in
onset, inadequate in extent or quality, or a total
failure. There may be time constraints, and the
reactions of the patient must be considered.

Slow onset. 'Tincture of time' is one of the
most useful supplements to any block, and the
author would not abandon any spinal or epidural
for at least 30 minutes, especially in the elderly.
Peripheral nerve blocks with long-acting agents
may take up to 45 minutes to develop. Where a
block has only partially developed, or where the
need for the list to proceed is becoming para-
mount, peripheral supplementation or local
infiltration by the surgeon can be employed.
Note should be made of the dose of local
anaesthetic added and it must be remembered
that the original dose of local anaesthetic drug
will only be partially metabolized when the additional drug is injected.

Inadequate block. The easiest way of coping
with an inadequate block is to induce general
anaesthesia, but having spent time explaining that
regional anaesthesia was the best anaesthetic for
the intended procedure, it may be frustrating and

annoying to the patient to have an alternative thrust upon him. Some patients prefer to remain awake despite some discomfort and there are various methods of making the situation tolerable. Small amounts of *intravenous opioids* can be given. These can be short-acting (for example, fentanyl) if it is anticipated that the block will develop further, or longer-acting (phenoperidine). Care should be taken in the use of these drugs because of their well known side-effects. *Intravenous sedation* may be sufficient to relieve minor discomfort but, if large doses are required, general anaesthesia should be induced without delay. Excessive use of parenteral sedatives and analgesics will lead to respiratory obstruction and depression, and will delay recovery. Inhalation of 50% nitrous oxide in oxygen may also relieve the discomfort associated with a partial block.

Complete failure. If there are compelling reasons for avoiding general anaesthesia, the block can be repeated. Time must be allowed for some of the first dose of local anaesthetic drug to be metabolized and modifications made in both technique and dosage to allow for this. Rearrangement of the list will be necessary and explanations should be offered to both the patient and staff.

PEROPERATIVE MANAGEMENT

Prevention and treatment of toxicity

Systemic toxicity of local anaesthetic drugs

Local anaesthetic drugs possess the ability to stabilize all excitable membranes, an effect which is not confined to peripheral nerves. Given sufficient tissue concentration, they will depress the function of both the central nervous and cardiovascular systems. Properly performed regional anaesthesia should not result in blood concentrations of local anaesthetic sufficient to cause systemic effects, but since these are life-threatening and usually of sudden onset (see Ch. 4), rapid action is necessary to counteract them.

Prevention. A thorough understanding of pharmacokinetics, especially those factors affecting absorption, distribution and elimination, is essential. A knowledge of the blood concentration

profile for the agent and technique employed will help the anaesthetist to be most vigilant at the time of greatest risk. For this reason it is suggested that the inexperienced anaesthetist limits his range of drugs and techniques until confidence in these is established. The two main causes of toxicity are overdosage and accidental intravascular injection. Overdose can be avoided simply by paying attention to toxic limits appropriate to the solution used and the site of injection. Inadvertent intravascular injection can be minimized by careful technique and selection of the appropriate equipment. Sufficient time should be allowed for blood to become visible in the catheter or needle after aspiration. Aspiration should be gentle, as the vessel wall may occlude the needle opening, but a negative test should not be regarded as absolute proof that the needle is correctly placed. Particular vigilance is required with injections into the head and neck, and with intravenous regional anaesthesia. In the former, accidental intra-arterial injection of a very small dose of local anaesthetic can cause convulsions and, in the latter, faulty equipment, slipshod technique or early release of the tourniquet may result in a large amount of drug entering the circulation.

Test doses. It is obvious that the needle or catheter has entered a vein or punctured the dura when blood or cerebrospinal fluid appears spontaneously or after aspiration. Unfortunately, intravenous, intra-arterial and subarachnoid injections can occur despite negative aspiration tests, and test doses are commonly employed to help exclude these possibilities. The 'test' solution will depend on the hazards to be excluded, but three criteria must be satisfied:

1. The test solution must be capable of producing unequivocal and easily observable evidence of intravenous, intra-arterial and subarachnoid injection within a reasonably short time
2. The solution used for the test dose should be unlikely to produce any detectable effect if injected into the right place
3. Sufficient time must be allowed for the test dose to produce an effect before the full dose is administered.

Local anaesthetic (3 ml) with 15 µg of adrenaline (1:200 000 adrenaline) will increase the heart rate by at least 30% within a minute of intravenous injection (Moore & Batra 1981). In patients receiving β adrenoceptor blocking agents, tachycardia is an unreliable sign of intravascular injection, but 10 µg of adrenaline will almost always cause an increase in systolic blood pressure of greater than 15 mmHg within 4 minutes (Guinard et al 1990). Intrathecal effects will appear in conscious patients within 5 minutes of the subarachnoid injection of 3–4 ml of 2% lignocaine. Local anaesthetic injected into the carotid and vertebral arteries produces instantaneous cerebral signs and, for blocks of the head and neck, slow injection together with close observation and communication with the patient is the best way to detect this serious complication. Epidural test doses are considered further in Chapter 8.

Treatment. It is not usually necessary to treat the signs and symptoms of toxicity, with the exception of convulsions, provided that respiration and circulation are maintained. The avoidance of hypoxia is the most important aspect of treatment of local anaesthetic toxicity. This requires scrupulous monitoring, the administration of oxygen, encouragement to breathe normally and constant verbal contact with the patient. Cardiovascular depression should be treated by elevation of the legs, intravenous fluids and the administration of a vasopressor such as ephedrine (5–30 mg). Major collapse requires full resuscitative measures.

If convulsions occur, the aim of treatment is to stop them as quickly as possible and to treat any accompanying respiratory or cardiovascular depression before cerebral hypoxia and acidosis compound the situation. Convulsions may be treated in one of three ways. *Intravenous barbiturates*, such as thiopentone, will rapidly abort local anaesthetic-induced convulsions. Their use has been criticised on the grounds that they may increase respiratory and cardiovascular depression, so it is important that only small increments, e.g. thiopentone 50–100 mg, are given. They have the advantages of being short-acting, readily available and familiar to all anaesthetists. *Benzodiazepines*, such as diazepam, have been shown

to prevent, and also to abort, local anaesthetic-induced seizures (de Jong & Heavner 1974, Munson et al 1977). Again, incremental dosage should be small, e.g. 2.5 mg. Convulsions induced by the more potent, longer-acting agents such as etidocaine and bupivacaine are more resistant to benzodiazepine treatment than those induced by lignocaine (de Jong & De Rosa 1981). *Suxamethonium*, 50 mg intravenously, will stop the physical manifestations of convulsive activity, but not the seizure activity within the brain, and the administration of suxamethonium to a hypoxic patient carries the risk of cardiac arrest.

After successful treatment of a reaction to an intravascular injection of local anaesthetic, it is wise to examine the patient to ascertain the extent of block. If a substantial area is affected, it is reasonable to assume only a small proportion of the solution was injected intravenously. If there is little or no evidence of anaesthesia it must be assumed that most, if not all, of the injection was intravascular.

Other adverse drug reactions

Treatment of allergy. True allergic reactions to local anaesthetic drugs are rare (see Ch. 4). If anaphylaxis occurs it is vital to give oxygen immediately, followed by adrenaline 50–100 µg (0.5–1.0 ml of 1:10 000 solution) intravenously, especially if bronchospasm is present (Nimmo et al 1990). Additional supportive measures include steroids, other bronchodilators and the infusion of fluids, preferably colloid, to restore the blood volume (Fisher 1977). Antihistamines are only of value in the milder reactions.

Adrenaline overdose. Treatment is symptomatic and will depend upon the patient's cardiovascular status. Oxygen and sublingual glyceryl trinitrate should be administered if angina develops. If tachycardia is the chief feature, β adrenoceptor blocking agents may be indicated, but they should be avoided where hypertension is the presenting clinical sign. In this circumstance a short-acting vasodilator such as nitroprusside may be given, but with great care because hypotension can rapidly follow the initial hypertension.

Methaemoglobinaemia. Some of the metabolites of prilocaine can reduce haemoglobin to methaemoglobin. Hjelm & Holmdahl (1965) have shown that 600 mg of prilocaine will produce a methaemoglobin concentration of 5.3%. This dose is far in excess of the amounts normally used, but does cause cyanosis which is just detectable clinically. In spite of this, prilocaine remains the safest of the amide local anaesthetics, because the cyanosis is of little significance in the healthy individual and can be reversed within 30 minutes by the intravenous administration of 1–2 mg kg^{-1} of methylene blue.

Hypotension and regional anaesthesia

Most research on the cardiovascular effects of central blocks has been performed on unpremedicated, healthy volunteers and patients. It may therefore be inappropriate to rely heavily upon the data from these studies when dealing with the surgical patient, who may be hypovolaemic, have cardiac disease, autonomic dysfunction or other conditions affecting his response. Cardiovascular depression can occur after both spinal and epidural block and is largely related to the level of sympathectomy produced, though there are minor differences between the two types of block. Epidural anaesthesia usually develops more slowly than spinal, so there is time for compensation to occur and the initial hypotension may therefore be less dramatic. The cardiovascular response to epidural block may be modified by the systemic effects of both local anaesthetic and vasoconstrictor drugs.

Peripheral vasodilatation caused by sympathetic block decreases left ventricular afterload. Peripheral venous dilatation will decrease venous return and hence cardiac output, but only if the denervated veins are below the level of the right atrium. Mean arterial pressure will decrease in proportion to the decrease in cardiac output and, less importantly, to the decrease in peripheral vascular resistance. As the mean arterial pressure falls there is a reduction in coronary blood flow but, fortunately, this is accompanied by a similar decrease in myocardial oxygen requirement. The latter is reduced because of decreased left ventricular afterload, decreased preload and bradycardia (Hackel et al 1956).

The bradycardia may be due to the Bainbridge reflex, because right atrial pressure receptors respond to decreased venous return. It may also be due to block of the cardio-accelerator fibres from T_1 to T_5. Scott (1975) has suggested that high sympathetic block may lead to an increase in parasympathetic activity, and there is the possibility that severe bradycardia and hypotension in susceptible patients are caused by vasovagal attacks (Wetstone & Wong 1974).

Sympathetic block below T_4 results in dilatation of the splanchnic, pelvic and lower limb vessels. In healthy patients various mechanisms come into play to compensate for this. Vasoconstriction above the level of the block occurs, mediated by unblocked sympathetic vasoconstrictor fibres (T_1–T_4), and release of catecholamines may be mediated by any unblocked fibres to the adrenal medulla. In addition, vascular tone below the level of the block may return because of autoregulation of flow by the precapillary sphincters (Granger & Guyton 1969). Unblocked cardiac sympathetic fibres mediate an increase in myocardial contractility and heart rate, and it has been suggested that low plasma concentrations of local anaesthetic drug also cause cardiovascular stimulation (Bonica et al 1970).

Sympathetic block above T_4 reduces or abolishes compensatory vasoconstriction in the head, neck and upper limb, as well as the ability of the cardiac sympathetic fibres to stimulate the heart. It is therefore surprising that the cardiovascular changes noted with high thoracic blocks have been relatively modest. McLean and colleagues (1967) found a 15–20% reduction in cardiac output and an increase in central venous pressure (CVP). Bonica and colleagues (1970, 1971) also demonstrated an increase in CVP and found that mean arterial pressure and peripheral resistance decreased by about 20%, but they observed no change in cardiac output or heart rate. Any adverse changes in cardiovascular state in a patient deprived of compensatory mechanisms requires prompt and efficient treatment from the anaesthetist.

Other risk factors

Hypovolaemia. Sympathetic block is particularly dangerous in the hypovolaemic patient. Massive cardiovascular changes have been observed in volunteers who had been volume depleted by over 10% (Kennedy et al 1968, Bonica et al 1972). In a study of spinal block to T_5, substantial decreases in mean arterial pressure, CVP and peripheral resistance were seen (Kennedy et al 1968). Despite minimal changes in cardiac output and rate, two subjects showed a transient asystole accompanied by a marked decrease in blood pressure when the block level rose to T_2–T_3. Similar effects were seen in an epidural study (Bonica et al 1972) in which plain solutions of lignocaine were used to produce a block to T_5. In five out of seven subjects vigorous resuscitation was required. The hypovolaemia was much better tolerated when the local anaesthetic solution contained adrenaline. Lignocaine–adrenaline mixtures cause an increase in cardiac output and heart rate with a decrease in peripheral resistance and mean arterial pressure. The increased heart rate may provide some protection against increased vagal activity.

The practical lessons are clear – spinal and epidural block should be avoided in any patient with uncorrected hypovolaemia, and blood lost during surgery must be replaced immediately.

Concomitant general anaesthesia. Three studies have investigated the combination of epidural block with general anaesthesia and spontaneous ventilation. Stephen and colleagues (1969) studied epidural anaesthesia administered about 20 minutes after the induction of a light general anaesthetic. In six of the 11 patients in the study there were no significant changes in cardiovascular status after the injection of 30 ml of 2% lignocaine. The remaining five patients all showed marked decreases in mean arterial blood pressure, but in only one was this associated with reduced cardiac output and bradycardia. The level of the block was thought to be around T_5. Scott and colleagues (1977) studied the effects of lignocaine with 1:200 000 adrenaline. The haemodynamic changes were quite variable, but this combination was associated with lower peripheral resistance

and larger decreases in mean arterial pressure than when plain solutions were employed – findings not dissimilar from those of Bonica in a study of conscious volunteers (Bonica et al 1970).

The effect of performance of epidural block, either before or after light general anaesthesia (thiopentone–nitrous oxide–oxygen) upon haemodynamics has been studied by Germann and colleagues (1979). Epidural block was carried out using 15–20 mg of 1.5% lignocaine through an indwelling catheter. This established analgesia to a level of T_6. When general anaesthesia was induced first, mean arterial pressure decreased by less than 9% from control values with a further reduction of 13% after the epidural block. In patients who received epidural block first, the mean arterial pressure decreased by 20% from control values, with a further 15% reduction after the induction of general anaesthesia. Heart rate and cardiac output were not changed.

It appears from these three studies that light general anaesthesia combined with epidural block may cause slightly greater cardiovascular depression than epidural alone. The sequence of performance of epidural block and general anaesthesia does not affect haemodynamic variables.

Reduced venous return. Any condition which causes a reduction in venous return, such as a gravid uterus, an intra-abdominal mass or ascites may lead to problems with epidural or spinal block. The anaesthetist should be aware that poor positioning and overenthusiastic use of packs and retractors may also reduce venous return.

Intermittent positive-pressure ventilation (IPPV). Very little information is available on the effect of spinal or epidural block combined with IPPV. Animal work has shown very marked cardiovascular depression with IPPV and high spinals (Lynn et al 1952). In a study of epidural block combined with IPPV in humans, the arterial pressure was 25% lower than in patients who breathed spontaneously (Jensen et al 1977). This decrease in blood pressure occurs because the sympathetic block associated with the regional technique prevents the vasoconstriction which normally compensates for reduced venous return and cardiac output seen with increased intrathoracic pressure.

Autonomic dysfunction. Some degree of autonomic dysfunction may occur with diabetes, alcoholism, rheumatoid arthritis, Guillain–Barré syndrome and in the elderly. In addition, there are the specific, but extremely rare conditions with autonomic dysfunction, such as the Riley–Day or Shy–Drager syndromes. Postural hypotension and high resting heart rates are common in all these conditions and the response of these patients to any form of anaesthesia is unpredictable (Page & Watkins 1978).

Significance of hypotension

A decrease in blood pressure is often considered undesirable, if not dangerous, but its beneficial effects include decreased surgical blood loss, improved operating conditions and decreased myocardial work. Even in patients with ischaemic heart disease modest levels of hypotension are well tolerated. Hypotension in spinal and epidural anaesthesia can be regarded as a physiological effect rather than a complication, and Lund (1971) has suggested that 'it may be a desirable phenomenon under certain circumstances'.

In general, the surest way to anticipate hypotension is to monitor the circulation. This not only means measurement of pulse and blood pressure, but also observation of the peripheral circulation. The level of analgesia should be recorded in some detail during continuous epidural block. After each top-up the level should be noted so that if the catheter migrates into the cerebrospinal fluid the sudden development of a more extensive block will draw attention to the patient *before* the hypotension becomes catastrophic.

Prevention of excessive hypotension

The most obvious way of preventing hypotension is to limit the extent of sympathetic block. A block to T_{10} results in very little sympathetic paralysis, yet a wide range of surgical procedures can be carried out. A more extensive block will result in a greater degree of sympathetic paralysis. *Prophylactic fluid loading* is only logical in those situations where acute blood loss is anticipated, as in obstetrics (Wollman & Marx 1968). In such cases, expansion of the intravascular volume compensates for the dilated vascular bed caused by sympathetic block. The accompanying decrease in haematocrit may cause temporary improvement in blood flow and the delivery of oxygen to the tissues. However, *routine* preloading with fluid assumes that hypotension will always occur. In fact, this is not the case, even with blocks to the upper thoracic region, since many conscious patients are able to compensate without the need for volume expansion.

Preloading can also lead to problems. Because most central blocks regress from above downwards, sympathetic tone returns before bladder sensation, and catheterization is often necessary. In the elderly patient there is also the risk that the fluid may overload the pulmonary circulation.

Routine *prophylactic vasopressor therapy* is unnecessary in most patients and so has little to commend it (Smith & Corbascia 1970). Engberg & Wiklund (1978a) studied the effects of ephedrine 50 mg administered subcutaneously before high epidural block in middle-aged and elderly patients. They found that although the haemodynamic effects of the block were minimized and cardiac work was unaltered from preinduction levels, arterial pressure and peripheral resistance *increased*. The addition of 1:20 000 phenylephrine to the local anaesthetic solution for epidural analgesia has been shown to maintain arterial pressure, but to reduce cardiac output slightly (Stanton-Hicks et al 1973).

Prophylactic fluid loading is wise for those patients in whom significant blood loss is anticipated, and prophylactic vasopressors may be indicated for patients in whom a sudden and dramatic decrease in blood pressure is likely, or for whom this is particularly undesirable. For example, carefully adjusted infusions of adrenaline may be used to maintain the circulation in the presence of a deliberately extensive epidural block for major orthopaedic surgery (Sharrock et al 1990).

Treatment of excessive hypotension

Before performing spinal or epidural block it is important to decide what degree of hypotension is unacceptable. Treatment is rarely required in a healthy patient before mean arterial pressure decreases by more than 30% of the resting control level but, in patients with one or more of the previously discussed risk factors, intervention may be indicated earlier.

Oxygen. While additional oxygen is not essential for all patients having regional anaesthesia, many anaesthetists feel that it is beneficial and it should certainly be administered to those at risk of developing hypotension. This will include the majority of patients over the age of 60 years. Supplementary oxygen should be given to all patients receiving sedation if a pulse oximeter is not available (Smith & Crul 1989).

Posture. The simplest and safest way to restore the blood pressure during spinal anaesthesia is to raise the legs. This restores cardiac output by increasing venous return to the heart. A steep head-down tilt has the same effect and, contrary to common belief, has relatively litttle effect on cephalad spread of local anaesthetic (Sinclair et al 1982). In any case cardiac output remains normal even during spinal anaesthesia high enough to produce total preganglionic sympathetic block, provided the patients are normovolaemic and kept in a head-down position (Greene 1982). Bromage states that patients with high epidural blocks should be kept horizontal or slightly head-down to ensure an adequate venous return. He further suggests that patients with blocks that involve both the lumbar and thoracic outflows are more sensitive to postural changes than those with analgesia confined to the thoracic segments alone (Bromage 1978).

Fluids. The rapid infusion of 500–1000 ml of balanced salt solution is often sufficient to restore arterial blood pressure to a satisfactory level, but carries the same risks as preloading (see above). If postural adjustments and reasonable fluid therapy fail to restore blood pressure to acceptable levels, vasopressors should be used.

Vasopressors. The detailed pharmacology of vasopressors has been extensively reviewed by Smith & Corbascia (1970). Only a handful of healthy patients will require vasopressors, but they should never be withheld when rapid restoration of blood pressure is urgently indicated. These drugs should be used sparingly and in minimum incremental doses until the vasomotor tone, lost by sympathetic block, has been restored. The vasopressors most commonly used in the treatment of hypotension caused by spinal or epidural analgesia are ephedrine and methoxamine.

Ephedrine is both a direct and an indirectly acting α and β adrenoceptor agonist which increases heart rate, stroke volume, cardiac output and peripheral vascular resistance. The latter may increase cardiac work without excessive increases in blood pressure or heart rate (Engberg & Wiklund 1978b). It is the drug of choice in obstetrics (Eng et al 1971) as its effect upon uterine blood flow appears to be less than that seen with other vasopressors (Ralston et al 1974). Incremental doses of 3–7.5 mg are satisfactory; larger doses may cause tachycardia or hypertension. It has the advantage of being relatively short-acting when given intravenously.

Methoxamine is a pure α adrenoceptor agonist. It increases peripheral resistance and has little effect upon cardiac output (Li et al 1965). It does not increase (but usually slows) heart rate, causes few dysrhythmias and has been recommended as the drug of choice in patients with ischaemic heart disease (Gilbert et al 1958). However, its pure α adrenoceptor action may result in pressure being maintained at the expense of flow. It may be preferred to ephedrine when hypotension and tachycardia coexist and is given in increments of 1–2 mg intravenously. *Phenylephrine* is a suitable alternative.

In some countries *dihydroergotamine* 0.5 mg is used to prevent and treat hypotension. It is particularly appropriate as it acts mainly on venous capacitance vessels, but may cause nausea and vomiting, and is obviously contraindicated in antepartum obstetric patients.

Vagolytics. Atropine is not a vasopressor and is not the drug of choice for hypotension due to sympathetic block. Nonetheless it has a role to play in the management of cardiovascular problems during regional anaesthesia. A heart rate of less than 60 beats per minute may be associated with an inadequate cardiac output. This is usually due to vagal overactivity combined with a high sympathetic block. Intravenous atropine, in increments of 0.3 mg, will increase the heart rate. However, vagal overactivity may be treated as effectively by the cautious administration of intravenous sedatives (e.g. thiopentone 50 mg), which will not produce a subsequent tachycardia.

Respiratory effects

Respiratory function is not usually affected by regional anaesthesia, and even extensive thoracic epidural block does not normally make any difference to ventilation or the ability to cough (McCarthy 1976). However, epidural and spinal anaesthesia may cause some paralysis of the respiratory muscles, and Freund and colleagues (1967) showed there was a marked decrease in the expiratory reserve volume with high spinal block. This may make it difficult for the patient to cough effectively. The concomitant use of other forms of analgesia, such as NSAIDs or small doses of opioids, will allow weaker concentrations of local anaesthetic, having less effect on motor nerves, to be used.

Respiratory depression and arrest may be due to extensive sympathetic block, reduced cardiac output and cerebral hypoxaemia. Pneumothorax must always be considered when respiratory distress occurs in a patient who has received intercostal, interpleural, supraclavicular or stellate ganglion block.

Sedative and anaesthetic supplements

The advantages and disadvantages of having the patient awake during surgery have been discussed in Chapter 2 and decisions about supplementation should be made, where possible, at the preoperative visit. It is important that this issue should be considered before consent is obtained. The block may be used alone, with light sedation and preservation of consciousness, with sedation sufficient to produce sleep, or with a full general anaesthetic. Many factors influence the choice of supplement, including: the preference of the patient; the presence of systemic disease or airway problems; the type and duration of the surgery; the facilities available, expecially for recovery; the experience of all the staff involved; and training requirements.

Light sedation

Most sedatives, anxiolytics and analgesics may be used to sedate patients undergoing regional anaesthesia. Longer-acting agents such as diazepam and morphine may not be as appropriate as their newer shorter-acting derivatives, especially in the outpatient. Temazepam (10–20 mg orally), midazolam (1–2 mg increments intravenously), propofol (by intravenous infusion), fentanyl (25 µg increments intravenously) and the inhalation of nitrous oxide (25–50%) are all widely used.

During elective surgery, these different methods may be used singly or in combination to promote sleep. Many patients will fall asleep under the influence of oral premedication alone once the block is effective.

Deep sedation

This is often preferred for major surgery where it is the intention that the patient should be asleep throughout the procedure. Methohexitone (10–20 mg increments) or thiopentone (25–50 mg increments), given intravenously to a patient who has received a benzodiazepine premedication, will often produce sleep for as long as 30 minutes. Alternatively, the agents mentioned in the previous subsection may be used in greater dosage. However, continuing dosage may lead to cumulation with delayed recovery and profound cardiorespiratory effects. Where prolonged unconsciousness is required, a general anaesthetic supplement may be more suitable.

General anaesthesia

It is sometimes argued that the administration of a general anaesthetic to a patient who has received regional anaesthesia is an unnecessary complication, but it has a number of advantages. No regional technique can be guaranteed to block all possible sources of discomfort in every patient undergoing surgery, and the conscious patient may interpret unblocked sensations from the operative field as pain. This is particularly true of abdominal surgery in which the viscera may be supplied by autonomic nerves from well above the level of the block. The discomfort of lying on an operating table for long operations may be intolerable despite the measures previously recommended.

Hypotension due to sympathetic block is a feature of spinal and epidural anaesthesia. For many procedures it greatly enhances the surgical field, and may contribute to the success of the operation. However, the level of hypotension required for this effect is below that which is well tolerated by the conscious patient, since the low pressure may reflexly trigger a vasovagal attack. General anaesthesia inhibits this reflex and allows the hypotensive effect of the block to become an advantage, rather than a 'complication' requiring prevention or treatment.

Supplementary general anaesthesia also allows the patient to be positioned and prepared for surgery while the block is becoming effective. In the conscious patient, these preparations may have to be delayed while the block develops. Furthermore, the atmosphere in the operating theatre is more relaxed, allowing surgeon and anaesthetist to discuss any problems – and enabling trainee staff to be taught – without inhibition. General anaesthesia will also eliminate any overt toxic reactions to the local anaesthetic agent.

Early experience of the problems associated with the conscious patient often deters anaesthetists from persisting with regional anaesthesia. The planned administration of a light supplementary general anaesthetic ensures success in almost every case. Any of the standard agents is suitable for induction, but nitrous oxide is the staple agent of maintenance. Given in concentrations of 65–70%, it is often sufficient on its own for body surface and limb operations. For abdominal procedures, halothane 0.5% or its equivalent is usually needed in addition. For body surface, limb and pelvic operations, the anaesthetic may be administered through a face or laryngeal mask, but endotracheal intubation is required for other abdominal and thoracic procedures. IPPV may produce a 'quieter' surgical field in operations near the diaphragm, but muscle relaxants are often only needed for intubation.

Monitoring

Monitoring of the patient should start before the procedure with recording of pulse and blood pressure. The type of monitoring will depend on the block, the patient, the anaesthetic supplement, if any, the operation, and the preference and experience of the anaesthetist. Wherever possible the electrocardiogram should be monitored continuously throughout the patient's stay in the anaesthetic room and theatre, particularly during test dose injection and the subsequent delivery of the full dose. If blood pressure recordings are required during injection, these should be performed by an assistant. At the time of the test dose injection, injection of the full dose and subsequent development of the block, the patient must be observed most carefully and communication with him is at its most valuable. Pulse oximetry is a useful adjunct and should be employed wherever sedation or general anaesthesia are used as supplements, because desaturation can occur readily (Smith & Crul 1989).

The patient is the most sensitive indicator of potential or actual problems. Observation of colour, pulse, respiratory pattern and the presence or absence of sweating will often give a quicker indication of problems than any machine. A knowledge of the likely time course of the onset of the block performed, and of the development of possible side-effects, will help the intelligent anticipation and treatment of complications. During long procedures, top-up doses will be necessary and their effects should be monitored as closely as those of the original injection.

Block level (see under 'Testing the block', p.59)

The level of block and anaesthesia of the surgical site should be monitored for as long as possible prior to surgery where a central block is being used. With careful planning the block should be established and stable before the patient is taken into theatre or anaesthetized. This is not always possible and further checks on a developing block can be made under the 'ether screen' which should be erected as soon as the patient is settled in position for surgery. Only the upper thoracic segments are available for testing, but these are the most important because extension of the block to this level will forewarn the anaesthetist of possible problems. Testing at this late stage will not give any warning of 'missed' segments and the surgeon should be asked to check discreetly the operative site for evidence of this before commencing his incision. It is the author's practice to inflate the blood pressure cuff well in excess of the systolic pressure to divert the patient's attention as the incision is made.

Positioning

Attention must be given to the position of the patient on the operating table. All anaesthetized areas should be padded and supported and unanaesthetized parts of the body should be positioned carefully. If the patient is awake, he should be shown how much movement he is allowed. Uncomfortable positions may be indications for supplementary general anaesthesia, but this may only become obvious after the operation has started.

POSTOPERATIVE CARE

The quality of personnel and facilities required for postoperative care should be the same whatever form of anaesthesia has been used. However, the emphasis will be different because of the particular features of regional anaesthesia. The patient recovering from regional anaesthesia supplemented with mild sedation or a light general anaesthetic will have few of the problems associated with recovery from full general anaesthesia, and residual neuromuscular block, central depression of ventilation, respiratory obstruction, and inadequate clearance of secretions occur less frequently. Patients who have had regional anaesthesia have a much lower risk of postoperative hypoxaemia than those who have received a general anaesthetic (Moller et al 1990).

The major hazard during recovery from regional anaesthesia is hypotension, particularly after spinal or epidural block. It is not uncommon for this to occur, due to redistribu-tion of blood flow, when the patient is moved from the operating table and transported to the recovery area. Blood pressure limits should be set, beyond which the anaesthetist or other medical staff should be informed. Written instructions for continuation of fluid therapy and action to be taken in the event of hypotension should be given at this time.

The frequency of recordings of vital signs will depend on the patient's condition, but particular attention must be directed to measurement of blood pressure until the block has obviously started to regress. Recordings may be required more frequently than after general anaesthesia. Severe hypotension has been reported up to 2 hours after the induction of spinal anaesthesia (Moore & Bridenbaugh 1966) and noted up to 90 minutes after the induction of epidural block (personal observation).

Particular vigilance is required if vasopressors have been needed to maintain blood pressure perioperatively. Their action is relatively short when given intravenously and hypotension may occur as the effects wear off. The recovery room staff must be told if vasopressors have been used and instructed to be particularly assiduous in measuring blood pressure.

Hypotension should be managed as described earlier and it is important that the staff looking after the patient should realize that surgical bleeding, as well as the block, may be responsible. This should be suspected when postoperative hypotension occurs suddenly in a patient in whom the block is regressing satisfactorily. Patients who have had spinal or epidural anaesthesia which extended to the thoracic segments may still have residual autonomic block for some time after the procedure. This may cause hypotension if the patient's posture is changed suddenly. Such patients should be mobilized gradually as the block regresses and should be attended when they first stand up.

Pressure areas

Positioning of the patient is just as important during recovery as it is in the operating theatre.

It is possible for the anaesthetized lower limb to fall off the side of the bed and for the patient to be unaware of this. Stretching or compression may then result in neural damage. Lofstrom and colleagues (1966) have shown similar problems with the upper limb. Sensory block prevents the patient from appreciating pressure over bony prominences. When analgesia is extended into the postoperative period by means of catheter techniques, skin necrosis may occur unless the patient's position is changed regularly.

Urinary retention

The bladder is innervated by the sacral autonomic fibres and these may be among the last to regain function after central blocks. Any patient who has received large volumes of fluid during surgery and who does not have a catheter in place should be regarded as being at risk of urinary retention. If the bladder is obviously distended, it should be catheterized, but there is no need to leave the catheter in place if prompt recovery of normal neural function is expected. If, on the other hand, the analgesia is to be continued into the postoperative period, an indwelling urinary catheter may be needed.

Regression of the block

Medical and nursing staff should be given an approximate indication of how long the block will last. The patient should be encouraged to report any subjective feelings. Failure to do this may mean that potentially serious side-effects of the block, such as epidural haematoma, go unnoticed and early treatment may be delayed. Good rapport between the patient and staff aids the detection of genuine complications and the tolerance of minor discomforts unconnected with the regional anaesthesia.

Postoperative analgesia

The provision of profound analgesia during the early postoperative period is a major benefit of regional anaesthesia. However, small doses of conventional parenteral analgesia may also be required to alleviate discomforts which lie outside the range of the block, and to encourage the sleep which all patients require after major surgery. In cases where the block is not to be continued into the postoperative period, parenteral analgesia should be given before the block wears off, rather than when the pain is fully established. There is evidence that the use of regional anaesthetic techniques reduces the requirement for postoperative analgesia (McQuay et al 1988), and may even reduce the incidence of chronic pain (Bach et al 1988).

Complications

Neurological sequelae

These can be caused by intraneural injection, incorrect use of the tourniquet, and faulty positioning during or after surgery, as well as by damage when eliciting paraesthesiae (Wooley & Vandam 1959, Lofstrom et al 1966, Barutell et al 1980, Kroll et al 1990). A note should be made whenever paraesthesiae are elicited as this may help an exact diagnosis to be made if problems persist (Lim & Pereira 1984). The symptoms of neural damage can vary (Selander et al 1979b). Any such case should be reviewed and investigated to try to establish the cause. The possibility of inadvertent injection of some neurolytic agent mixed with or in mistake for the local anaesthetic drug must never be forgotten.

Backache

This is a common complaint in the postoperative period. Lund (1971) found an incidence varying from 2 to 25% after spinal anaesthesia. There is no evidence for the commonly held belief that epidural block causes more backache because of the larger needles used, although there is an increase in the amount of backache suffered by obstetric patients who have had an epidural when compared to those who have not (McArthur et al 1990). The most likely cause of postoperative backache is positional and related to the relaxation of the muscles and ligaments of the back, with loss of the normal lumbar lordosis, secondary to the block. Patients who receive general anaesthesia involving muscle relaxants also complain of backache occasionally. The use of NSAIDs may be helpful.

Headache

The vast majority of postoperative headaches occur in patients who have not had a dural puncture. These are often caused by stress and anxiety and are usually ill-defined in site. They are not related to posture and are rarely incapacitating. Reassurance and symptomatic treatment is all that is required. Anaesthetists should be aware of the characteristic features of postlumbar puncture headache: it is postural, being first noticed when the patient sits or stands, and diminishing or disappearing when he lies down; it is usually occipital with cervical radiation. Severe postlumbar puncture headache may be accompanied by visual and auditory disturbances. Hearing loss is less when smaller needles are used (Fog et al 1990). Postlumbar puncture headache must not be left untreated (see Ch. 8) because an intracranial haematoma can result (Macon et al 1990).

Pain at the injection site

There is sometimes pain and local tenderness at the site of injection. This is due to the mild trauma which inevitably occurs when a needle is inserted into tissues. It usually settles down in a day or so. If it fails to do so, other causes, such as local infection, contamination with antiseptic or a neurolytic agent or nerve damage, should be considered.

Haematoma

This can occur after any nerve block, but is more common where nerves are closely related to blood vessels. At peripheral sites it usually resolves in a couple of weeks and gives rise to few problems. This should be explained to the patient. Where puncture of a blood vessel is part of the technique, as in the transarterial approach to the axillary brachial plexus, a haematoma is more common and long-lasting paresthesiae frequent (Hartung & Rupprecht 1989).

A spinal or epidural haematoma may be followed by serious and permanent neurological sequelae if not treated immediately. Any patient with prolonged neural deficit and complaining of pain must be treated very seriously. Early help should be sought from neurological, radiological and neurosurgical colleagues where there is the slightest doubt. The same applies to the diagnosis and treatment of the isolated nerve palsies which occasionally occur.

Nausea and vomiting

The commonest causes of postoperative nausea and vomiting are general anaesthesia, the use of opioid drugs and the ingestion of blood after ear, nose and throat surgery and oral surgery. It is much less common after regional anaesthesia, but the incidence increases if the systolic blood pressure falls below 80 mm Hg. The administration of oxygen is helpful (Ratra et al 1972), as is intravenous atropine if the symptoms are accompanied by bradycardia.

REFERENCES

Abouleish E, Orig T, Amortegui A J 1980 Bacteriologic comparison between epidural and caudal techniques. Anesthesiology 53: 511–514

Alleman B H, Gerber H, Gruber U F 1983 Spinal conduction anaesthesia in the face of subcutaneously administered heparin–dihydroergot for thromboembolism prophylaxis. Anaesthetist 35: 80–83

Bach S, Noreng M F, Tjellden N U 1988 Phantom limb pain in amputees during the first 12 months following limb amputation, after preoperative lumbar epidural blockade. Pain 33: 297–301

Ballin N C 1981 Paraplegia following epidural analgesia. Anaesthesia 36: 952–953

Bamford C R 1978 Spinal epidural hematoma due to

heparin. Archives of Neurology 35: 693–694

Barutell C, Vidal F, Raich M, Montero A 1980 A neurological complication following interscalene brachial plexus block. Anaesthesia 35: 365–367

Bashein G, Ready L B, Haschke R 1984 Electrolocation: insulated versus non-insulated needles. Regional Anesthesia 9: 31

Beechey A P G, Eltringham R J, Studd C 1981 Temazepam as premedication in day surgery. Anaesthesia 36: 10–16

Bieter R N 1936 Applied pharmacology of local anaesthetics. American Journal of Surgery 34: 500–510

Blomberg S, Emanuelsson H, Ricksten S-E 1989 Thoracic epidural anesthesia and central hemodynamics in patients with unstable angina pectoris. Anesthesia and Analgesia 69: 558–562

Bonica J J, Berges P U, Morikawa K 1970 Circulatory effects of peridural block: I. Effects of level of analgesia and dose of lidocaine. Anesthesiology 33: 619–626

Bonica J J, Akamatsu T J, Berges P U, Morikawa K, Kennedy W F 1971 Circulatory effects of peridural block: II. Effects of epinephrine. Anesthesiology 34: 514–522

Bonica J J, Kennedy W F, Akamatsu T J, Gerbershagen H U 1972 Circulatory effects of peridural block: III. Effects of acute blood loss. Anesthesiology 36: 219–227

Bromage P R 1978 Epidural analgesia. W B Saunders, Philadelphia

Bromage P R, Gertel M 1972 Brachial plexus anesthesia in chronic renal failure. Anesthesiology 36: 488–493

Buckley F P, Robinson N B, Simonowitz D A, Dellinger E P 1983 Anaesthesia in the morbidly obese. A comparison of anaesthetic and analgesic regimens for upper abdominal surgery. Anaesthesia 38: 840–851

Butler A B, Green C D 1970 Haematoma following epidural anaesthesia. Canadian Anaesthetists' Society Journal 17: 635–639

Chaudhari L S, Kop B R, Dhruva A J 1978 Paraplegia and epidural analgesia. Anaesthesia 33: 722–725

Cooper D W 1967 Spontaneous spinal epidural hematoma. Journal of Neurosurgery 26: 343–345

Cousins M J 1972 Hematoma following epidural block. Anesthesiology 37: 263

Crawford J S, James F M, Nolte H, Van Steenberge A, Shah J L 1981 Regional anaesthesia for patients with chronic neurological disease and similar conditions. Anaesthesia 36: 821

Dehring D J, Ahrens J F 1990 Pulmonary thromboembolism: disease recognition and patient management. Anesthesiology 73: 146–164

de Jong R H, De Rosa R A 1981 Benzodiazepine treatment of seizures from supraconvulsant doses of local anesthetics. Regional Anesthesia 6: 51–54

de Jong R H, Heavner J E 1974 Diazepam prevents and aborts lidocaine convulsions in monkeys. Anesthesiology 41: 226–230

Eng M, Berges P U, Ueland K, Bonica J J, Parer J T 1971 The effects of methoxamine and ephedrine in normotensive pregnant primates. Anesthesiology 35: 354–360

Engberg G, Wiklund L 1978a The use of ephedrine for prevention of arterial hypotension during epidural blockade. A study of the central circulation after subcutaneous premedication. Acta Anaesthesiologica Scandinavica 66(Supplement): 1–26

Engberg G, Wiklund L 1978b The circulatory effects of intravenously administered ephedrine during epidural blockade. Acta Anaesthesiologica Scandinavica 66(Supplement): 27–36

Fisher A, Waterhouse T D, Adams A P 1975 Obesity: its relation to anaesthesia. Anaesthesia 24: 208–216

Fisher M M 1977 Blood volume replacement in acute anaphylactic cardiovascular collapse related to anaesthesia. British Journal of Anaesthesia 49: 1023–1026

Fisher M M 1984 Intradermal testing to anaesthetic drugs: practical aspects of performance and interpretation. Anaesthesia and Intensive Care 12: 115–120

Fog J, Wang L P, Sundberg A, Mucchiano C 1990 Hearing loss after spinal anesthesia is related to needle size. Anesthesia and Analgesia 70: 517–520

Frankhouser P L 1983 Hazard of a new epidural catheter. Anesthesiology 58: 593–594

Freund F G, Bonica J J, Ward R J, Akamatsu T J, Kennedy W F 1967 Ventilatory reserve and level of motor block during high spinal and epidural anesthesia. Anesthesiology 28: 834–837

Galindo A 1982 Illustrated regional anesthesia. RM Scientific Publications, Miami

Galindo A, Galindo A 1980 Special needle for nerve blocks. Regional Anesthesia 5: 12–13

Gerard J L, Edouard A, Berdeaux A, Duranteau J, Ahmad R 1989 Interaction of intravenous diazepam and bupivacaine in conscious dogs. Regional Anesthesia 14: 298–303

Germann P A S, Roberts J G, Prys-Roberts C 1979 The combination of general anaesthesia and epidural block I. The effects of sequence of induction on haemodynamic variables and blood gas measurements in healthy patients. Anaesthesia and Intensive Care 7: 229–238

Gilbert J L, Lange G, Poleroy I, Brooks C M 1958 Effects of vasoconstrictor agents on cardiac irritability. Journal of Pharmacology and Experimental Therapeutics 123: 9–15

Granger H J, Guyton A C 1969 Autoregulation of the total systemic circulation following destruction of the central nervous system in the dog. Circulation Research 25: 379–388

Grant I S, Nimmo W S, Clements J A 1981 Pharmacokinetics and analgesic effect of i.m. and oral ketamine. British Journal of Anaesthesia 53: 805–809

Greene N M 1982 Physiologic responses to spinal anesthesia. American Society of Anesthesiologists Annual Refresher Course Lectures, p 129

Gregg R V, Turner P A, Denson D D, Stuebing R C, Selhorst C S, Forsberg T 1988 Does diazepam really reduce the cardiotoxic effects of intravenous bupivacaine? Anesthesia and Analgesia 67: 9–14

Griffiths H W C, Gillies J 1948 Thoracolumbar splanchnicectomy and sympathectomy. Anaesthesia 3: 134–136

Gringrich T F 1968 Spinal epidural hematoma following continuous epidural anesthesia. Anesthesiology 29: 162–163

Gronert G A 1980 Malignant hyperthermia. Anesthesiology 53: 395–423

Guinard J-P, Mulroy M F Carpenter R L, Knopes K D 1990 Test doses: optimal epinephrine content with and without acute beta-adrenergic blockade. Anesthesiology 73: 386–392

Hackel D B, Sancetta S M, Kleinerman J 1956 Effect of hypotension due to spinal anesthesia on coronary blood flow and myocardial metabolism in man. Circulation 13: 92–97

Hartung H J, Rupprecht A 1989 Die axillare Plexus brachialis – Blockade. Eine Studie an 178 Patienten. Regional-Anaesthesie 12: 21–24

Helperin S W, Cohen D D 1971 Hematoma following epidural anesthesia: report of a case. Anesthesiology 35: 641–644

Henderson J J, Macrae W A 1983 Complications. In: Henderson J J, Nimmo W S (eds) Practical regional anaesthesia. Blackwell, Oxford

Hindman B J, Koka B V 1986 Usefulness of the post-aspirin bleeding time. Anesthesiology 64: 368–370

Hirlekar G 1980 Paraplegia after epidural analgesia associated with an extradural spinal tumour. Anaesthesia 35: 363–364

Hjelm M, Holmdahl M H 1965 Biochemical effects of aromatic amines. II Cyanosis, methaemoglobinaemia and Heinz-body formation induced by a local anaesthetic agent (prilocaine). Acta Anaesthesiologica Scandinavica 9: 99–120

Howells T H, Huntsman R G, Boys J E, Mahmood A 1972 Anaesthesia and sickle-cell haemoglobin, with a case report. British Journal of Anaesthesia 44, 975–987

Janis K M 1972 Epidural hematoma following postoperative epidural analgesia: case report. Anesthesia and Analgesia 51: 689–692

Jensen B D, Berthelsen P, Brochner-Mortensen J 1977 Glomerular filtration rate during halothane anaesthesia and epidural anaesthesia in combination with halothane anaesthesia. Acta Anaesthesiologica Scandinavica 21: 395–399

Kakkar V V, Corrigan T P, Fossard D P et al 1975 Prevention of fatal postoperative pulmonary embolism by low doses of heparin. An international multicentre trial. Lancet ii: 45–51

Katz J D, Krich L B 1976 Acute febrile reaction complicating spinal anaesthesia in a survivor of malignant hyperthermia. Canadian Anaesthetists' Society Journal 23: 285–289

Kennedy W F, Bonica J J, Akamatsu T J, Ward R J, Martin W E, Grinstein A 1968 Cardiovascular and respiratory effects of subarachnoid block in the presence of acute blood loss. Anesthesiology 29: 29–35

Klassen G A, Bramwell R S, Bromage P R, Zborowska-Sluis D T 1980 Effect of acute sympathectomy by epidural anesthesia on the canine coronary circulation. Anesthesiology 52: 8–15

Kock M, Blomberg S, Emanuelsson H, Lomsky M, Stromblad S-O, Ricksten S-E 1990 Thoracic epidural anesthesia improves global and regional ventricular function during stress-induced myocardial ischemia in patients with coronary artery disease. Anesthesia and Analgesia 71: 625–630

Kroll D A, Caplan R A, Posner K, Ward R J, Cheney F W 1990 Nerve injury associated with anesthesia. Anesthesiology 73: 202–207

Lambert D H, Deane R S, Mazuzan J E 1982 Anesthesia and the control of blood pressure in patients with spinal cord injury. Anesthesia and Analgesia 61: 344–348

Li T-H, Shimosato S, Etsten B 1965 Methoxamine and cardiac output in non-anesthetized man and during spinal anesthesia. Anesthesiology 26: 21–30

Lim E K, Pereira E 1984 Brachial plexus injury following brachial plexus block. Anaesthesia 39: 691–694

Lingenfelter R W 1983 Hazard of a new epidural catheter. Anesthesiology 58: 292–293

Lofstrom J B 1975 Ulnar nerve blockade for the evaluation of local anaesthetic agents. British Journal of Anaesthesia. 47: 297–300

Lofstrom J B, Wennberg A, Widen L 1966 Late disturbance in nerve function after block with local anaesthetic agents. Acta Anaesthesiologica Scandinavica 10: 111–122

Lund P C 1971 Principles and practice of spinal anesthesia. Thomas, Springfield

Lynn R B, Sancetta S M, Simeone F A, Scott R W 1952 Observations on the circulation in high spinal anesthesia. Surgery 22: 195–213

McArthur C, Lewis M, Knox E G, Crawford J S 1990 Epidural anaesthesia and long term backache after childbirth. British Medical Journal 301: 9–12

McCarthy G J 1976 The effect of thoracic extradural analgesia on pulmonary gas distribution, functional residual capacity and airway closure. British Journal of Anaesthesia 48: 243–248

McDonald R 1991 Aspirin and epidural blocks. British Journal of Anaesthesia 66: 1–3

McEvedy P G (1946) Local anaesthesia. Manchester University Medical School Gazette 15: 2–8

McLaren A P H, Mulligan G W, Otton P E, McLean L D 1967 Hemodynamic alterations associated with epidural anesthesia. Surgery 62: 79–87

McQuay H J, Carroll D, Moore R A 1988 Postoperative orthopaedic pain – the effect of opiate premedication and local anaesthetic blocks. Pain 33: 291–295

Marinacci A A, Courville C B 1958 Electromyogram in evaluation of neurological complications of spinal anesthesia. Journal of the American Medical Association 168: 1337–1345

Markham J W, Lynge H N, Stahlman G E B 1967 The syndrome of spontaneous spinal epidural hematoma. Report of three cases. Journal of Neurosurgery 26: 334–342

Mauney F M, Ebert P A, Sabiston D C 1970 Postoperative myocardial infarction. A study of predisposing factors, diagnosis and mortality rate in a high risk group of surgical patients. Annals of Surgery 172: 497–502

Moller J T, Wittrup M, Johansen S H 1990 Hypoxemia in the postanesthetic care unit: An observer study. Anesthesiology 73: 890–895

Montgomery S J, Raj P P, Nettles D, Jenkins M T 1973 The use of the nerve stimulator with standard unsheathed needles in nerve blockade. Anesthesia and Analgesia 52: 827–831

Moore D C 1976 Regional block, 4th edn. Thomas, Springfield

Moore D C, Batra M 1981 The components of an effective test dose prior to epidural block. Anesthesiology 55: 693–696

Moore D C, Bridenbaugh L D 1966 Spinal (subarachnoid) block. A review of 11, 574 cases. Journal of the American Medical Association 195: 907–912

Muller H, Sarges R, Jouaux J, Runte W, Lampante L 1990 Intraoperative suppression of spasticity by intrathecal baclofen. Anaesthetist 39: 22–29

Munson E S, Paul W S, Embro W J 1977 Central-nervous-system toxicity of local anesthetic mixtures in monkeys. Anesthesiology 46: 179–183

Nielsen C H 1989 Bleeding after intercostal nerve block in a patient anticoagulated with heparin. Anesthesiology 71: 162–164

Nimmo W S, Aitkenhead A R, Clarke R S J, Weller R M 1990 Anaphylactic reactions associated with anaesthesia. Association of Anaesthetists of Great Britain and Ireland, London.

Odoom J A, Sih I L 1983 Epidural analgesia and anticoagulant therapy; experience with one thousand cases of continuous epidurals. Anaesthesia 38: 254–259

Page M M, Watkins P J 1978 Cardiorespiratory arrest and diabetic autonomic neuropathy. Lancet i: 14–16

Perel A, Reches A, Davidson J T 1977 Anaesthesia in the Guillain–Barré syndrome. A case report and recommendations. Anaesthesia 32: 257–260

Pither C E, Ford D J, Raj P P 1984 Peripheral nerve stimulation with insulated and uninsulated needles: Efficacy and characteristics. Regional Anesthesia 9: 42–43

Racz G B, Sabonghy M, Gintautas J, Kline W M 1982 Intractable pain therapy using a new epidural catheter. Journal of the American Medical Association 248: 579–581

Raj P P, Rosenblatt R, Montgomery S J 1980 Use of the nerve stimulator for peripheral blocks. Regional Anesthesia 5: 14–21

Ralston D H, Shnider S M, De Lorimier A A 1974 Effects of equipotent ephedrine, metaraminol, mephentermine and methoxamine on uterine blood flow in the pregnant ewe. Anesthesiology 40: 354–370

Ramanathan J, Sibai B M, Vu T, Chauhan D 1989 Correlation between bleeding times and platelet counts in women with pre-eclampsia undergoing cesarean section. Anesthesiology 71: 188–191

Rao T L K, El-Etr A A 1981 Anticoagulation following placement of epidural and subarachnoid catheters: An evaluation of neurologic sequelae. Anesthesiology 55: 618–620

Ratra C K, Badola R P, Bhargava K P 1972 A study of factors concerned in emesis during spinal anaesthesia. British Journal of Anaesthesia 44: 1208–1211

Reiz S 1989 Circulatory effects of epidural anesthesia in patients with cardiac disease. Acta Anaesthesiologica Belgica 30: 21–27

Reiz S, Nath S, Rais O 1980 Effects of thoracic epidural block and prenalterol on coronary vascular resistance and myocardial metabolism in patients with coronary artery disease. Acta Anaesthesiologica Scandinavica 24: 11–16

Rosenblatt R M and Shal R 1984 The design and function of a regional anesthesia block room. Regional Anesthesia 9: 12–16

Sage D J 1990 Epidurals, spinals and bleeding disorders in pregnancy: a review. Anaesthesia and Intensive Care 18: 319–326

Schonwald G, Fish K J, Perkash I 1981 Cardiovascular complications during anesthesia in chronic spinal cord injured patients. Anesthesiology 55: 550–558

Scott D B 1975 Management of extradural block during surgery. British Journal of Anaesthesia 47: 271–272

Scott D B, Littlewood D G, Drummond G B, Buckley F P, Covino B G 1977 Modification of the circulatory effects of extradural block combined with general anaesthesia by the addition of adrenaline to lignocaine solutions. British Journal of Anaesthesia 49: 917–925

Selander D, Dhuner K-G, Lundborg G 1977 Peripheral nerve injury due to injection needles used for regional anaesthesia. Acta Anaesthesiologica Scandinavica 21: 182–188

Selander D, Edshage S, Wolff S 1979a Paraesthesia or no paraesthesia? Nerve lesions after axillary blocks. Acta Anaesthesiologica Scandinavica 23: 27–33

Selander D, Brattsand R, Lundborg G, Nordborg C, Olsson Y 1979b Local anesthetics: importance of mode of application, concentration and adrenaline for the appearance of nerve lesions. Acta Anaesthesiologica Scandinavica 23: 127–136

Seltzer J L, Porretta J C, Jackson B G 1977 Plastic particulate contaminants in the medicine cups of disposable non-spinal regional anesthesia sets. Anesthesiology 47: 378–379

Seropian R, Reynolds B M 1971 Wound infections after preoperative depilatory versus razor preparation. American Journal of Surgery 121: 251–254

Sharrock N E, Mineo R, Urquhart B 1990 Hemodynamic response to low-dose epinephrine infusion during hypotensive epidural anesthesia for total hip replacement. Regional Anesthesia 15: 295–299

Sinclair C J, Scott D B, Edstrom H H 1982 Effect of the Trendelenberg position on spinal anaesthesia with hyperbaric bupivacaine. British Journal of Anaesthesia 54: 497–500

Smith D C, Crul J F 1989 Oxygen desaturation following sedation for regional anaesthesia. British Journal of Anaesthesia 62: 206–209

Smith N J, Corbascia A N 1970 The use and misuse of pressor agents. Anesthesiology 33: 58–101

Somerville T G, Gibson M 1973 Particulate contamination in ampoules: a comparative study. Pharmaceutical Journal 211: 128–131

Stanton-Hicks M d'A, Berges P U, Bonica J J 1973 Circulatory effects of peridural block. IV. Comparison of the effects of epinephrine and phenylephrine. Anesthesiology 39: 308–314

Steen P A, Tinker J H, Tarhan S 1978 Myocardial infarction after anesthesia and surgery. Journal of the American Medical Association 239: 2566–2570

Stephen G W, Lees M M, Scott D B 1969 Cardiovascular effects of epidural block combined with general anaesthesia. British Journal of Anaesthesia 41: 933–938

Tucker G T 1983 Pharmacokinetics of local anaesthetic drugs. In: Henderson J J, Nimmo W S (eds) Practical regional anaesthesia. Blackwell, Oxford

Varkey G P, Brindle G F 1974 Peridural anaesthesia and anticoagulant therapy. Canadian Anaesthetists' Society Journal 21: 106–109

Wadhwa R K 1977 Obstetric anesthesia for a patient with malignant hyperthermia susceptibility. Anesthesiology 46: 63–64

Weiss M G, Adkinson N F, Hirshman C A 1989 Evaluation of allergic drug reactions in the peri-operative period. Anesthesiology 71: 483–486

Wetstone D L, Wong K C 1974 Sinus bradycardia and asystole during spinal anesthesia. Anesthesiology 41: 87–89

Wildsmith J A W, McClure J H 1991 Editorial: anticoagulant drugs and central nerve blockade. Anaesthesia 46: 613–614

Winnie A P 1969 'An immobile needle' for nerve blocks. Anesthesiology 31: 577–578

Winnie A P 1983 Plexus anesthesia Vol. 1 Churchill Livingstone, Edinburgh, p 211

Wollman S B, Marx G F 1968 Acute hydration for prevention of hypotension of spinal anesthesia in parturients. Anesthesiology 29: 374–380

Wooley E J, Vandam L D 1959 Neurological sequelae of brachial plexus nerve block. Annals of Surgery 149: 53–60

6. Anatomy of the spine

W. A. Chambers

THE VERTEBRAL COLUMN

The human spine or vertebral column is a strong curved pillar (Fig. 6.1). It is formed by a series of vertebrae which are united by intervertebral discs of cartilage and the sum of small movements between adjacent vertebrae confers considerable mobility. The vertebral canal (which contains the spinal cord) is formed by the successive vertebral foramina of the individual vertebrae and by the ligaments and discs connecting them. There are seven cervical, 12 thoracic and five lumbar vertebrae. The sacrum comprises five, and the coccyx four, fused segments, respectively.

The vertebrae

Although the vertebrae show regional differences they all conform to a basic pattern (Fig. 6.2): the body, through which the weight of the subject is transmitted, and the vertebral (or neural) arch, which surrounds and protects the spinal cord lying in the vertebral foramen. The arch consists of a pedicle and a lamina on each side, and a dorsal spine. Each lamina carries a transverse process and a superior and inferior articular process. The pedicles are notched and the notches of each adjacent pair together form an intervertebral foramen which is traversed by a spinal nerve.

The lumbar vertebrae

The bodies of the lumbar vertebrae are large and kidney shaped. The vertebral foramina are triangular and intermediate in size between those in the thoracic and cervical regions. The relatively large wedge-shaped discs account for the mobility of this region. The pedicles are thick, with shallow superior notches. The transverse processes are slender, increasing in length from L_1 to L_3 and then becoming shorter again. The laminae are short and do not overlap each other and the lumbar spines are horizontal and oblong. The fifth lumbar vertebra, being considerably longer anteriorly, is wedge shaped and produces the lumbosacral angle. Its transverse processes, although short and thick, are strong and arise not only from the arch but also from the side of the vertebral body.

The thoracic vertebrae

The bodies, flattened in front and behind, are small but increase in size from above downwards. The intervertebral discs are thicker in front and contribute substantially to the length of this region. The vertebral foramina are large and triangular, freely accommodating the relatively thick spinal cord. From T_2 to T_8 the vertebrae bear upper and lower demi-facets for the rib heads. The pedicles pass directly backwards and, except for T_1, have virtually no superior notch, but a very deep inferior notch. The transverse processes are large, pass backwards as much as laterally and, typically, bear a facet for articulation with the tubercle of the corresponding rib. The spines are long in the thoracic region, each one overlapping the spine below.

It should be noted that the general features change gradually and that the transition between

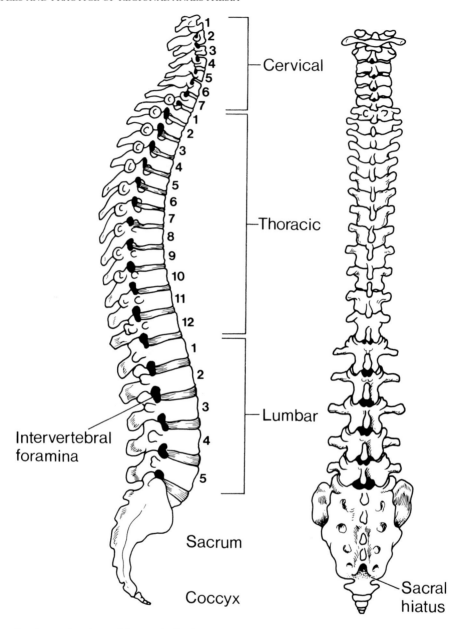

1
2
3
4
5
6
7

—Cervical

1
2
3
4
5
6
7
8
9
10
11
12

—Thoracic

1
2
3
4
5

—Lumbar

Intervertebral
foramina

Sacrum

Coccyx

Sacral
hiatus

Fig. 6.1 Lateral and posterior views of the vertebral column.

regions is by no means abrupt. Thus the lower thoracic vertebrae show a tendency to lumbar characteristics in the body, spine and inferior articular processes and conversely the first lumbar vertebra may occasionally carry a rib.

Intervertebral ligaments

The individual vertebrae are linked to each other by a complicated system of intervertebral articular facets and ligaments (Fig. 6.3). Of all the parts of a vertebra only the pedicles are without ligaments.

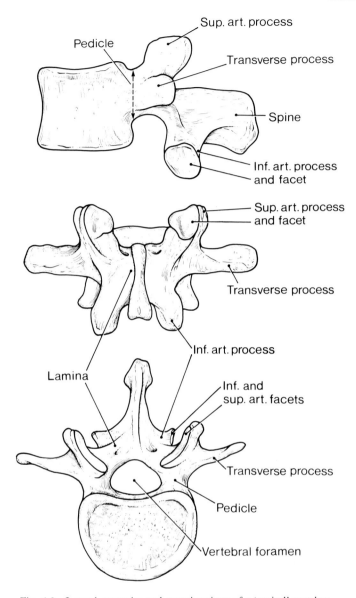

Fig. 6.2 Lateral, posterior and superior views of a 'typical' vertebra.

The *anterior longitudinal ligament* runs along the front of the vertebral bodies from C_2 to the sacrum, becoming wider as it descends. The *posterior longitudinal ligament* extends along the posterior surfaces of the vertebral bodies. The laminae are united by the broad highly elastic *ligamentum flavum* which becomes thicker from above downwards. It stretches from the lower border and adjacent inner surface of one lamina to the upper border and outer surface of the lamina below. This gives the epidural space a 'saw tooth' pattern (Reynolds et al 1985) and means that at each interspace the distance from the ligamentum flavum to the dura is greater caudally (Fig. 6.3). In elderly patients the elasticity of the ligamentum flavum tends to be lost and calcification may occur. The *interspinous ligament*s connect the shafts of adjacent spines and are thin flimsy

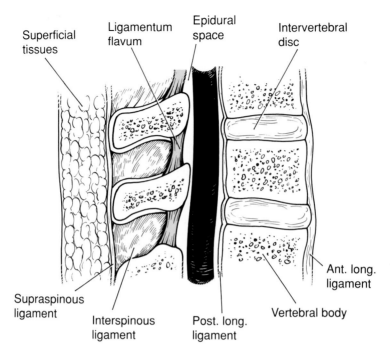

Fig. 6.3 Sagittal section of lumbar vertebrae to show the principal ligaments.

structures. The *supraspinous ligament* is a powerful fibrous structure which connects the tips of the spines from C_7 to the sacrum. This may become ossified in old age and render penetration with a thin needle impossible.

Other ligaments which are of less importance to the anaesthetist in the context of regional anaesthesia include the ligamentum nuchae (the upward continuation of the supraspinous ligament) and the occipito-atlanto-axial ligaments.

The intervertebral discs

These fibrocartilaginous discs are adherent to a thin layer of hyaline cartilage which covers the upper and lower parts of each vertebral body. In the peripheral part of the disc (annulus fibrosus) fibrous tissue predominates. The softer core of the discs (nucleus pulposus) is normally under pressure and expands when this is relieved. The nucleus gradually changes until in old age it cannot be distinguished from the annulus, the discs becoming thinner and less resilient. Whatever an individual's height, the length of the vertebral column is about 70 cm in the male and 60 cm in the female, with the intervertebral discs accounting for about one-fifth of this total length. However, atrophy of the discs in the elderly together with osteoporosis of the vertebrae leads to the decreased height and kyphotic deformity of old age.

Spinal curves

In the embryo the spine is curved into a gentle 'C' shape, concave forwards, and this primary curvature persists in the thoracic and pelvic regions. Extension of the head when it is held up and the extension of the lower limbs which occurs with standing erect produce secondary curvatures in the cervical and lumbar regions which are concave backwards (Fig. 6.1). The curves are produced largely by moulding of the discs. The cervical curve usually includes the first two thoracic vertebrae and the lumbar curve is more marked in women, particularly in pregnancy. In the thoracic region the column may deviate somewhat laterally, usually towards the right, the line being restored by compensatory curves above and below.

The intervertebral discs allow the vertebrae to rock upon one another, compressing one side of the disc and expanding the opposite side. The small movements taken together allow free bending of the column forwards (flexion), backwards (extension) and to the side (lateral flexion). In addition the discs allow slight rotation to a degree dependent on the nature of the synovial joints at different levels.

Movement of the spine

Extension is the freer movement and is greatest in the lumbar and least in the thoracic regions. Flexion, which is largely restrained by tension in the extensor muscles, is most marked in the thoracic region and almost absent in the lumbar. It should be noted that natural forward bending is largely flexion at the hip joints and is not really flexion of the trunk. The ligamentum flavum stretches freely on flexion and its elastic recoil avoids the formation of folds which might be nipped between the bones on extension. Because of the ribs, lateral flexion is very limited in the thoracic region, but rotation is freest. Lateral flexion is greatest in the lumbar region, but slight rotation is also possible.

If the vertebral column is viewed from behind, the laminae and spines can be seen to overlap each other in such a fashion that the spinal canal is completely hidden except in the lower lumbar region. The gap between the lumbar spinous processes can be widened by flexion of the spine (Fig. 6.4), although this manoeuvre has a more limited effect in the thoracic region. Rotation may distort the bony structures so that a direct approach to the vertebral canal is not possible from the midline. This is more likely to be a problem in the thoracic region where a greater degree of rotation is possible.

The sacrum

The sacrum, consisting of five fused sacral vertebrae, forms a curved wedge between the hip bones and has markedly concave anterior and convex posterior surfaces. The anterior surface (Fig. 6.5) bears four transverse ridges at the sites

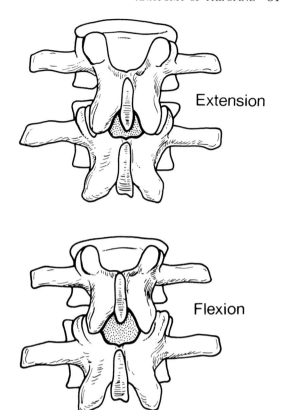

Fig. 6.4   Effect of flexion and extension on the interlaminar gap in the lumbar region.

of the obliterated discs which end on each side in the four anterior sacral foramina. Lateral to these lie the fused lateral masses. The anterior primary rami of the upper four sacral nerves pass through the anterior foramina. Posteriorly (Fig. 6.6) the vertebral laminae form a rough plate which bears a median crest composed of three or four fused spinous tubercles and intermediate crests of small articular tubercles derived from the fusion of the articular processes. Below, the lowest articular processes form small blunt horns, the sacral cornua, which are connected to the coccyx by ligaments. The last laminar arch (and occasionally two or more) fails to fuse in the midline and leaves a triangular gap, the sacral hiatus. This usually lies about 5 cm above the tip of the coccyx and directly above the uppermost limit of the natal cleft. The fifth sacral nerve and the filum terminale traverse the sacral hiatus. Lateral to the articular tubercles

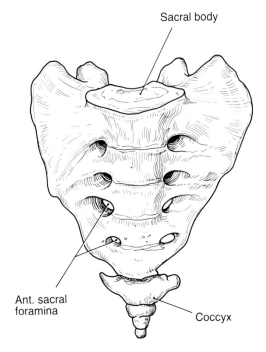

Fig. 6.5   Anterior surface of the sacrum.

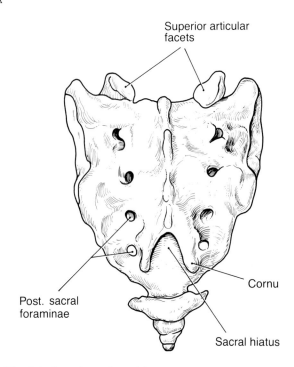

Fig. 6.6   Posterior surface of the sacrum.

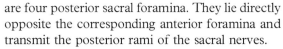

are four posterior sacral foramina. They lie directly opposite the corresponding anterior foramina and transmit the posterior rami of the sacral nerves.

The sacral canal is triangular. The horizontal margins of its upper opening give attachments to the lowest ligamentum flavum, and the sacral hiatus is roofed by a membrane which stretches to the coccyx. The canal contains the lower part of the cauda equina, meninges and a quantity of fat.

Vertebral anomalies

Variations in the anatomy of the vertebral column are of more than passing interest since they may make the performance of a spinal or epidural block difficult or even impossible. Recognized abnormalities include absence of single vertebrae or of the lower sacrum and coccyx, fusion of two or more vertebrae, the development of additional vertebrae or hemivertebrae and spina bifida. Spina bifida results from a failure of fusion of the two developmental centres in the arch. This is not usually associated with any neurological defect, but there may be an overlying dimple, lipoma or

tuft of hair to warn of an underlying bony anomaly. Rarely there is a gross defect of one or more of the arches with protrusion of the cord or its coverings. Fusion of two or more vertebrae may occur, particularly in the region of the sacrum where the fifth lumbar vertebra may be wholly or partly fused to it. In contrast, the first sacral segment may be wholly or partly separated from the rest of the sacrum. Variations in the structure of the sacrum are dealt with in Chapter 9.

CONTENTS OF THE VERTEBRAL CANAL

Spinal cord

The spinal cord is about 45 cm long and is slightly thicker than a pencil. It is somewhat flattened anteroposteriorly, especially in the lumbar region, and has cervical and lumbar enlargements. It is continuous with the medulla oblongata above and tapers into the conus medullaris below, from which a thread-like structure, the filum terminale, continues to be attached to the coccyx. Up to the third month of intrauterine life the cord extends

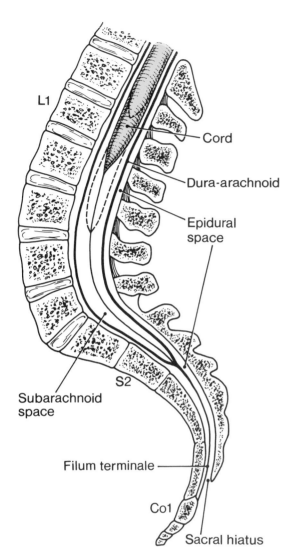

L1

Cord

Dura-arachnoid

Epidural space

Subarachnoid space

S2

Filum terminale

Co1

Sacral hiatus

Fig. 6.7 Sagittal section of lumbar and sacral regions of the spine. The dotted lines indicate the range for the termination of the spinal cord.

contrast the upper thoracic roots pass much more horizontally.

The meninges

The spinal cord has three covering membranes (the meninges) – the dura mater, the arachnoid mater and the pia mater (Fig. 6.8). The *dura mater* covering of the brain is a double membrane which encloses the cerebral venous sinuses. The dura which encloses the spinal cord is a continuation of the inner layer of the cerebral dura and is composed of dense fibrous tissue. The endosteal (outer) layer of cerebral dura terminates at the foramen magnum and below this level is represented by the periosteal lining of the spinal canal. The dural sac usually extends to the second sacral segment; occasionally it extends to the third sacral segment or it may end as high as the fifth lumbar segment. It then continues as the covering of the filum terminale. It lies rather loosely within the canal, supported in the extradural fat, and is attached to the following: the edge of the foramen magnum above; the posterior longitudinal ligament anteriorly; and the coccyx by the filum terminale inferiorly. Laterally there are prolongations along the dorsal and ventral nerve roots which are continuous with the epineurium of the spinal nerves. Posteriorly the dural sac is quite free.

The *arachnoid mater* is a thin membrane which lines the dural sac and sends prolongations along each nerve root. The *pia mater,* the innermost membrane, is a vascular sheath which closely invests the brain and spinal cord.

The spinal meninges divide the vertebral canal into several distinct compartments; the subarachnoid, subdural and epidural spaces. The *subarachnoid space* contains the cerebrospinal fluid (CSF) and the spinal cord and is crossed by incomplete trabeculae. The pattern of these is somewhat variable (Nauta et al 1983), but in most cases a midline dorsal septum, the septicum posticum, extends from the mid-cervical to the lumbar region (Fig. 6.8). It has irregular perforations and tends to thicken with increasing age (Key & Retzius 1879). The dorsolateral septi are more fenestrated, tend to atrophy with age, and attach the dorsal rootlets to the arachnoid. More

the full length of the canal, but thereafter the vertebrae grow much more rapidly and in the newborn the cord usually terminates at the lower border of the third lumbar vertebra. In adult life the cord usually ends at the level of the disc between the first and second lumbar vertebrae, although there is some variation (Fig. 6.7).

The difference in growth results in the lumbar and sacral roots being elongated to reach their foramina, thus forming the cauda equina. In laterally still, the substantial dentate ligaments support the spinal cord by attaching it to the dura mater (Key & Retzius 1879). Anterior trabeculae in the subarachnoid space are less common, but if they and the septicum porticum are complete they can result in a unilateral spinal (Armstrong 1989).

The *subdural space* is really only a potential space – the arachnoid is normally in close contact with the dural sheath and is separated from it by a thin film of serous fluid. The *epidural space* lies between the dural sheath and the spinal canal. It extends from the foramen magnum to the sacral hiatus and is filled with semi-liquid fat, lymphatics, arteries and veins. In young children the epidural fat is very fluid (Tretjakoff 1926), allowing local anaesthetic solutions to spread extensively. The epidural veins are valveless and run mainly vertically in four principal trunks which communicate freely by

venous rings at each vertebral level. The increase in CSF pressure which accompanies coughing results partly from the shunting of blood from veins in the trunk to these veins. The arteries are relatively small. They enter at each vertebral foramen and lie mainly in the lateral part of the space. They supply adjacent vertebrae and ligaments, and contribute to the supply of the spinal cord.

The dural sac normally lies eccentrically towards the anterior aspect of the vertebral canal and thus the epidural space consists of a smaller anterior compartment and two larger posterolateral compartments. The depth of the posterior epidural space varies from as little as 1 mm in the cervical region to 6 mm in the lumbar region and is widest in the sacral region because of the absence of the dural sac.

Dorsal midline strands have been demonstrated in the epidural space (Blomberg 1986). These

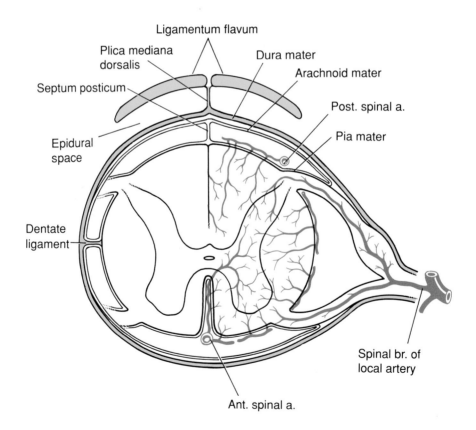

Fig. 6.8 Transverse section to show the spinal meninges and arterial blood supply. The nerve roots have been omitted on the left for clarity.

connect the ligamentum flavum to the dura and can cause a fold in the dura mater, the plica mediana dorsalis (Fig. 6.8), thus narrowing the epidural space in the midline. The strands can alter the direction of a catheter, especially as increased lengths are inserted. In some cases a complete midline membrane may be present which can prevent a catheter and injected solution crossing from one side to the other. Connective tissue bands may also originate from the plica mediana dorsalis and extend laterally, thus subdividing the posterolateral compartment of the epidural space into anterior and posterior sections (Savolaine et al 1988).

Cerebrospinal fluid

The CSF, normally clear and colourless, fills all the cavities in, and spaces around, the central nervous system. It is isotonic with plasma, but contains only traces of protein. It is secreted mainly by the choroid plexuses of the lateral ventricles, but also by plexuses in the third and fourth ventricles and on the surface of the brain. The fluid is reabsorbed by the arachnoid villi and granulations, and a considerable amount also drains into the connective tissue spaces of the nerves. Its normal composition is shown in Table 7.1.

Blood supply

The blood supply of the spinal cord is from the anterior and posterior spinal arteries (Fig. 6.8). The anterior spinal artery is a single midline vessel and is formed at the foramen magnum by the union of a branch from each vertebral artery. It is the largest of the vessels and supplies a large anterior portion of the cord. The posterior spinal arteries consist of one or two vessels on each side and are derived from the posterior inferior cerebellar arteries. This supply is augmented by spinal branches of the vertebral, ascending cervical, posterior intercostal, lumbar and lateral sacral arteries, which pass through the intervertebral foramina. Most of these are insignificant, but some, such as those at T_4 and T_{11}, contribute substantially.

The arterial supply to the cord is somewhat vulnerable and occlusion of these vessels may follow trauma, hypotension or the use of vasoconstrictors. Blockage of a posterior vessel may have little effect, but occlusion of the anterior spinal artery has serious consequences.

Venous drainage is through a plexus of anterior and posterior veins which drain along the nerve roots into segmental veins – the vertebral veins in the neck, the azygos veins in the thorax, lumbar veins in the abdomen and lateral sacral veins in the pelvis.

REFERENCES

Armstrong P J 1989 Unilateral subarachnoid anaesthesia. Anaesthesia 44: 918–919
Blomberg R 1986 The dorsomedian connective tissue band in the lumbar epidural space of humans. Anesthesia Analgesia (Cleveland) 65: 747–752.
Key E A H, Retzius M G 1879 Studien in der Nervensystems und des Bindegewebs. Samson and Wallin, Stockholm
Nauta H J E, Dolan E, Yasargil M G 1983 Microsurgical anatomy of the spinal subarachnoid space. Surgical Neurology 19: 431–437

Reynolds A F, Roberts P A, Pollay M, Stratmeier P H 1985 Quantitative anatomy of the thoracolumbar epidural space. Neurosurgery 17: 905–907
Savolaine E R, Pandaya J B, Greenblatt S H, Conover S R 1988 Anatomy of the human lumbar epidural space. Anesthesiology 68: 217–220
Tretjakoff D 1926 Das Epidurale Fett gewabe. Zeitschrift für Anatomische 79: 100

7. Spinal anaesthesia

A. P. Rubin

Spinal anaesthesia is induced by the injection of local anaesthetic into the subarachnoid space. It is used most commonly to produce anaesthesia for surgery and obstetrics, and less frequently in the assessment and treatment of chronic pain states.

The technique became very popular in the early 20th century, as the method is simple and a very small dose of local anaesthetic produces excellent analgesia, profound muscle relaxation and a reduction in bleeding. However, the introduction of specific neuromuscular blocking agents and other improvements in general anaesthesia, together with adverse publicity surrounding the Woolley and Roe case (Cope 1954), accounted for a dramatic decrease in its use in the UK. It is only in the last decade that it has regained popularity and that many of the classical ideas have been re-evaluated.

Cerebrospinal fluid

Formation (Fig. 7.1)

Cerebrospinal fluid (CSF) is formed by the choroid plexuses which consist of small tufts of capillaries in direct contact with the lining of the lateral ventricles. Normally about 150 ml is produced per day, but when the volume is low, this may increase to 450 ml. The CSF passes through the interventricular foramina of Munro to the third ventricle, then through the cerebral aqueduct (aqueduct of Sylvius) to the fourth ventricle. It leaves the fourth ventricle by the lateral and median apertures (foramina of Luschka and Magendie) to reach the subarachnoid space, which lies between the pia and arachnoid mater, and

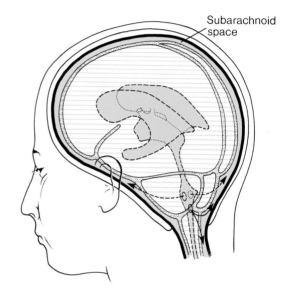

Fig. 7.1 Circulation of cerebrospinal fluid.

extends superficially over the whole surface of the brain and spinal cord. Extensions of the subarachnoid space may be found a variable distance along peripheral nerves and also enter the substance of the brain and spinal cord in the perivascular Virchow–Robin spaces. The CSF is absorbed by microscopic arachnoid villi which project from the subarachnoid space. Some absorption probably takes place directly by the venous plexuses, and some within the perivascular spaces.

Composition (Table 7.1)

CSF is a clear, colourless fluid. Compared with plasma the sodium and chloride content are slightly higher, and the protein content is consid-

Table 7.1   Composition of cerebrospinal fluid

H^+	32–36 nmol l^{-1}
Glucose	1.5–4.0 nmol l^{-1}
Sodium	140–150 mmol l^{-1}
Chloride	120–130 mmol l^{-1}
Bicarbonate	25–30 mmol l^{-1}
Protein	0.15–0.3 g l^{-1}

erably lower. The normal pressure of CSF in the lumbar region is 60–100 mm H_2O with the patient in the lateral position, rising to 200–250 mm H_2O in the sitting position. The volume is usually about 130 ml, of which approximately 35 ml is in the spinal subarachnoid space.

Specific gravity

The specific gravity is about 1.006–1.008 (taking water as 1.000 at 25°C). It probably increases with age, and with some systemic disease states, such as uraemia and hyperglycaemia. The specific gravity decreases 0.001 for each 5°C rise in temperature, so that at 37°C it is usually 1.004–1.006. Any injected solution reaches body temperature within 60 seconds and it is the specific gravity at body temperature which determines baricity relative to the CSF. Thus, a solution of specific gravity greater than 1.006 at 37°C is hyperbaric, and one less than 1.003 at 37°C is likely to be hypobaric. Between these two values, solutions can be considered to be isobaric. Osmolality may be important, and the osmolality of CSF at 37°C is about 280 mOsm. The ideal spinal solution would be isotonic, but most are hypertonic. Any potentially hazardous effect is decreased by the immediate dilution of the solution by the CSF.

INDICATIONS AND CONTRAINDICATIONS

Spinal anaesthesia is restricted largely to operations performed below the level of the umbilicus. The likely duration of surgery is important, since a single-shot spinal will not regularly produce surgical anaesthesia for much longer than 2–3

hours. There is currently renewed interest in continuous spinals now that the technology is available for the production of fine-gauge catheters (28–32 g). Theoretically, a continuous technique allows both the extent and duration of block to be matched more precisely to the operation. Spinal anaesthesia is particularly suitable for older and poor risk patients, such as those suffering from chronic respiratory, diffuse hepatic and renal disease, diabetes mellitus and some forms of cardiovascular disease. The higher the sensory block, the more extensive will be the sympathetic block and the greater the degree of vasodilatation produced. Compensation occurs due to vasoconstriction above the level of the block and an increase in cardiac rate and stroke volume. Sympathetic effects (reduced afterload and cardiac work) may be beneficial in patients with congestive cardiac failure or ischaemic heart disease, but reduced perfusion pressure could be disastrous in a patient with aortic stenosis.

The advantages and disadvantages to the individual patient must be balanced, and only when the risks outweigh the benefits is the technique contraindicated. Many of the *contraindications* to spinal anaesthesia apply equally to other forms of regional block (Ch. 5) and these include anticoagulant therapy and other coagulation disorders, unwillingness of the patient, disease or severe deformity of the vertebral column, active neurological disease, localized or systemic infection, severe hypovolaemia and other forms of shock. Contraindications specific to spinal anaesthesia include pre-existing headache and raised intracranial pressure. In the patient with headache, the small but significant risk of a postlumbar puncture headache may complicate the situation. A lumbar puncture in the presence of raised intracranial pressure may lead to a sudden reduction in CSF pressure and coning of the brain in the foramen magnum.

TECHNIQUE OF LUMBAR PUNCTURE

The patient should be on a tilting table or trolley. An intravenous line must be established, blood pressure apparatus connected and resuscitation equipment available and checked. An under-

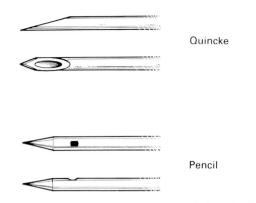

Fig. 7.2 Quincke and pencil point pattern spinal needle tips.

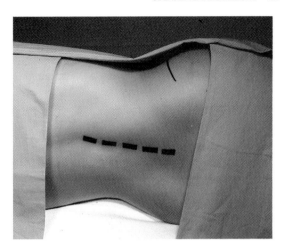

Fig. 7.3 Position for lumbar puncture in the lateral position. The hips and shoulders are vertical to eliminate rotation. A sandbag has been placed beneath the patient's loin to prevent lateral curvature of the spine.

standing of the anatomy of the lumbar spine (Ch. 6) and a scrupulous aseptic technique are essential (Ch. 5).

Spinal needles (Fig. 7.2)

Spinal needles are usually 9 cm (3.5 inches) long, and should have a close-fitting stilette, a smooth lining and, ideally, a transparent hub so that the flow of CSF is rapid and can be identified quickly (Messahel et al 1983). The needle should produce minimal trauma and the smallest possible hole in the dura mater. The traditional needle for a spinal anaesthetic has a Quincke tip, but pencil-point designs, such as the Whitacre or Sprotte, are becoming increasingly popular for use in younger patients because they decrease markedly the incidence of headache (Hart & Whitacre 1951).

Position

Various factors should be considered in choosing the position for lumbar puncture, including the subject's general condition and anatomy, and the baricity of the solution to be used.

Lateral horizontal position (Fig. 7.3)

This is the usual position as it is the most comfortable, and is easier in the less cooperative or sedated patient. Flexion of the lumbar spine is necessary to open the spaces between the spines and laminae and to facilitate the passage of the needle into the subarachnoid space. The patient is

placed on his side, with the legs acutely flexed at the hip and knees. Further flexion may be achieved by curvature of the upper spine, and encouraging the patient to tuck his chin on to his chest. The back should be near the edge of the table, that is, at right angles to the line of vision of the anaesthetist positioned behind the patient. The

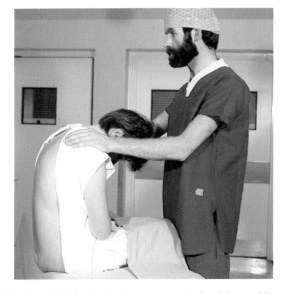

Fig. 7.4 Position for lumbar puncture in the sitting position.

back must be truly vertical at both hips and shoulder level so that a needle entering in the midline will continue in the midline as long as it is kept parallel to the top of the table or floor.

Sitting position (Fig. 7.4)

This position is helpful in the obese and in other patients in whom the spines are difficult to palpate as it is easier to identify the midline and assess the angles. However, it may be dangerous in the sedated patient as the blood pressure may fall due to pooling of blood in the lower extremities.

The patient is placed with the buttocks near the edge of the table, and the legs over the opposite edge with the feet supported on a stool. The patient rests his elbow on his thighs, or folds his arms forwards over pillows, and flexes the neck. An assistant should support the patient from the front, and every effort should be made to see that the back remains vertical.

The midline approach (Fig. 7.5)

The midline approach is recommended as it is easier than the paramedian, the space between the laminae is widest and the ligaments are relatively insensitive. A line drawn between the highest points of the iliac crests will cross the fourth lumbar spine of the space between the fourth and fifth spines. Other vertebral levels may be identified from this point and marked. As the spinal cord ends at about the lower border of the first lumbar vertebra, punctures are made below the level. The widest interspinous space is usually selected, although the intended area of block may influence the choice. The skin is carefully prepared with

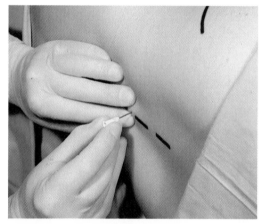

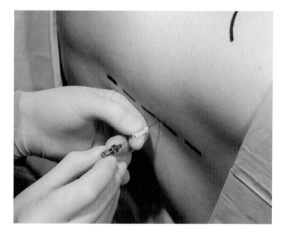

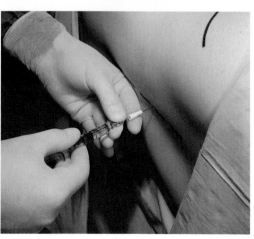

Fig. 7.5 Midline insertion of a 25 g spinal needle. The fingers of the left hand straddle the spine and a wide bore needle is inserted into the supraspinous ligament with a very slight cephalad angulation. The guide needle is then held steady and the spinal needle is passed through it. Once the dura has been penetrated the spinal needle is immobilized between thumb and second finger and a syringe is attached.

antiseptic which is allowed to dry so that there is no risk of carrying antiseptic into the epidural or subarachnoid spaces, and sterile drapes are applied. The local anaesthetic for infiltration is drawn up into one syringe, and the exact volume of the spinal solution drawn into a different size syringe to avoid confusion. The index and middle fingers of the non-dominant hand are placed on either side of the interspace so that only the spines, interspace and supraspinous ligament (the midline ridge) remain between the fingers. The infiltrating local anaesthetic – usually 1% lignocaine – is injected slowly in the midline of the chosen interspace. The subcutaneous tissues and the supraspinous ligament should be infiltrated as well as the skin, so that the patient does not move during insertion of the spinal needle. Care should be taken to ensure that the spinal needle is inserted through the anaesthetic area by keeping the 'straddling' fingers in place.

Use of 22 g needle

The 22 g needle is relatively rigid and an introducer is not required. The needle, with stilette in place and the *bevel facing laterally* if it has a Quincke tip, is inserted through the puncture site. It is advanced in the midline in a slightly cephalad direction (100–150°), as the interlaminar space is cephalad to the interspinous space. If the needle leaves the midline it enters the paraspinal muscles where it may be felt by the fingers straddling the spine and it will tend to drop rather than be gripped by the midline ligaments. Once the grip is felt, the midline and cephalad direction should be verified and the needle advanced further. The increasing resistance of the ligamentum flavum can be appreciated, as well as a loss of resistance as the needle enters the epidural space. A further loss of resistance, often accompanied by slight discomfort, is noticed as the needle pierces the dura and arachnoid to enter the subarachnoid space. If bone is contacted, this is likely to be the lamina of the vertebra, and the needle will need to be redirected. Usually a more cephalad direction is necessary, but the midline position of the needle should be checked first.

Use of 25 g, 26 g or 29 g needle

These needles are very flexible and it may be difficult to direct them accurately, so it is usual to insert an introducer first. The introducer may be designed specifically (e.g. the Sise), but a disposable 19 g or 20 g needle is equally satisfactory. Its use prevents contact of the spinal needle with the skin, and lessens the risks of infection and implantation of epidermis in deeper tissues. The direction of the guide needle, which should not be long enough to traverse the ligaments completely, must be verified. The fine needle is then inserted through it until the dura and arachnoid have been pierced.

Confirmation of dural puncture

The correct position of the needle is confirmed by a flow of CSF when the stilette is withdrawn. This will take time with fine needles and occasionally aspiration will be necessary. If no flow is obtained, but it is felt that the needle is in the subarachnoid space, the needle may be rotated through 90 or 180° and further attempts made to obtain fluid. If the fluid is blood stained, time must be allowed for it to clear before injecting the solution. If it does not clear quickly, another puncture should be made. Once there is a free flow of clear CSF, the syringe containing the spinal solution is attached, care being taken not to move the needle. A small quantity (0.1 ml) of CSF is aspirated to ensure that the needle tip is still in the subarachnoid space and the solution is then injected at a rate of about 1 ml 10s^{-1}. A further aspiration may be performed halfway through the injection and again at the end, to confirm that all the local anaesthetic has been injected correctly. This final aspirate should be reinjected as it contains a high concentration of local anaesthetic. The needle is withdrawn and an adhesive plaster or plastic spray is applied to the puncture site.

Lateral and paramedian approaches

Both these approaches involve insertion of the needle some distance from the midline. Although the terms are often used interchangeably, some anaesthetists make a distinction between them. With the paramedian approach the needle is inserted just caudad to the interspinous space and directed both cephalad and medially. With the lateral approach the needle is inserted level with the interspinous space and has no cephalad angulation.

These approaches may be used if there is little space in the midline, if the ligaments are very calcified or if the anaesthetist prefers one of them. It should be understood that the approach is lateral or paramedian at the skin, but that the needle should still enter the subarachnoid space in the midline. This means that more complex angles are involved and that the techniques are more difficult to understand and practise. The paramedian approach is considered further in Chapter 8.

FACTORS AFFECTING SPREAD

Once local anaesthetic has been injected, the block develops very quickly, so the patient should be placed immediately in the appropriate position and cardiovascular monitoring started. The patient's position will depend on the baricity of the injected solution and the desired extent of anaesthesia. Posture may be used to aid the attainment of the desired level of block, but this is only likely to help during the first 20 minutes.

Since the pioneering work of Barker (1907), it has been thought that the spread of solution within the subarachnoid space depended mainly on its baricity in relation to CSF, and the posture of the patient. There has also been a firm belief that further spread could be achieved by increasing the volume of solution injected, and that the curves of the vertebral column might limit spread. These concepts have been the subject of much recent clinical research and new ideas can now be advanced (McClure & Wildsmith 1988).

Effect of baricity

The specific gravity of a local anaesthetic solution may be adjusted by the addition of water, normal saline or glucose so that it becomes hypobaric, isobaric or hyperbaric in relation to CSF (Brown et al 1980). A specific gravity from 1.008 to 1.035

may be produced, depending on the amount of glucose added. It should be remembered that 5% glucose is isotonic with body fluids, and that any increase in concentration above this will raise the tonicity of the solution above that of CSF with some risk of neural damage. The glucose may have other effects besides increasing the baricity. It may help to 'hold' the solution together by making it more viscous, so decreasing its tendency to diffuse into, and be diluted by, the CSF. Hence the glucose encourages the spread of a bolus of concentrated anaesthetic. The addition of glucose results in decreased absorption of local anaesthetic from the subarachnoid space, and blood concentrations (which are indeed detectable after subarachnoid block) are lower (Burm et al 1983).

When equal volumes of solution are injected into supine patients, it is apparent that hyperbaric solutions spread very much higher than isobaric or hypobaric ones (Chambers et al 1981a). Hyperbaric and isobaric solutions tend to produce blocks of good quality and spread, whereas hypobaric solutions often result in poor-quality, patchy blocks of variable extent. If higher blocks are required, they are much more reliably obtained with hyperbaric solutions, perhaps with a head-down position, than with glucose-free solutions. Glucose-free solutions such as 3 ml of 0.5% bupivacaine produce some blocks above T_9, but the majority are below T_{10} and a few below T_{12} (Cummings et al 1984). The use of glucose-free solutions should be restricted to patients having surgery of the lower limb, hip and perineum. The higher blocks produced by hyperbaric solutions tend to have a shorter duration of action than those produced by isobaric or hypobaric solutions.

Posture

When mildly hypobaric solutions such as glucose-free bupivacaine are injected with the patient maintained in the sitting position for 2 minutes, the resulting block is two to three segments higher than when the lateral position is used (Kalso et al 1982). Posture is often used to manipulate the spread of hyperbaric solutions, but such an approach has limitations. For example, a classical saddle block can only be produced if the patient is kept sitting for several minutes after the injection of a small volume of a hyperbaric solution. Even then there may be some upward spread when the patient is placed supine. Similarly, it is possible to produce unilateral blocks with hyperbaric solutions injected in the lateral position, but once the patient is placed supine, the block will spread to the same height on both sides (Wildsmith et al 1981).

Effect of dose and volume

There is a critical dose below which a reasonable block cannot be expected. Increasing the dose may increase the spread to a small extent, but the most marked effects are to improve the quality of anaesthesia and to prolong the duration (Axelsson et al 1982, 1984, Chambers et al 1982a). Thus, large volumes of solutions may be used to ensure an adequate block with a long duration of action.

Level of injection

The level of injection plays a part in determining the height of block achieved by a given volume, but since spinal anaesthesia is performed over a very restricted portion of the lumbar vertebral column, this is not an important practical factor.

Barbotage

Barbotage involves the repeated aspiration and reinjection of CSF, during the injection of the spinal solution. It has been said to increase the spread, although it is more likely merely to increase unpredictability.

Speed of injection

Slower injections (1 ml $10s^{-1}$) tend to produce more predictable spread than rapid injections. Rapid injections may be considered as a form of barbotage.

FACTORS AFFECTING DURATION

The duration of action depends on:

1. Individual drug properties;
2. The dose injected;
3. The total spread achieved;
4. The addition of vasoconstrictors;
5. The general condition of the patient.

Individual drug properties

Many drugs might be used, but at the present time only bupivacaine is commercially available in the UK in a range of suitable solutions (0.5% and 0.75% glucose-free and 0.5% with 8% glucose). At low segmental levels the longest duration of sensory and motor block results from the use of glucose-free bupivacaine (Cummings et al 1984). Preservative- and glucose-free 2% lignocaine may be used, and 5% lignocaine with 7.5% glucose and 1% amethocaine (which can be mixed with glucose, saline or water) can be obtained by special arrangement. Lignocaine produces a shorter duration of action than amethocaine or bupivacaine (120 versus 170 minutes at L_2). Amethocaine 0.5% in 5% glucose lasts 90–120 minutes.

Dose

Larger doses are likely to increase the duration of action – an effect which is useful for long operations. Increasing the dose of amethocaine from 10 to 15 mg increases the duration of block at the level of T_{12} by about 50% (Wildsmith & Rocco 1985).

Spread

While the individual features of the drug and the dose injected are the most important factors in determining duration, the greater the spread achieved with a given dose of drug, the shorter will be the duration of action. A drug limited to a small segmental area will last longer because the concentration in each nerve will be higher.

Vasoconstrictors

Vasoconstrictors have been thought to increase the duration of anaesthesia and phenylephrine and adrenaline have been used widely, particularly in the United States. The addition of vasoconstrictors to solutions of lignocaine, bupivacaine and amethocaine has no effect on the total spread of block (Chambers et al 1981b, 1982a,b). The same studies showed that adrenaline does not significantly prolong the duration of hyperbaric lignocaine, amethocaine or bupivacaine. Phenylephrine did produce a significant increase in the duration of amethocaine, but not of lignocaine or bupivacaine. While it is apparent that the addition of vasoconstrictors will occasionally result in prolonged block, the effect is often minimal (Racle et al 1988) and the practice cannot be recommended. Longer duration of action should be achieved by using an appropriate drug in larger dose, or by using a continuous technique.

General condition of the patient

It is likely that in patients in poor physical condition the spread will be greater and the duration prolonged. Neither the age of the patient (Pitkanen et al 1984) nor the pH of the CSF (Park et al 1975) seems to affect spread.

TECHNIQUES

A technique should be chosen which is likely to produce a block of sufficient quality, extent and duration for the proposed surgery, without the risk of unnecessary spread to the upper thoracic sympathetic outflow (Fig. 7.6). When a single-shot technique is used it is wise to give generous doses to ensure satisfactory anaesthesia.

Saddle (perineal) block

When the maximum height of block required is S_1, a low volume of hyperbaric solution, for example up to 1 ml, may be injected, with the sitting position maintained for 5 minutes. A disadvantage is that there is a risk of venous pooling, reduction in cardiac output and a decrease in blood pressure. The hip joint will not be blocked and this may lead to discomfort in the patient placed in the lithotomy position. Alternatively 3 ml of 0.5% glucose-free bupivacaine may be administered to the supine patient, but it may produce a *much* higher level of block than is needed for perineal surgery.

Upper lumbar block

For blocks up to L_1, 3 ml of 0.5% glucose-free bupivacaine is usually sufficient whatever posture is used. This has a particular advantage if the patient has a painful condition such as a fractured neck of femur, because the spinal may be induced with the painful side uppermost. As has been mentioned, some high blocks will follow the use of glucose-free bupivacaine, and isobaric amethocaine is much more predictable (Wildsmith & Rocco 1985), but it is not so readily available in the UK. For procedures of shorter duration, 2% glucose-free lignocaine (3–4 ml) may be used but, like plain bupivacaine, it is less predictable.

Mid-thoracic block

For all lower abdominal operations, including herniorrhaphy, a block extending into the mid-thoracic region is needed, and hyperbaric solutions are preferred. Heavy bupivacaine (2–3 ml) may be injected, with the patient first in the lateral position and then turned supine. Hypotension is inevitable in a significant percentage of patients and measures for its prevention and treatment must be available.

With the above method, a large proportion of blocks will be more extensive than is required. A somewhat lower level of block would be adequate for the surgery and reduce the incidence of hypotension. One strategy for achieving this is to inject a standard hyperbaric solution with the patient sitting for about 2 minutes prior to placement in the supine position (Wildsmith et al 1981). An alternative is to inject in a horizontal patient a solution containing a lower concentration of glucose than is usual (Bannister et al 1990). An appropriate glucose concentration is produced by 1 ml of the hyperbaric preparation of bupivacaine mixed with 8–9 ml of the plain solution, and a dose of 3 ml of the mixture is usually given.

Continuous spinal anaesthesia

At the time of writing, continuous spinal anaesthesia, made feasible by developments in fine-bore plastic tubing technology, is undergoing close evaluation. The general principles are the same as

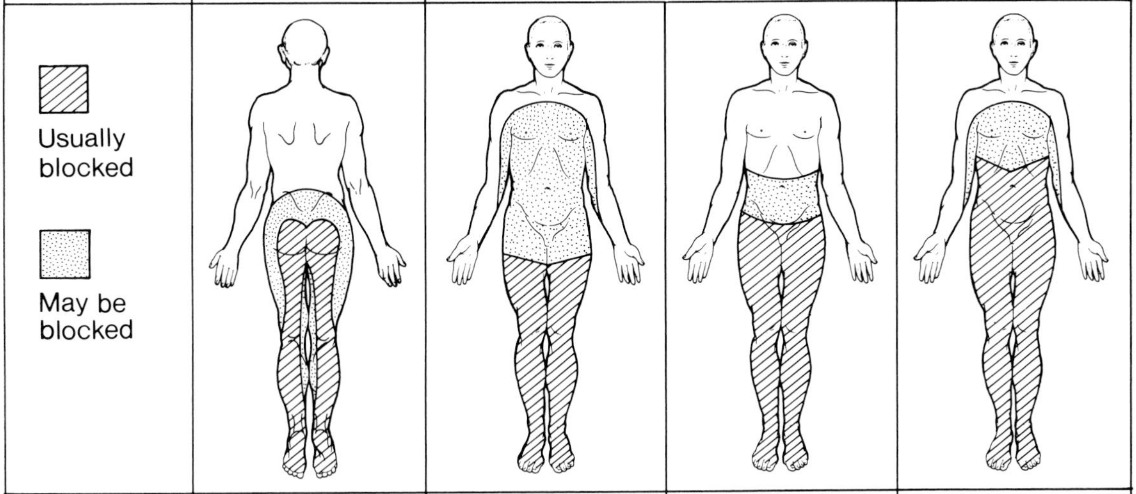

	Saddle block	Upper lumbar blocks		Mid-thoracic block
Usually blocked ▨ May be blocked ▦				
SOLUTION	Any hyperbaric	Plain Bupivacaine	Plain Amethocaine	Any hyperbaric
VOLUME (ml)	1	3	2	2-3
POSTURE	Sitting for 5 min	Patient placed supine after injection		

Fig. 7.6   Techniques of spinal anaesthesia.

for a single-injection technique, but only small increments (approximately 1 ml) of solution are given to allow titration of both the extent and duration of block. The concept is attractive, but there are practical difficulties. Fine-gauge catheters are not easy to manipulate and require careful handling if they are not to kink or break. Occasionally very unusual distributions of block are seen (Morrison et al 1991) and repeated injections with the aim of extending the recalcitrant blocks have resulted in cauda equina injury (Rigler et al 1991). It is claimed (Denny et al 1987) that the incidence of headache is less when a catheter is used, but this is the only study to find this to date.

Intrathecal opioids

The general principles behind the use of spinal opioids have been discussed in Chapter 3. The direct injection of these drugs into the CSF is obviously more rapidly effective than their initial epidural injection, but the risks of respiratory depression are also greater. This is not a technique for the occasional user, but the more lipid-soluble opioids can be used to good effect, particularly in patients who may be expected to have severe pain when the spinal local anaesthetic finally regresses. There seems little point in making single injections of a shorter-acting drug such as fentanyl, but both morphine and diamorphine have been used successfully (Paterson et al 1984). Where it is available, diamorphine, being the more lipid-soluble drug, is preferred and there is evidence that it is cleared more rapidly from the CSF (Kotob et al 1986). A dose of 0.5–1 mg is usually sufficient.

Now that fine-bore catheters are available it seems likely that techniques involving the continuous intrathecal infusion of opioid drugs will be developed, but these are at present experimental.

SIDE-EFFECTS

Cardiovascular

The sympathetic outflow extends from T_1 to L_2, and the height of block is an important factor in determining the degree of peripheral vasodilatation, and the degree of hypotension. However, if venous return, or the sympathetic stimulation to the heart decreases, unopposed parasympathetic overactivity may lead to sudden extreme hypotension and asystole. This can occur even with low blocks and is more likely in the conscious patient. Unlike epidural block, the amount of local anaesthetic or vasoconstrictor absorbed is too small to modify the cardiovascular changes. The prevention and treatment of hypotension have been discussed in Chapter 5.

Respiratory

Spinal anaesthesia is unlikely to affect resting ventilation or produce changes in blood gases. However, high spinals result in a 20% decrease in inspiratory capacity, and a marked reduction in expiratory reserve volume (Egbert et al 1961, Freund 1969). The patient may find it difficult to take a deep breath and cough effectively, and may develop the sensation of dyspnoea. Apnoea is rare and is usually secondary to hypotension and brain stem ischaemia, although if the block reaches upper cervical levels, apnoea due to bilateral phrenic nerve root involvement may occur. Management of a 'total spinal' is discussed in Chapter 8.

Gastrointestinal system

The small intestine becomes contracted, peristalsis continues and the sphincters relax. Upper abdominal and intraperitoneal visceral stimuli transmitted by unblocked vagal afferent fibres may be perceived as pain, and this may produce nausea and vomiting (Ratra et al 1972). Oxygen and atropine may help to prevent or treat nausea, which may also be an early symptom of hypotension.

Other effects

Blood loss is reduced and the stress response delayed. It is likely that the incidence of deep venous thrombosis is also reduced, and early morbidity and mortality diminished, when compared with general anaesthesia.

COMPLICATIONS

Most of the complications, with the exception of headache, are extremely rare, and usually preventable.

Headache

Headache is a very common symptom after surgery and it must not be assumed that all headaches following lumbar puncture are due to it.

Dural puncture

This is the most important cause of headache and is due to a leak of CSF from the subarachnoid to the epidural space. Low CSF pressure allows descent of the brain and this stretches the dura, tentorium, venous sinuses, and dural and cerebral blood vessels as well as the nerve endings. It results in the classic headache, which is primarily occipital radiating to the frontal and orbital regions, and is often associated with cervical muscle spasm. The headache is postural, becoming worse when the head is raised and better when the patient is supine or head-down. It may be associated with nausea, vomiting, photophobia, dizziness and cranial nerve palsies, especially of the sixth nerve. It may be very severe, and last for several days. Very rarely an intracranial subdural haematoma has followed prolonged CSF leak (Newrick & Read 1982).

The incidence can be reduced by using fine needles. An 18 g needle may produce an incidence as high as 24% whereas a 26 g should reduce it to less than 1%. The likelihood of headache is increased by multiple punctures of the dura, and by the bevel being inserted transversely rather than longitudinally, so that dural fibres are cut rather than separated (Mihic 1985). It has been suggested that extreme flexion of the spine stretches the dura and increases the size of the puncture hole. Extension of the head during lumbar puncture may reduce the tension on the dura mater.

Age decreases the incidence, possibly because decreased elasticity of the tissues allows less stretching of intracranial structures. Dehydration from any cause results in low CSF pressure, which increases the severity of the headache. Young women, and especially obstetric patients, seem to have a rather higher incidence, but the use of pencil-point-type needles would appear to reduce quite considerably the risk of this complication occurring even in these patients. Such needles are several times the price of a traditional spinal needle, but this expense is more than justified in patients at high risk of this distressing complication.

Management of dural puncture. All patients who have had a spinal anaesthetic must be kept fully hydrated and should avoid straining in the early postoperative period. It has been shown that adoption of the supine position for 24 hours *does not reduce the incidence of headache* (Caarbaat & Van Crevel 1981), although it is accepted that if the patients have dural puncture headaches they will prefer to lie flat to obtain relief. Methods which raise the epidural pressure, such as the prone position or the use of tight abdominal binders, may help to reverse the pressure gradient and reduce the CSF leak. Patients should be encouraged to drink freely, and should be given a mild analgesic. If the headache does not resolve within 1 or 2 days and is incapacitating, an epidural blood patch should be considered and the technique is described in Chapter 8. A blood patch may be associated with a low incidence of transient neurological problems, such as backache, paraesthesiae, numbness and signs of meningeal irritation. However, it should be free from long-lasting sequelae, and subsequent epidural anaesthesia is said to be uneventful.

Other causes of headache

Other very rare causes of headache include meningitis. This is usually aseptic (chemical), and associated with the adhesive arachnoiditis which follows injection of the wrong solution, or one contaminated with skin preparation solution. The headache is felt all over, is bursting in character, constant, and unaffected by posture. There are usually associated signs of meningism or meningitis. Reports of bacterial meningitis do occasionally appear and serve to emphasize the importance of a scrupulous aseptic technique (Wildsmith 1991).

More commonly, headache is incidental and is due to causes unrelated to the spinal anaesthetic. Anxious patients, especially those prone to migraine, frequently develop headaches in the immediate postoperative period.

Urinary retention

The sacral autonomic fibres are among the last to recover function and detrusor muscle contractions return very late. This may prevent micturition (Axelsson et al 1974). It is also difficult to micturate lying supine in bed – a position which the patient should maintain until the risk of postural hypotension has passed. Fluid preload is a potent cause of overdistension of the bladder and should be avoided unless a urinary catheter is to be inserted for other reasons.

Backache

This is a common postoperative symptom and it has been shown to be as frequent after general anaesthesia as spinal anaesthesia (Brown & Elman 1961). Careful attention must be paid to avoiding an abnormal posture while the block is in place, because it may predispose to subsequent backache.

Neurological complications

These are extremely rare (Dripps & Vandam 1954). All neurological problems following spinal anaesthesia should be identified and investigated carefully by a competent neurologist. The vast majority will be found to be unrelated to the technique (Marinacci 1960). They may arise from the injection of inappropriate chemicals or drugs, or from the introduction of infection. This may result in an adhesive, proliferative arachnoiditis or transverse myelitis, usually affecting the cauda equina initially ('cauda equina syndrome'), but often spreading higher. There will be pain, sphincter disturbances, sacral analgesia and perhaps some numbness and weakness of the legs. The onset may be rapid or slow, and the clinical course may be static, or progress towards recovery or deterioration.

Urgent surgical treatment is required for haematoma, abscess or tumours producing neurological signs. Epidural abscesses are due more often to haematogenous spread than to the local introduction of infection. Trauma to nerve roots may follow spinal anaesthesia, but is much more commonly due to incorrect posture, pressure or trauma during surgery.

Complications may be due to vascular problems – classically causing the 'anterior spinal artery syndrome'. Failure of the supply to this vessel at T_{11} (see Ch. 6) causes a painless paralysis of the legs and sphincters due to infarction of the anterior segments of the spinal cord. This syndrome may follow periods of hypotension, especially in elderly patients, but may be due to ligation of vessels at surgery.

An important neurological complication which is being reported more frequently is permanent brain damage due to a prolonged period of hypotension. While this is more likely with a total spinal after inadvertent dural puncture in an attempted epidural, it can occur with deliberate spinal anaesthesia (Caplan et al 1988). Careful monitoring and appropriate treatment of the blood pressure should prevent its occurrence.

REFERENCES

Axelsson K H, Mollefors K, Olsson J O, Lingardh G, Widman B 1974 Bladder function in spinal anaesthesia. Linkoping University Medical Dissertation 184: v3–v21

Axelsson K H, Edstrom H H, Sundberg A E A, Widman G B 1982 Spinal anaesthesia with hyperbaric 0.5% bupivacaine: effects of volume. Acta Anaesthesiologica Scandinavica 26: 439–445

Axelsson K H, Edstrom H H, Widman G B 1984 Spinal anaesthesia with glucose-free 0.5% bupivacaine: effects of different volumes. British Journal of Anaesthesia 56: 271–278

Bannister J, McClure J H, Wildsmith J A W 1990 Effect of glucose concentration on the intrathecal spread of 0.5% bupivacaine. British Journal of Anaesthesia 64: 232–234

Barker A E 1907 A report on clinical experiences with spinal analgesia in 100 cases. British Medical Journal i: 665–674

Brown E M, Elman D S 1961 Postoperative backache. Anesthesia and Analgesia; Current Researches (Cleveland) 40: 683–685

Brown D T, Wildsmith J A W, Covino B G, Scott D B 1980 Effect of baricity on spinal anaesthesia with amethocaine. British Journal of Anaesthesia 52: 589–596

Burm A G, Van Kleef J W, Gladines M P 1983 Plasma concentrations of lidocaine and bupivacaine after subarachnoid administration. Anesthesiology 59: 191–195

Caarbaat P A T, Van Crevel H 1981 Lumbar puncture headache: controlled study on the preventive effects of 24 hours bed rest. Lancet ii: 1133–1134

Caplan R A, Ward R J, Pawsner J, Cheney F W 1988 Unexpected cardiac arrest during spinal anesthesia: a closed claims analysis of predisposing factors. Anesthesiology 68: 5–11

Chambers W A, Edstrom H H, Scott D B 1981a Effect of baricity on spinal anaesthesia with bupivacaine. British Journal of Anaesthesia 53: 279–282

Chambers W A, Littlewood D G, Logan M R, Scott D B 1981b Effect of added epinephrine on spinal anesthesia with lidocaine. Anesthesia and Analgesia 60: 417–420

Chambers W A, Littlewood D G, Edstrom H H, Scott D B 1982a Spinal anaesthesia with hyperbaric bupivacaine. Effects of concentration and volume administered. British Journal of Anaesthesia 54: 75–80

Chambers W A, Littlewood D G, Scott D B 1982b Spinal anesthesia with hyperbaric bupivacaine: effect of added vasoconstrictors. Anesthesia and Analgesia 61: 49–52

Cope R W 1954 The Woolley and Roe case: Woolley and Roe versus Ministry of Health and others. Anaesthesia 9: 249–270

Cummings G C, Bamber D B, Edstrom H H, Rubin A P 1984 Subarachnoid block with bupivacaine. A comparison with cinchocaine. British Journal of Anaesthesia 56: 573–579

Denny N, Masters R, Pearson D, Read J, Sihota M, Selander D, 1987 Post dural puncture headache after continuous spinal anesthesia. Anesthesia and Analgesia 66: 791–794

Dripps R D, Vandam L D 1954 Longterm follow-up of patients who received 10 098 spinal anesthetics. I: failure to discover major neurological sequelae. Journal of the American Medical Association 156: 1486–1491

Egbert L D, Tamersoy K, Deas T C 1961 Pulmonary function during spinal anesthesia: the mechanism of cough depression. Anesthesiology 22: 882–885

Freund P G 1969 Respiratory effects of subarachnoid and epidural block. In: Bonica J J (ed) Clinical anesthesia 2 Regional anesthesia: recent advances and current status, pp 98–107. FA Davis, Philadelphia

Hart J R, Whiteacre R J 1951 Pencil point needle in prevention of postspinal headache. Journal of the American Medical Association 147: 657–658

Kalso E, Tuominen M, Rosenberg P H 1982 Effect of posture and some CSF characteristics on spinal anaesthesia with isobaric 0.5% bupivacaine. British Journal of Anaesthesia 54: 1179–1184

Kotob H I M, Hand C W, Moore R A et al 1986 Intrathecal morphine and heroin in humans: 6-hour drug levels in spinal fluid and plasma, Anesthesia and Analgesia 65: 718–722

McClure J H, Wildsmith J A W 1988 Aspects of spinal anaesthesia. In: Kaufman L (ed) Anaesthesia review 5, ch 5, pp 269–285. Churchill Livingstone, Edinburgh

Marinacci A A 1960 Neurological aspects of complications of spinal anesthesia with medicolegal implications. Bulletin of the Los Angeles Neurological Society 24: 170–192

Messahel F M, Robinson J J, Mathews E T 1983 Factors affecting cerebrospinal fluid flow in two spinal needles. British Journal of Anaesthesia 55: 169–175

Mihic D N 1985 Postspinal headache and relationship of needle bevel to longitudinal dural fibres. Regional Anesthesia 10: 76–81

Morrison L M M, McClure J H, Wildsmith J A W 1991 Clinical evaluation of a spinal catheter technique in femoro-popliteal graft surgery. Anaesthesia 46: 576–578

Newrick P, Read D 1982 Subdural haematoma as a complication of spinal anaesthetic. British Medical Journal 285: 341–342

Park W Y, Balingit P E, Macnamara T E 1975 Effects of patient age, pH of cerebrospinal fluid and vasopressors on onset and duration of spinal anesthesia. Anesthesia and Analgesia, Current Researches (Cleveland) 54: 455–463

Paterson G M C, McQuay H J, Bullingham R E S, Moore R A 1984 Intradural morphine and diamorphine. Dose response studies. Anaesthesia 39: 113–117

Pitkanen M, Haapaniemi L, Tuominen M, Rosenberg P H 1984 Influence of age on spinal anaesthesia with isobaric 0.5% bupivacaine. British Journal of Anaesthesia 56: 279–284

Racle J P, Benkhadra A, Poy J Y 1988 Subarachnoid anaesthesia produced by hyperbaric lignocaine in elderly patients. Prolongation of effect with adrenaline. British Journal of Anaesthesia 60: 831–835

Ratra C K, Badola R P, Bhargave K P 1972 A study of factors concerned in emesis during spinal anaesthesia. British Journal of Anaesthesia 44: 1208–1211

Rigler M L, Drasner K, Krejcie T C et al 1991 Cauda equina syndrome after continuous spinal anesthesia. Anesthesia and Analgesia 72: 275–281

Wildsmith J A W 1991 Regional anaesthesia requires attention to detail. British Journal of Anaesthesia 67: 224–225

Wildsmith J A W, Rocco A G 1985 Current concepts in spinal anesthesia. Regional Anesthesia 10: 117–121

Wildsmith J A W, McClure J H, Brown D T, Scott D B 1981 Effects of posture on the spread of isobaric and hyperbaric amethocaine. British Journal of Anaesthesia 53: 273–278

8. Lumbar and thoracic epidural anaesthesia

E. N. Armitage

Although it is over 40 years since the first epidural block was performed in the UK, it is only in recent years that the technique has become firmly established as a substitute for, or an adjunct to, general anaesthesia for operative surgery. The development of long-acting local anaesthetic drugs and increasing knowledge of the physiology of regional anaesthesia have ensured that epidural block can be practical and safe. However, the technique owes its popularity to two other factors which, while not exclusive to epidural block, apply particularly to it.

Firstly, epidural block at the lumbar and lower thoracic level is suitable for most gynaecological and urological work, and for some general abdominal and orthopaedic surgery. The anaesthetist capable of performing it can therefore supply anaesthesia for a wide range of surgery as well as for obstetrics. Secondly, the insertion of a catheter into the epidural space and its subsequent maintenance are both comparatively easy. The benefits of the block can therefore be extended into the postoperative period by either repeated injections or continuous infusion of local anaesthetic.

This does not mean that the method has no disadvantages. Pre-existing neurological conditions, coagulation disorders and low-dose heparin therapy may be weightier contraindications to epidural block than to other regional techniques; and although epidural anaesthesia is very useful for a great deal of major surgery, visceral sensation remains unblocked. General anaesthesia – unnecessary with many peripheral blocks – is required as a supplement in these cases.

Equipment

The basic requirements for a regional block have been described in Chapter 5. More equipment (much of it specifically designed) is needed for an epidural block than for most others and anaesthetists vary in their preference for these items.

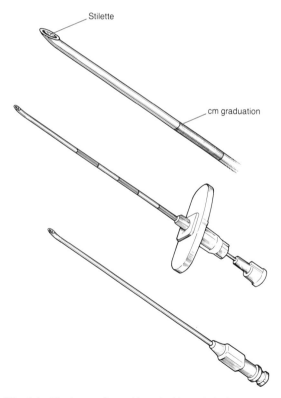

Stilette

cm graduation

Fig. 8.1 Tuohy needles, with and without 'wing' attachment.

Needles

The *Tuohy* needle (Fig. 8.1) is widely used in the UK. The shaft is usually 8 cm (3 inches) long, graduated in centimetres and available in both 16 g and 18 g sizes. The needle wall is thin so that the lumen will admit a catheter of reasonable size. A stilette prevents coring of superficial tissues and increases rigidity so that the needle does not bend when redirected. The point is relatively blunt and is contoured so that a catheter emerges at an angle of about 20°, but this design does have the important disadvantage that the catheter cannot be withdrawn through the needle without the risk of it being transected (Fig. 8.2). If it is necessary to withdraw the catheter, the needle must be withdrawn simultaneously. Some anaesthetists feel that the version of the needle with a 'winged' hub provides better control during insertion.

The *Crawford* needle (Fig. 8.3) has a short bevel of conventional design. Since the catheter emerges straight from the tip, it will impinge on the dura unless the needle is introduced at an angle. This, and other epidural needles of similar design, are better suited to the paramedian approach, which gives greater angulation than can be obtained from the midline.

Disposable needles are available from several manufacturers (e.g. Portex, Steriseal, Abbott). They are of consistently high quality, are guaranteed sterile and are used by the majority of anaesthetists. However, some practitioners find tissue planes easier to identify if the needle is not too sharp and they prefer a blunter, reusable needle.

Syringes

If the epidural space is to be located by the loss of resistance technique, it is essential that the plunger should run smoothly along the entire length of the barrel. Traditionally, reusable glass syringes have been used and are excellent if scrupulously maintained. If the syringe is autoclaved as one unit, the plunger tends to stick in the barrel, so these two components should be separated before being placed in epidural packs which are prepared locally. Glove powder can also cause friction and the ground-glass surface of the plunger should not be handled when the syringe is assembled. It can be very difficult to ensure that glass syringes are properly looked after and many anaesthetists prefer high-quality, disposable products. These have a very consistent feel and are free of the idiosyncrasies of glass.

Catheters

These are made in two sizes for adults, to fit either a 16 g or 18 g needle. Their design and manufacture represent a compromise between conflicting

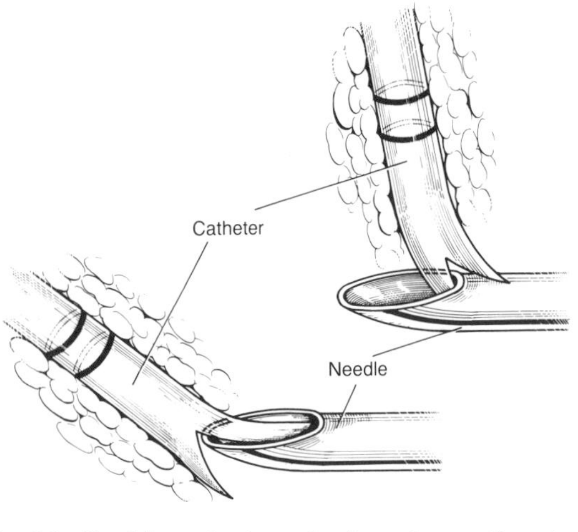

Catheter

Needle

Fig. 8.2 Possible mechanisms of catheter damage if one is withdrawn through a Tuohy needle.

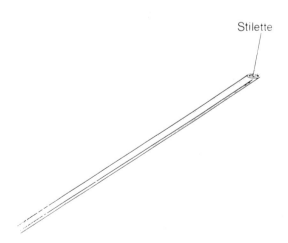

Stilette

Fig. 8.3 The Crawford needle.

requirements. The internal diameter of the catheter should be as large as possible to minimize the resistance to injection down its 90 cm length, but the wall must not be so thin that it buckles or kinks where it enters the epidural space or emerges from the skin. Early epidural catheters were open ended and, being rather sharp, tended to puncture blood vessels and, occasionally, the dura. Later, catheters with a closed, rounded tip and two or more side holes within 2 cm of the end became available. This design reduces the risk of venous and dural puncture and is still widely used, but the side holes are points of weakness at which the catheter may kink or break. Now that the quality of medical plastics has improved, there is much to be said for the use of end-hole catheters because intravenous and subarachnoid placement will be more easily recognized. However, there is some evidence that their use is associated with a higher incidence of unilateral block and missed segments (Michael et at 1989).

Most catheters are marked at 5 cm intervals from the tip, and some also have marks every centimetre up to 10 cm (Fig. 8.4). The anaesthetist should be familiar with the marking pattern since it enables him to know how much catheter has been inserted and whether it is intact on removal. At the distal end, the Luer hub is detachable and allows the needle to be removed.

Filters

The prime function of a filter is to exclude bacteria. Several makes are capable of excluding particles as small as 0.22 μm. The injection of small fragments of ampoule glass is also prevented. As debris collects on a filter, its resistance increases and it should be changed every 24 hours when it forms part of an infusion system.

Testing of equipment

It is rare to encounter malfunction in modern sterile disposable products, but it is much better that it should be discovered before the procedure commences. The syringe plunger should run freely in the barrel and the nozzle should fit the hub of the needle and the epidural catheter. The stilette of the needle should be flush with the bevel. The

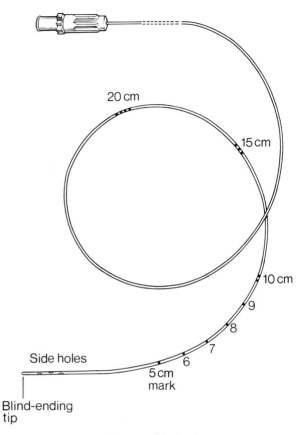

Fig. 8.4   Typical markings on epidural catheter.

catheter should pass easily through the needle, and its patency and that of the filter should be tested by the prior injection of saline or local anaesthetic.

IDENTIFICATION OF THE EPIDURAL SPACE

This is obviously the key to epidural anaesthesia. Several methods have been described, but the commonest and simplest is the midline approach in the lumbar region using loss of resistance to saline. This basic technique will be described first and alternatives will be discussed later.

Standard method

Position of the patient

If the patient is anaesthetized or heavily sedated he should be placed in the lateral position, with knees

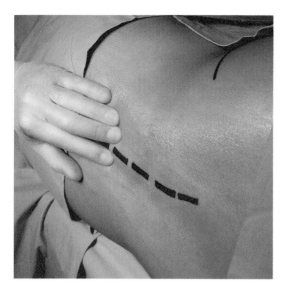

Fig. 8.5 Position of the fingers to immobilize the skin over the vertebral spines.

bent and spine flexed. The less experienced anaesthetist will find it helpful to place a pillow under the patient's loin to correct lateral flexion of the spine (Fig. 7.3). The right-handed anaesthetist usually prefers the patient to be lying on his left side and the following detailed description of an epidural block assumes this position.

If the patient is conscious, the procedure may be performed with him sitting. This is often preferred by obese and bronchitic patients who may find the flexed, lateral position intolerable.

Identification of vertebral level. A line drawn between the iliac crests crosses either the fourth lumbar spine or interspace. Spines of other vertebrae can be palpated, numbered and, if necessary, marked from this reference point.

Needle insertion

A lumbar space between two easily palpable spines (usually L_3–L_4) is chosen and, in the conscious patient, the skin and subcutaneous tissues are infiltrated with local anaesthetic. The skin is pierced with a large, sharp needle, at a point equidistant between the spines and in the midline. The vertebral spines, bridged by the interspinous ligaments, form a midline ridge and the needle will

tend to slip to right or left unless the skin is immobilized. This is done by straddling the ridge with the second and third fingers of the left hand and pressing firmly (Fig. 8.5). The Tuohy needle is introduced through the skin puncture with the bevel facing upwards, that is, towards the patient's right. As it is advanced into the superficial tissues, it is kept at right angles to the patient in both skin planes (Fig. 8.6). The fingers of the left hand

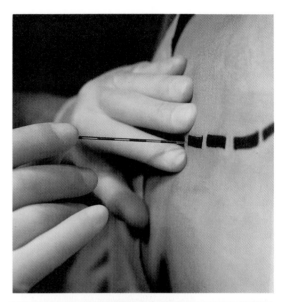

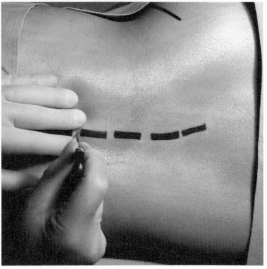

Fig. 8.6 Correct angulation of the needle for midline insertion in the lumbar region.

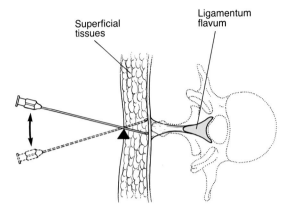

Fig. 8.7 While the tip of the needle is in the superficial tissues, the hub is very mobile. It behaves like a see-saw.

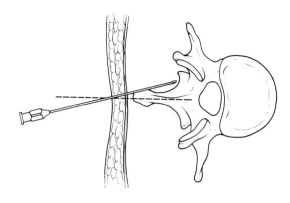

Fig. 8.9 The commonest error is for the anaesthetist to lower his hands so that the needle deviates from the midline as it is advanced.

maintain their position astride the midline until the needle tip has entered the ligamentum flavum.

With the needle inserted perhaps 2 cm, it is useful to test its 'feel' in the tissues by moving the hub up and down. Since the tip is able to move relatively freely in the superficial tissues, the needle behaves like a see-saw, the fulcrum being its point of entry at the skin (Fig. 8.7). When the needle is advanced further, the tip eventually engages in the ligamentum flavum and if the hub is again moved up and down, the 'feel' is very different since the needle is now fixed at two points along its length and behaves like a springboard (Fig. 8.8). When

this sign has been elicited, it is worth checking again that the correct angles have been maintained during the deeper insertion of the needle. There is a tendency to allow the hub to drop slightly as the needle is advanced, with the result that the tip is directed upwards, to the patient's right (Fig. 8.9). If this has happened the needle should be removed and reinserted.

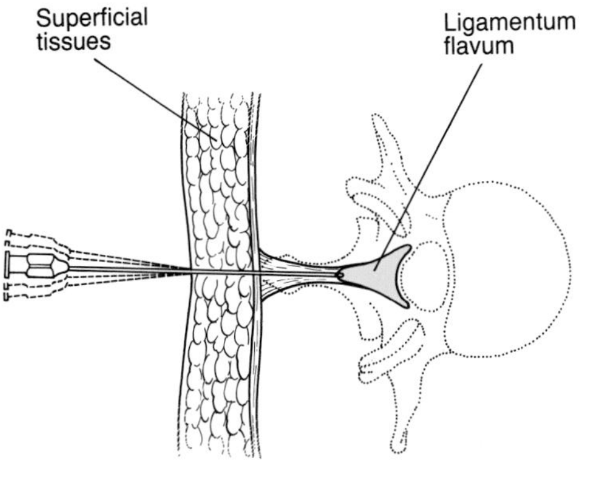

With the needle at the correct angle and the tip engaged in the ligamentum flavum, the stilette is removed and a syringe containing saline is attached to the needle. In order to avoid accidentally advancing the needle at this stage, the hub is held between the thumb and first finger of the left hand while the dorsum of the hand is steadied against the patient's back.

Location of the epidural space

Because of their densities, the intervertebral ligaments offer varying degrees of resistance to both the advance of a needle and to the injection of liquid. Identification of the space depends on the fact that saline, being incompressible, cannot be injected if the needle tip is in the ligament. Once the epidural space is entered, both advance of the needle and injection of saline become easier since the space contains only loose tissue.

The whole needle–syringe assembly is advanced slowly while steady pressure is applied to the plunger with the right thumb. It is essential that the

Fig. 8.8 Once the tip is firmly embedded in the ligamentum flavum, very little hub movement is possible. The hub behaves like a springboard.

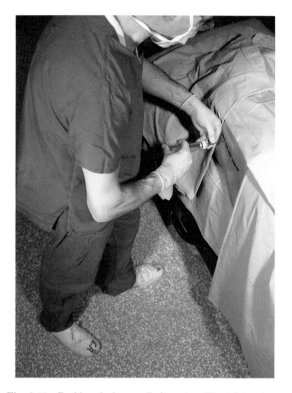

Fig. 8.10 Position during needle insertion. The left hand, pressed against the patient, steadies the needle and controls its angulation while the right provides the driving force. Balance is maintained by the forward position of the left foot.

anaesthetist should be properly balanced and comfortable if he is to control the needle and syringe. This is best achieved if he stands with one foot ahead of the other, as though walking in the direction of needle movement (Fig. 8.10).

Entry to the epidural space is marked by the sudden ability to inject saline, 5 ml of which is usually sufficient to establish without doubt that the needle is correctly placed. During this injection, the needle–syringe assembly is rotated 90° anticlockwise so that the bevel of the needle (which until now has been facing laterally to the patient's right) faces cephalad. With the first finger and thumb of the left hand stabilizing the needle, the syringe is detached. Some fluid may appear at the hub. Cerebrospinal fluid (CSF) can quickly be distinguished from injected saline by allowing it to drop on to the anaesthetist's forearm. CSF will be at body temperature; injected saline will still be appreciably colder.

The use of liquid for locating the epidural space has the advantage that the loss of resistance sign is clear-cut, the ease of injection when the needle enters the space being in marked contrast to the total inability to inject when it is in the ligamentum flavum. In addition, the jet of liquid injected as the space is entered tends to push the dura away from the needle point. Some anaesthetists feel that this liquid also facilitates the subsequent passage of the epidural catheter by 'lubricating' the space, and there is evidence that it also reduces the risk of blood vessel puncture (Verniquet 1980).

Insertion of the catheter

When the catheter has been inserted 9 cm, the tip will have reached the end of the needle and there is almost always some resistance to its emergence into the epidural space. This can usually be overcome by gripping centimetre-long lengths of catheter close to the needle hub and inserting the catheter a little at a time. If the catheter refuses to pass, the needle may be carefully advanced a further millimetre because part of the bevel may still be in the ligamentum flavum (Fig. 8.11). Obviously a catheter will not pass until all the bevel is clear of the ligament. A second injection of 5 ml of saline or local anaesthetic may also help a catheter to pass by 'opening up' the epidural space.

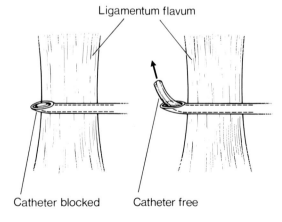

Fig. 8.11 The catheter will not pass into the epidural space unless the entire bevel is through the ligamentum flavum.

Although this description of the midline approach has stressed the importance of keeping the needle at right angles to the skin in both planes, this can be modified in cases in which there is difficulty in advancing the catheter. It is usually possible to re-introduce the needle with a degree of cephalad inclination and this, together with the manoeuvres described above, generally results in the catheter passing easily. If it does not, another interspace should be selected.

The epidural space is vascular, and blood is occasionally seen running back down the catheter. If this happens, the catheter is withdrawn until the flow stops and then flushed with saline to prevent it becoming occluded with blood clot. Clear fluid appearing in the catheter may be either CSF or injected saline. CSF usually flows briskly and can be aspirated easily. A catheter which has punctured the dura or which, despite slow withdrawal, remains in a vein should be removed and inserted at an adjacent interspace.

When the catheter has been suitably positioned, a small amount of saline or local anaesthetic should be injected to ensure that it is still patent and has not kinked in the epidural space. The catheter must be firmly fixed so that it cannot be accidentally dislodged on the operating table or during nursing procedures on the ward, but it should not be so closely applied to the back that it kinks at its entry point. Dressings (which should not be too bulky) must be secured with two strips of wide, waterproof adhesive plaster (Sleek), and the catheter led up the back to the shoulder under a *thin* strip of adhesive tape (Fig. 8.12). Sleek is unnecessary for this as well as being uncomfortable to remove. When the patient is returned to the supine position, the patency of the catheter should be tested again to make sure that it has not been occluded by resumption of the supine position. A catheter inserted with the patient in the flexed position occasionally becomes kinked at its point of entry into the supraspinous ligament when the back is straightened.

The test dose

The object of a test dose is to exclude intrathecal or intravascular placement of a catheter. The

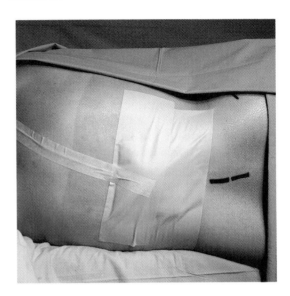

Fig. 8.12 Protective dressing for an epidural catheter.

general principles have been discussed in Chapter 5, but it is worth re-emphasizing here that the test dose must be capable of exerting the desired 'test' effect and must be given in a dose large enough to produce it. The effect must be allowed sufficient time to develop, and should be easily observable. There have been cases in which test doses of 2 or 3 ml of 0.25% bupivacaine failed to produce any sign of intrathecal injection, and only after the full dose had been given did extensive spinal anaesthesia develop.

There is disagreement about the value of test doses. Certainly they will be of no help and may actually be misleading if the above criteria are not applied. They are unlikely to detect an intrathecal injection if the patient is under general anaesthesia since it is impossible to obtain adequate neurological information. On the other hand, adrenaline-containing solutions quickly give warning of intravascular injections and it is these which most often need to be excluded. For example, blood appearing in a catheter indicates that an epidural vessel has been damaged, and it should not be assumed that intravascular injection cannot occur just because the catheter has been withdrawn until blood no longer flows. A negative cardiovascular response to the epidural injection of an adrenaline-containing solution is reassuring under these circumstances.

If the patient is conscious and is to undergo major surgery with an epidural block unsupplemented by general anaesthesia, concentrated solutions of local anaesthetic will be required. In that situation, a small volume will contain sufficient drug to cause cerebral symptoms after intravenous injection. Any numbness or tingling of the tongue, light-headedness or tinnitus is an indication that this has occurred. Scott (1983) has argued that the test dose is a ritual rather than a practical exercise and he suggests that injections should be made slowly (10 ml min^{-1}) with frequent aspiration tests. Continuous rapport with the patient is maintained and if signs or symptoms of toxicity appear, the injection should be stopped before a dose likely to cause a major reaction is given.

ALTERNATIVE METHODS

Location of the epidural space

Loss of resistance to air

Advocates of this method point out that if at any stage clear fluid appears from the epidural needle, it must be CSF, but this assumption is not valid if generous amounts of local anaesthetic have been used to infiltrate the skin and deeper tissues prior to insertion of the epidural needle. It is possible for this fluid to track back when the stilette is removed and, if it is mistaken for CSF, the patient may receive treatment for a dural puncture which did not in fact occur.

The disadvantage of using loss of resistance to air is that air, unlike saline, is compressible, and it is possible to 'spring' the plunger in the barrel even when the epidural needle is in the ligamentum flavum. Indeed, advance of the needle–syringe assembly tends to be punctuated by such intermittent springing of the plunger when air is used, so that it is not a smooth, steady movement. Those who regularly use liquid find the end-point much more definite than with air and there is evidence that, in obstetric patients at least, the use of air is more likely to be associated with unblocked segments than liquid (Valentine et al 1991).

The Doughty method

This method is important because it has been successfully taught by Doughty for several years and is now widely practised and taught by anaesthetists who were trained by him. It is probably the only technique which has been rigorously assessed for use by anaesthetists learning epidural anaesthesia. The anaesthetist stands sideways on to the patient and faces caudad.

There are three components to the technique (Fig. 8.13). The thumb and first and second fingers of the right hand grip the rim of the syringe barrel and are responsible for advancing the needle–syringe assembly through the ligamentum flavum and into the epidural space. The thumb and first finger of the left hand grip the hub of the needle to control its forward progress, the stability necessary for this important function being obtained by firmly pressing the left forearm and hand against the patient's back. Loss of resistance is detected by pressure exerted on the syringe plunger by the base of the right index finger or by the palm of the right hand. This pressure is separate from that applied by the thumb and fingers of the right hand and does not contribute to the advance of the needle.

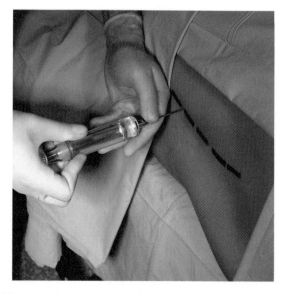

Fig. 8.13   Position of the hands for the Doughty method.

The amount of liquid in the syringe must be such that the plunger 'fits' the anaesthetist's hand and is in comfortable contact with the base of the index finger or, if preferred, the palm of the hand. The optimal volume of liquid therefore depends on the size of the anaesthetist's hand. The method, didactically taught and carefully supervised, results in inadvertent puncture of the dura in only about 0.4% of cases.

Subatmospheric pressure

Traditionally, it has been believed that there is a subatmospheric pressure within the epidural space due to transmission of the intrapleural pressure through the intervertebral foramina (Macintosh & Mushin 1947). It has also been suggested that the pressure is due simply to 'tenting' of the dura by the point of the needle (Aitkenhead et al 1979). Whichever is the case, air or liquid will tend to be sucked in through the needle when its tip enters the epidural space. Two techniques have been described to take advantage of this.

In the *hanging drop* method (Soresi 1932), a drop of fluid is applied to the hub of the needle once its tip is embedded in the ligaments. As the tip enters the space, the drop of fluid is sucked in. In the *balloon* method (Macintosh 1950), a small balloon is attached to the needle and is inflated through a side port. As the needle tip enters the space the balloon deflates. Both techniques have been widely and successfully used, but they are more complicated than the loss-of-resistance method and are now mainly of historical interest.

Paramedian (lateral or oblique) approach

The midline approach, being relatively easy, is the method recommended for the beginner and it will provide satisfactory access to the epidural space in most patients. It does, however, have some disadvantages which may be overcome by use of the paramedian approach.

Advantages

The 'paramedian' needle passes between the laminae of adjacent vertebrae. Calcified interspi-nous ligaments are therefore avoided and, since the track of the needle is not dictated by the amount of space between adjacent vertebral spines, there is more room for manoeuvre. The cephalad angle at which the needle is inserted can be selected by the anaesthetist – it is not dependent on the position or angle of the vertebral spines. These factors make the paramedian approach the method of choice for thoracic epidural block.

The needle is less likely to puncture the dura since it traverses the epidural space obliquely, so that the distance from the needle's point of emergence from the ligamentum flavum to its contact with the dura is greater than with the midline approach (Fig. 8.14). The chances of dural puncture can be further reduced if a Crawford needle is inserted with its bevel facing anteriorly (Fig. 8.14).

Insertion of the catheter is usually very easy because the cephalad angle of the needle directs the catheter along the long axis of the epidural space. The deflection of the catheter from the tip of a Tuohy needle further assists this process. Blomberg (1988), using epiduroscopy in cadavers, found that all catheters introduced by the para-median approach followed a straight cephalad path. In the clinical situation, the final position of the tip cannot be precisely known unless it is verified radiographically, but the catheter is obvi-ously less likely to impinge on the dura or form loops and knots.

With the paramedian approach, the vertebral lamina is deliberately located and the needle 'walked' off it superiorly into the ligamentum flavum. This bony landmark is very reassuring in the obese and, once found, it allows the needle to be re-angled and further advanced with confi-dence. It is unnerving for an anaesthetist to preside over the steady disappearance of a needle by the midline route into the back of an obese patient with no sign of loss of resistance and no information as to where the tip is in relation to the epidural space.

Technique

The approach to the epidural space by the paramedian route differs from the midline ap-proach in that neither of the final angles required

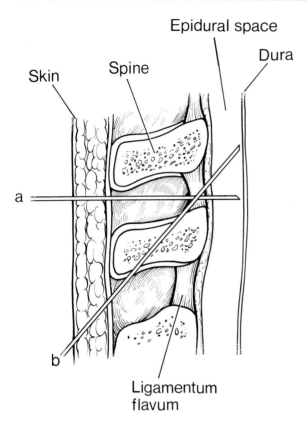

Fig. 8.14 Needle angles for the midline (a) and paramedian (b) approaches. Note that the distance from the ligamentum flavum to the dura with the paramedian approach is almost twice that of the midline.

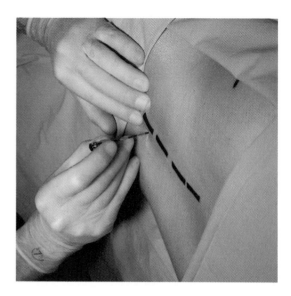

Fig. 8.15 Initial needle position for the paramedian approach. The tip is about 1 cm from the midline.

are right angles. The skin over the vertebral spines is immobilized with the second and third fingers of the left hand (Fig. 8.5), but the skin is pierced about 1 cm to the left of the midline (Fig. 8.15). The needle is then inserted perpendicular to the skin until it strikes the left vertebral lamina and the depth at which this occurs is noted from the centimetre graduations. It is now necessary to redirect the needle in both cephalad and medial directions (Fig. 8.16), and each angulation will be considered separately.

Firstly, the needle tip must be 'walked' along the lamina in a cephalad direction so that it eventually clears it and enters the ligamentum flavum between the chosen lamina and the one above it. When performing this manoeuvre, it is essential that the needle be withdrawn about 1 cm before each cephalad probe on to the lamina. Attempts to

realign the needle without withdrawal will cause it to bend and this will greatly increase the force required to advance it through the tissues. It will be apparent that the more caudad the initial position of the needle in relation to the vertebral lamina, the greater will be the cephalad inclination when it eventually clears the lamina. Establishment of this important angle will not, however, alter the paramedian position of the needle tip. If advanced without any other change of angle, the tip would remain about 1 cm from the midline and would enter the lateral part of the epidural space (often rich in venous plexuses), or miss it altogether.

The second objective must therefore be to redirect the needle so that its tip passes 1 cm medially and enters the epidural space in the midline. Experience is required to judge this angle correctly. It will be greatest in lean patients in whom the distance between the skin and epidural space is short, and in cases in which the anaesthetist selects a generous paramedian approach and inserts the needle some distance from the midline. The angle will be smallest in obese patients where the 1 cm correction is made over a large distance, and in cases in which a narrow paramedian approach is selected and the needle is inserted close to the midline.

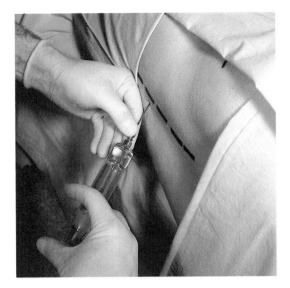

Fig. 8.16 Final needle angulation for the paramedian approach. Note that it is directed both cephalad and medially.

For descriptive purposes, these angles have been considered separately and the beginner will find it helpful to concentrate on one at a time. As experience and confidence increase, however, it is possible to create them simultaneously and to minimize probing of the lamina. In straightforward cases, the experienced anaesthetist can correctly angle the needle straight into the ligamentum flavum after the initial perpendicular location of the lamina.

Thoracic epidural anaesthesia

If upper abdominal or thoracic surgery is to be performed, the epidural needle and catheter must be inserted in the thoracic region so that the resulting area of anaesthesia 'matches' the operative field. Accurate determination of thoracic levels by counting vertebral spines from the lumbar region is not always easy and it is often simpler to count downwards from the prominent seventh cervical vertebra. The use of the paramedian approach allows the needle to be inserted with unrestricted cephalad inclination so that the catheter can emerge from its tip almost parallel to the longitudinal axis of the epidural space. There is therefore a good chance that a catheter inserted at,

say, the T_{11}–T_{12} interspace will pass easily to T_8 or above and a block adequate for abdominal surgery can be produced without recourse to large volumes of local anaesthetic. For this reason, the author prefers the paramedian to the midline approach because, in the latter, the interspinous space is narrow and the degree of cephalad inclination is limited by the obliquity of the vertebral spines.

Attempts to produce anaesthesia of the thoracic dermatomes by injecting at the lumbar level are anatomically illogical and may result in more complications than benefits. Even the injection of a large volume of drug does not guarantee adequate cephalad spread, so the patient may still find respiration and coughing painful in the postoperative period. In addition, there will almost certainly be side-effects due to extensive lumbosacral block – numbness and paralysis of the lower limbs and retention of urine. Finally, hypotension is more marked with a thoracolumbar block than with a block centred upon the midthoracic dermatomes (Holmdahl et al 1972).

Thoracic epidural anaesthesia should not be attempted until the anaesthetist has first mastered the lumbar route and become experienced in the management of major surgery.

FACTORS AFFECTING SPREAD OF SOLUTIONS

It is obviously important to identify any factors which may influence spread of a local anaesthetic in the epidural space, and to define their effects, where possible. Anatomical differences and physiological effects within the epidural space, the age, height, weight and posture of the patient, the rate of injection, the direction of the needle bevel at the time of injection, and the mass of drug injected have all been studied. However, in the individual patient, these factors interact, so that it is difficult to predict accurately the effect of a given dose of local anaesthetic.

Epidural anatomy

The vertebral canal is triangular in cross-section. Post-mortem resin studies have shown that in the lumbar region the dura tends to be closely applied to the 'angles' of the triangle so the epidural space is very narrow at these points. The space therefore consists of one ventral and two dorsolateral compartments, and is certainly not a uniform tube surrounding a cylindrical theca (Husemeyer & White 1980). In view of this and the fact that fibrous septa are sometimes present, it is perhaps surprising that local anaesthetics spread as evenly and consistently as they do.

In the cervical region, the relationship of the dura to the ligamentum flavum is closer than elsewhere, and the dura is even adherent to periosteum in places. Consequently, the cervical epidural space is very narrow and in some cases may be little more than a potential space. This may account for the clinical observation that, even when the thoracic segments are profoundly blocked, the cervical segments are rarely affected (Grundy et al 1978a).

Epidural physiology

Negative pressure in the epidural space, due to transmission of negative intrathoracic pressure through the intervertebral foramina, is greatest in the upper and middle thoracic regions and least in the lumbar and sacral regions as distance from the thorax increases. Greater negative pressure is produced in the sitting position than in the supine, and in the flexed spinal position than in the extended. On the other hand, there may be no negative epidural pressure in conditions such as chronic obstructive airway disease in which intrathoracic pressure is abnormal, and in patients with raised intra-abdominal pressure.

This negative pressure may influence the early spread of injected solutions, particularly their tendency to track through the intervertebral foramina. It has been suggested that the spread of injected solutions may be a biphasic process, consisting firstly of the effects of this negative pressure and, later, of the effects of the positive pressure generated by injection (Park et al 1982a).

Advanced pregnancy exerts marked effects on the epidural space, some of them attributable to the rise in venous pressure caused by the partial occlusion of the inferior vena cava by the gravid uterus. This causes engorgement not only of

epidural veins, but also of those surrounding the intervertebral foramina, so that the latter are effectively occluded. A given dose of local anaesthetic will therefore be less likely to escape from the epidural space. During labour itself, uterine contractions intensify epidural venous engorgement and produce a positive pressure rise in the epidural space of 10–20 cm H_2O.

Patient factors

Age

Bromage (1969) introduced the concept of the *segmental dose requirement*, which he defined as the mass of drug required to block one segment. He showed that this was greatest at about 19 years of age, when 1.5 ml per segment of 2% lignocaine was required, and found that the dose requirement declined linearly as age increased. However, Sharrock (1978), using 0.75% bupivacaine with adrenaline, found that the segmental dose requirement was virtually constant at about 1.3 ml per segment in patients between the ages of 20 and 40 years, but in patients over 60 years, the spread of anaesthesia did not correlate with the dose. Indeed in some cases in this age group, 10 ml or less, injected at L_2–L_3, produced blocks up to T_4 and higher, and the segmental dose requirement varied between 0.35 and 1.2 ml.

This difference between the young and the old may be due to the fact that the intervertebral foramina tend to become occluded with age. Radiopaque dye injected epidurally can be seen tracking laterally into the paravertebral region in young patients, and it is at least possible that a local anaesthetic may exert some of its action there. No such tracking is seen in the elderly and epidural spread is therefore likely to be more extensive. More drug is also available to diffuse through the dura into the CSF and this may explain why a comparatively small epidural dose sometimes results in an extensive block (Sharrock 1978).

Height

Although tall patients tend to require large doses of drug for block of a given number of segments, the correlation between dose and height is poor.

Indeed, it has been calculated that if two patients 30 cm different in height are given the same dose, the resulting block will only be one segment higher in the short patient (Grundy et al 1978a).

Weight

Obese patients carry most of their excess fat subcutaneously, but they also have increased deposits in all areas where fat normally occurs. Any such increase in fat in the epidural space might be expected to affect the spread of drugs. The spread of 20 ml of 0.75% bupivacaine was studied in patients about to undergo Caesarean section, some of whom were lean and some grossly obese. The drug was injected with patients in either the horizontal or the sitting position. It was found that although posture made no difference to the eventual height of the block in the lean group, the sitting position resulted in lower blocks in the obese (Hodgkinson & Husain 1981).

Posture

Posture and gravity are of limited value in controlling the spread of local anaesthetic in the epidural space. In patients who were given 2% lignocaine with adrenaline and maintained in the lateral position, the block developed earlier on the dependent side and lasted about 20 minutes longer, but it extended only one to two segments further than on the upper side (Apostolou et al 1981). Another study using 0.75% plain bupivacaine produced similar findings (Grundy et al 1978b). Nevertheless, the effect of posture is sufficient to be of some clinical use. For example, it occasionally happens that an area of skin, usually in the groin region, remains sensitive when areas above and below it are analgesic. If the patient is turned so that this 'missed' segment is dependent, and a further injection is given, anaesthesia often results. Posture can also be used to obtain perineal analgesia during lumbar epidural block.

Injection factors

Rate of injection

This exerts very little influence on the spread of local anaesthetic in the epidural space. A threefold increase in the rate of injection of 0.75% plain bupivacaine produced a mean block less than one segment higher (Grundy et al 1978a).

Direction of the needle bevel

In patients under the age of 40 years, the segmental spread of an epidural block is the same whether the needle bevel faces cephalad or caudad. In patients over 40 years, there is a tendency towards more cephalad spread when the bevel has faced cephalad, but the difference is slight and never more than two segments (Park et al 1982b).

Mass of drug

The extent of sensory block produced by a particular agent is in general determined by the mass of drug injected rather than by the volume. However, this principle does not hold for extremes of concentration and volume, nor does it apply to the degree of motor block, as this is very closely related to drug concentration. The characteristics of individual local anaesthetics are considered below.

CLINICAL PROFILE OF BLOCK

The onset, duration and quality of a block are determined by the intrinsic properties of the individual local anaesthetic agent, the concentration in which it is used and the effect of any vasoconstrictor. There is wide variation between agents regarding speed of onset, duration of action and density of motor block. Increase in the concentration of a drug and the addition of adrenaline usually increase the rate of onset of a block, prolong its duration, and improve its quality. Carbonation of the solution has similar effects (see Ch. 4).

Methods of clinical assessment

Much of the work designed to define and compare the characteristics of local anaesthetics has given inconclusive and sometimes conflicting results because different criteria have been used for assessment. However, the most important clinical features of a local anaesthetic may be established if the typical pattern of onset and regression of an epidural block is understood (Fig. 8.17).

Onset time

Any thorough assessment should take into account not only the time taken for the onset of analgesia (defined as inability to appreciate pinprick), but also anaesthesia (defined as inability to appreciate touch). These times, charted bilaterally for each spinal segment affected, give the *mean segmental latency profile* for a particular drug.

Duration of block

Determination of the time at which bilateral analgesia and anaesthesia were last detectable for each affected spinal segment provides a *mean*

segmental duration profile. A simpler assessment of duration can be made by measuring the *two-segment regression time*. The maximum spread of the block is noted, and the interval is measured from the time of injection to the time at which the block has regressed two segments from this maximum. The method is valid when applied to patients who have been conscious throughout the procedure. If, however, they have received a general anaesthetic in addition to the epidural, and have undergone major surgery, two segment regression may have occurred before the end of surgery or before the patient is sufficiently conscious to cooperate in the assessment. In such cases, four or six segment regression times may be used.

A wholly clinical approach to the assessment of duration of block is to note the time at which the patient first complains of pain. Comparison be-

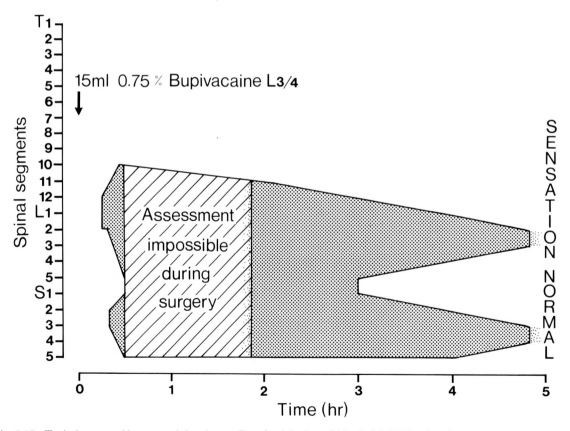

Fig. 8.17   Typical segmental latency and duration profiles after injection of 15 ml of 0.75% bupivacaine.

tween agents with this method is only valid if surgical factors, such as the type of incision and operation, are standardized, and the method lacks the precision of the duration profile and the segment regression assessments. It does, however, provide the clinical anaesthetist with the most valuable information of all – the time at which the patient may be expected to require a top-up or some alternative form of analgesia.

Density of motor block

The degree of motor block is usually assessed on a 0–3 scale: 0 being no motor block, 1 being inability to raise the extended leg, 2 being the additional inability to flex the knee, and 3 being the additional inability to flex the ankle. This last sign is taken to indicate total paralysis of the affected muscles.

Local anaesthetics in the epidural space

Lignocaine

Analgesia is provided by 1% lignocaine, but a 2% solution is required to produce acceptable muscle relaxation. Preservative-free 1.5% lignocaine in 25 ml ampoules is marketed especially for epidural use. This concentration provides anaesthesia as well as analgesia, but it cannot be relied upon to produce satisfactory muscle relaxation in every case.

The time of onset is short, and analgesia is detectable after about 6 minutes in dermatomes close to the site of injection when the 2% solution is used. Unfortunately the duration is also short, but can be prolonged by about 50% by the addition of adrenaline 1:200 000. Even then, two segment regression takes place between $1\frac{1}{2}$ and 2 hours after injection of the 2% solution.

Prilocaine

In some countries, prilocaine, the least toxic of the amide local anaesthetics, is available as a 2% solution. The onset time is slower than 2% lignocaine – a block is detectable after about 9 minutes and is complete within 20 minutes. The

duration exceeds that of lignocaine and the six segment regression time is between $2\frac{1}{2}$ and 3 hours. Motor block is clinically satisfactory, but rarely profound.

Bupivacaine

This long-acting agent is available as 0.25, 0.5 and 0.75% solutions. The 0.25 and 0.5% solutions can also be obtained containing adrenaline 1:200 000. The stronger solutions produce excellent analgesia, anaesthesia and muscle relaxation. The 0.75% solution is ideal for surgical anaesthesia in the conscious patient because it provides prolonged sensory and motor block (Fig. 8.17).

Plain bupivacaine is comparatively slow to act and since this is the only disadvantage of an otherwise excellent agent, attempts have been made to overcome it. Initial reports that carbonation resulted in a more rapid onset of anaesthesia and more profound sensory and motor block have not been confirmed (Brown et al 1980), but the addition of adrenaline to the 0.75% solution significantly decreases the onset time, and analgesia can be detected within 5 minutes (Sinclair & Scott 1984). Plain bupivacaine in 0.75% solution will provide 4–6 hours of analgesia and this pain-free period is increased to between $6\frac{1}{2}$ and 8 hours if adrenaline is added to the solution.

Effects of adrenaline

In addition to its effects on the clinical profile of the drug, adrenaline can also exert systemic effects in the concentrations commonly used in epidural block (20 ml of 1:200 000 contains 100 μg) and causes an increase in heart rate, cardiac output and stroke volume, and a decrease in mean arterial pressure and total peripheral resistance. These are the effects of β-adrenergic stimulation. The α-adrenergic effects of adrenaline are not seen systemically, presumably because higher concentrations are required to produce them (Goodman & Gilman 1975).

If the local anaesthetic used for the epidural contains adrenaline, the simultaneous use of a halogenated inhalational anaesthetic agent is theoretically contraindicated due to the risk of cardiac arrhythmias. In practice, these do not seem to occur, probably because, in the presence of an effective epidural block, minimal concentrations of inhalational agent are required. Sinclair and Scott (1984) used 0.5% halothane in a mixture of nitrous oxide and oxygen, and considered that 100 μg of adrenaline was unlikely to cause harmful systemic effects.

MANAGEMENT OF EPIDURAL ANAESTHESIA

The operative period

Epidural block in the conscious patient

If operations are to be performed on conscious patients, profound anaesthesia must be supplied for the operative field. Bupivacaine (0.75%) produces dense and reliable anaesthesia and is the agent of choice. The drug should be injected at the appropriate vertebral level so that the extent of anaesthesia 'matches' the operation. It is important that the anaesthetist takes into account not only the innervation of the skin incision, but also that of structures likely to be handled during surgery. For example, 10 ml of solution injected at L_1–L_2 is adequate for inguinal herniorrhaphy, but for abdominal hysterectomy 15–20 ml is required to ensure that perineal sensation is blocked. For surgery of the lower limb, 10–15 ml should be injected at L_3–L_4.

A knowledge of the principles, practice and limitations of epidural block and the behaviour of drugs in the epidural space is essential if the anaesthetist is to obtain satisfactory and consistent results, but supplementary sedation, general anaesthesia and systemic opioids may still be required at some stage in a patient's management. Their use, far from implying that the block has failed, acknowledges that it is the whole patient which must be managed and that there are some sources of discomfort which an epidural is intrinsically incapable of relieving. For example, afferent stimuli from the coeliac plexus may cause distress, and supplementary sedation or analgesia in these cases enhances rather than devalues the effect of

the block. The choice of agents has been discussed in Chapter 5.

'Balanced' epidural anaesthesia

Combining epidural block and general anaesthesia has several advantages, with the precise technique depending on the type and site of surgery.

For lower abdominal surgery and major orthopaedic surgery, Scott (1975a) argues persuasively in favour of a sleep dose of thiopentone, administered after the epidural injection of 20 ml of 2% lignocaine, followed by inhalation of nitrous oxide, oxygen and halothane 0.5% from a face-mask. Traditional fears that the superimposition of general anaesthesia on an extensive epidural block might cause profound hypotension do not appear to be justified. Significant decreases in both systolic and diastolic blood pressure do occur (see Ch. 5), but treatment with vasopressors is not generally required.

For upper abdominal and thoracic procedures, control of ventilation is essential, so general anaesthesia is induced and neuromuscular blocking agents are used to produce muscle relaxation. The object of the epidural block is then to provide only analgesia, for which 0.25% bupivacaine is injected in 5 ml increments. The technique has several advantages. The anaesthetist can be sure that the patient's airway is safe and pulmonary ventilation is adequate, and the fact that analgesia and muscle relaxation are obtained with two different drugs results in versatility and refinement. Considerably smaller amounts of local anaesthetic are required than if this one agent is expected to provide both effects. The technique is also suitable for patients in whom spontaneous ventilation may be undesirable because of obesity, severe respiratory disease, head-down tilt or the nature of the surgery.

The postoperative period

If the full potential of an epidural block is to be realized, it should, where possible, be continued into the postoperative period after major surgery and be used, either alone or in conjunction with other analgesic methods, to prevent pain for the next 2–3 days. The provision of complete analgesia for this length of time is difficult to achieve, and depends not only on the effectiveness of the method chosen, but also on the availability of medical and nursing personnel to supervise and monitor it.

It should be stressed that the object is to *prevent* pain rather than to relieve it. There is now good evidence that pretreatment is a more effective way of dealing with a variety of acute pain states than treatment after the pain has occurred (Bach et al 1988, Woolf 1989). *No system of analgesia will yield its full potential unless it is targeted at prevention rather than relief.* The continued use of the term 'pain relief' is probably doing more than anything else to retard progress in this field (Armitage 1989).

Personnel and organization

Intensive care and recovery units are well staffed and patients receiving epidural analgesia can be sure of prompt top-ups and efficient management of infusions from resident anaesthetists or experienced trained nurses. There is no doubt that the best results are obtained where these facilities are available. Unfortunately, it is not possible, in most district general hospitals in the UK, for all major surgical cases to be nursed in intensive-care units. As yet, few hospitals have adequate long-term recovery facilities, but the wider provision of high-dependency units would ease this situation (Report 1991).

The problem of how to control postoperative pain for general surgical patients has been addressed in the USA by Ready and colleagues (1988). They described the development of an acute pain team consisting of a senior anaesthetist, a trainee and a nurse. In the UK, interest has been stimulated by the Report of the Working Party on Pain after Surgery (Report 1990), and Wheatley and his colleagues (1991) have published the results of their first year's experience of running an acute pain service. The composition of such a group will depend on local circumstances, but there are two essentials. The group must be small

so that responsibility for pain control is not diluted and, in the case of an epidural, ultimate responsibility must remain with the anaesthetist who initiated it.

Methods of administration

The aim of a continuous epidural is to produce a band of analgesia which encompasses the dermatomal nerves supplying the area of the wound. In order to achieve this, the first requirement is that the catheter tip is positioned so that analgesic solution will spread to the appropriate nerves with minimal dosage. This solution may be administered by either repeated bolus injections or by continuous infusion. With a bolus, a relatively high pressure will be generated as the solution emerges into the epidural space and this will have an effect on spread. Burn and colleagues (1973) injected radiopaque solution by the lumbar route and showed that 20 ml spreads mostly cephalad, to the low- or mid-thoracic segments, and that this spread is not affected by the posture of the patient at the time of injection. With a continuous infusion, on the other hand, the patient's posture can influence the effect of gravity on spread. For example, Dawkins (1966) has shown that when local anaesthetic is infused into the epidural space of patients in the reclining position, gravity favours more caudad spread as the infusion progresses (Fig. 8.18) – an effect which tends to be more marked when comparatively low infusion rates are used. Thus, in order to produce block of a given extent, the catheter will need to be inserted higher if an infusion is to be used than if intermittent injections are given.

It is likely that intermittent injections of local anaesthetic alone will produce more consistent spread – and analgesia – than an infusion. However, intermittent injections are more demanding of staff time and they result in fluctuating levels of block. 'Break through' pain may occur if the administration of a bolus is delayed, yet cardiovascular instability may be seen after a bolus because of sudden extension of sympathetic block. Precise timing of injections is therefore essential. Continuous infusion minimizes these problems,

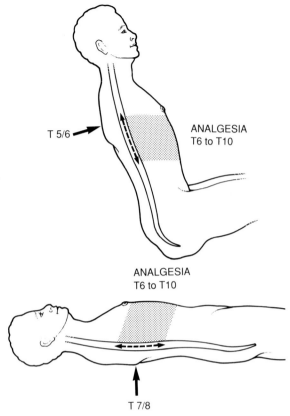

Fig. 8.18 Influence of posture on the distribution of analgesia during continuous epidural infusion in sitting and supine positions.

but significant regression of the block may occur when local anaesthetics are used alone. This is more likely to result in a failure of pain control with a vertical as opposed to a horizontal incision.

Local anaesthetic regimes

Bolus injections. Scott and colleagues (1982), using a pump capable of delivering bolus injections at variable time intervals, found that 8 ml of 0.5% plain bupivacaine, given 2-hourly, resulted in virtually complete analgesia in all cases, though this regime tended to cause some hypotension after the injections. Schweitzer & Morgan (1987) subsequently found that 3 ml of 0.5% bupivacaine with adrenaline, given hourly, produced smoother analgesia. Unfortunately, pumps capable of deliv-ering bolus injections at variable time intervals are not commercially available.

Infusions. Variable-rate infusion pumps can be used to administer a steady flow of local anaesthetic solution. The pump must be accurate and reliable, and must be powerful enough to overcome the resistance of the 90 cm length of narrow epidural catheter.

A suitable initial regime is the infusion of 0.1% plain bupivacaine at 20 ml h^{-1}, and it will usually be apparent after a few hours if this rate requires adjustment. If the block is regressing, a bolus must be given from the pump before it is reset at a higher rate – simply resetting the pump at a higher rate will be insufficient. Packs containing 500 ml of 0.1% bupivacaine in saline can be prepared in the hospital pharmacy and may become available commercially.

Opioid regimes

The discovery of opioid receptors in the spinal cord opened up an entirely new avenue for the treatment of postoperative pain (see Ch. 3). Unfortunately, the early promise of the technique was not confirmed, the transition from animal studies to widespread clinical use was far too rapid and anecdotal reports greatly outnumbered properly controlled trials. There is considerable variation in patient response and the risk of delayed respiratory depression remains significant.

Morphine was the first agent to be used epidurally in man and its relatively poor lipid solubility is probably responsible for both its long duration of action – the feature which, more than any other, marked out epidural opioids as a major clinical advance – and the occurrence of its more serious side-effects, delayed respiratory and central nervous system depression. Although initial reports claimed that 2 mg gave excellent analgesia, 10 mg in 10 ml was soon being used, but it requires 30 minutes to act and may not produce adequate pain control. It is more effective when given prophylactically. Chambers and colleagues (1981) found that 10 mg of morphine, given with bupivacaine, produced analgesia which lasted, on average, just under 12 hours, though the range was wide and the duration was spread fairly evenly from just over 4 hours to 19 hours. One of the patients in this study had delayed recovery of consciousness after anaesthesia and a respiratory rate of ten breaths per minute. She was unrousable until given naloxone. Pruritis is a side-effect of most epidural opioids, but is commonest with morphine and occurs even when preservative-free solutions are used (Weddell & Ritter 1980). Retention of urine is dose-dependent, with an incidence as high as 90% in one series (Bromage 1981).

Diamorphine and fentanyl are both highly lipid-soluble and have rapid onset times. Diamorphine produces its effect within 15 minutes of injection, and a dose of 0.1 mg kg^{-1} gives analgesia very similar in quality to the same dose given intramuscularly, though it lasts considerably longer (Jacobson et al 1983). Diamorphine, 5 mg in 10 ml of saline, has been shown to reduce the stress response to surgery as measured by plasma glucose and cortisol concentrations, an effect which could not have been due to plasma diamorphine concentrations and must therefore have been spinally mediated (Cowen et al 1982). In a study investigating the effects of different concentrations of fentanyl, Welchew (1983) concluded that 100 µg in 10 ml of saline was the optimal dose.

Buprenorphine, a partial agonist, is highly lipid-soluble, has a strong affinity for spinal receptors and dissociates from them slowly, so on theoretical grounds it should be very suitable for epidural use. Murphy and colleagues (1984) found that a dose of 60 µg in 10 ml of saline provided analgesia comparable with morphine given intramuscularly in a dose of 0.15 mg kg^{-1}, and no side-effects were observed.

Combination regimes

Where the quality of pain control provided by epidural opioids *or* local anaesthetics has been compared, the latter has proved superior (Torda & Pybus 1984). However, reliance on a single agent will not always guarantee success. Lee and colleagues (1988) studied the epidural infusion of bupivacaine, diamorphine or a mix-

ture of the two and found the last to be significantly more effective. As well as producing better analgesia, there is increasing evidence that the use of combinations will allow reduction in the dose of both opioid and local anaesthetic (Dahl et al 1990). Many combinations have been used, but bupivacaine with either diamorphine or fentanyl is the most popular. There are enthusiasts for both high-volume/low-concentration and low-volume/high-concentration infusions, but the hourly dosage of bupivacaine is usually in the region of 10–15 mg. Opioid is added to the solution so that up to 0.5 mg of diamorphine, 10 µg of fentanyl or 0.2 mg of morphine is given in each hour. Much more work is required to establish which combination, if any, has the optimal risk/benefit ratio.

Supplementary medication

This is sometimes required to treat symptoms which are beyond the scope of the epidural block. These include anxiety about the operation, sleeplessness, and discomfort from sites other than the wound, such as shoulder tip pain due to pneumoperitoneum. These problems are dealt with 'automatically' in patients receiving conventional opioid analgesics. In a patient receiving only epidural local anaesthetic, small doses of systemically administered opioids may be given safely and effectively. There may also be occasions, particularly in the first few hours after surgery, when similar treatment may be necessary in a patient receiving a combination of epidural drugs. Clearly, this increases the risk of respiratory depression. However, the need for such treatment can be reduced by the prior administration of a non-steroidal anti-inflammatory drug (NSAID) (Dahl & Kehlet 1991). Indeed, NSAIDs, continued into the postoperative period, can provide the third analgesic component in what has become known as multimodal or balanced analgesia for the treatment of postoperative pain (Dahl et al 1990).

Once the operation is over and pain is controlled, anxiety decreases in most patients. Nevertheless, some may benefit from the administration of a small amount of an anxiolytic agent, although it must be appreciated that this may contribute to cardio-respiratory depression and will have no analgesic action.

Aspects of management

A properly managed epidural block can provide excellent postoperative analgesia, but it is essential that its performance and management follow an established and *well-defined routine*. The procedure for the administration and monitoring of top-up doses, whether these are given by medical or nursing staff, must be thoroughly understood, and the importance of *preventing pain* rather than relieving it must be appreciated. If the epidural solution is given by infusion, nurses should be familiar with the operation of the pump and should check, at regular intervals, that it is delivering the correct volume. Whatever the title of the ward in which the patient is nursed, the important principle is that the *quality of supervision* must be high. Clear *management protocols* should be drawn up and there is much to be said for having them in written form at each patient's bedside. The anaesthetist carries overall responsibility and the best results will only be obtained if he is closely involved in the clinical management.

The nursing and surgical staff must be aware that epidural patients differ from those receiving conventional analgesia. In general, the circulation is more stable than many anaesthetists believe, but it is important to emphasize that continued bleeding can lead to significant hypotension *without* tachycardia. If *hypotension* is due simply to the block and is at the level which is causing concern, it should be treated as indicated below. Fears that the relative hypotension and complete analgesia may mask abdominal signs, causing delay in diagnosis of surgical complications, are groundless. Patients suffering from haemorrhage or an anastomotic leak look and feel unwell, in marked contrast to those running a normal postoperative course with an epidural.

When an epidural is used as the analgesic component of a balanced anaesthetic, significant *motor weakness* in the lower limbs is unlikely. If larger doses of local anaesthetic are used peri-operatively, some motor block may be produced. With the doses employed postoperatively, any motor block should regress, but if it does not – and especially if, having regressed, it returns – the catheter must be assumed to have *migrated intrathecally*.

One of the more difficult aspects of management is to decide whether a *patient who is in pain* requires supplementary medication or an increase in epidural dosage. If the pain is unilateral or associated with pinprick evidence of regression, it is more likely that the epidural needs reinforcing. The dose of the bolus top-up must take into account the fact that there is still a significant amount of drug in the epidural space, even though the block is inadequate. The administration of 5 ml of solution is usually sufficient; it is wise to increase the infusion rate thereafter.

The continued administration of bupivacaine into the epidural space for up to 48 hours will raise concerns about *systemic toxicity*. The systemic concentrations seen are relatively high (Griffiths et at 1975, Ross et al 1980), but the appearance of toxic symptoms does not depend solely on the plasma concentration. Scott (1975b) administered intravenous bupivacaine at different rates to conscious volunteers and found that symptoms appeared at low plasma concentrations when the infusion rate was high. The rate of increase tends to be very slow when dilute bupivacaine is given by epidural infusion and this may explain why Ross and colleagues (1980) observed no toxic symptoms in their patients. One advantage of an infusion technique is that, if a catheter migrates into an epidural vein, there will not be a sudden further increase in plasma concentration, as will happen when a bolus is given.

COMPLICATIONS OF EPIDURAL ANAESTHESIA

The side-effects of epidural anaesthesia, such as hypotension and shoulder tip pain, have already been mentioned and the general complications of regional anaesthesia have been dealt with in Chapter 5. There are, however, complications which arise specifically from epidurals.

Dural puncture

The incidence varies with the skill and experience of the anaesthetist, but if the technique is taught according to sound principles and is carefully performed, dural puncture should occur in less than 1% of cases. Dural puncture by the epidural needle is usually obvious. Puncture by the catheter may be harder to diagnose since flow of CSF down the catheter is comparatively slow and CSF may be mistaken for saline or local anaesthetic if the latter has been used to identify the epidural space. A catheter accurately positioned in the epidural space does not necessarily remain there. It can migrate through the dura so that subsequent injections are intrathecal rather than epidural.

If dural puncture occurs, it is usual to withdraw the needle or catheter and to attempt epidural puncture and cannulation at an adjacent interspace. This occasionally results in a widespread block, presumably due to local anaesthetic leaking through the hole in the dura and producing an intrathecal effect. An effective and carefully observed test dose is essential in these cases.

Total spinal. If dural puncture is not recognized and a full epidural dose is injected into the CSF, a profound and extensive block will result for which full cardiopulmonary resuscitation may be required. Covino and colleagues (1980) recommend that a volume of CSF equal to the volume of solution injected should be withdrawn through the catheter as soon as the error is discovered. Some of the drug will hopefully be present in the aspirate, and the remainder will eventually be diluted as more CSF is formed.

Symptoms

Headache occurs commonly after dural puncture. The traditional explanation – and probably the correct one – is that the leak of CSF into the epidural space causes reduction of CSF pressure in the theca, and the resulting tendency of the cord to descend puts increased tension on the supporting meninges. The headache classically comes on when the patient sits up or stands, disappears when he lies flat, and usually affects the occipital and nuchal areas. The incidence increases when large needles are used – a 16 g Tuohy needle produces symptoms in up to 18% of patients (Dripps et al 1961).

Treatment

The condition is self-limiting and will resolve completely, usually within a week. Mild cases should be treated with analgesics, a high fluid intake, laxatives to minimize straining at stool and bed rest. Severe cases, as well as being intolerable for the patient, carry the risk of intracranial haemorrhage, and active steps should be taken to prevent CSF leakage.

An *epidural blood patch* is the most effective method of sealing the dural puncture site. The patient's own blood is drawn under aseptic conditions, and a sample is sent for culture. The blood is injected in volumes of 15–20 ml epidurally, ideally at the interspace at which the dural puncture occurred. An indwelling epidural catheter should not be used for this since the distance of the catheter tip will be at least one interspace away from the dural hole and the blood clot may not extend far enough to cover it. The patient, after lying supine for 30 minutes, is allowed to be fully mobile, and Crawford (1980), reporting on 98 obstetric patients treated by this method, recorded only one whose headache was not relieved. Treatment with a blood patch does not appear to affect the success of subsequent epidural blocks and is certainly not a contraindication to them (Abouleish et al 1975).

An anaesthetist who has already punctured the dura and has, perhaps with difficulty, located the epidural space and passed a catheter at the second attempt, may be reluctant to perform an epidural blood patch in case he punctures the dural yet again. In these circumstances an *epidural infusion of saline* may be given through the epidural catheter. A bacterial filter should be incorporated in the system, and the infusion continued at a rate of 60 ml h^{-1} for 24 hours (Crawford 1972). The method results in a cure in over 70% of cases, but the patient must obviously remain in bed while the infusion is in progress.

Venous puncture

The insertion of a needle and catheter into the epidural space is a blind technique, so accidental venous puncture is a complication which all anaesthetists occasionally encounter. It is more likely to occur when the needle enters the epidural space a few millimetres from the midline, since the venous plexuses occupy the lateral parts of the space. The appearance of blood from the epidural needle is rare. Venous puncture with a catheter is more common and occurs in up to 10% of obstetric cases. The injection of 10 ml of fluid before insertion of the catheter reduces the incidence to about 3% (Verniquet 1980). Venous puncture occasionally occurs when the catheter tip migrates into an epidural vessel, and blood is discovered in the catheter when a top-up dose is about to be given. The catheter should be syringed with saline and withdrawn until blood can no longer be aspirated. A test dose of local anaesthetic containing adrenaline should then be given.

Epidural haematoma

Since any bleeding into the epidural space is impossible to control directly, haematoma formation can occur, and epidural block is contraindicated in patients with coagulopathies and those receiving anticoagulants (see Ch. 5). A haematoma which exerts pressure on spinal nerves may cause neurological symptoms and signs very similar to those of epidural block. If sensory loss or lower limb weakness outlast the expected duration of the block, neurological advice should be sought, and investigations commenced, at an early stage.

Hypotension

The discussion in Chapters 2 and 5 on the physiology and significance of hypotension resulting from regional block provides a basis for deciding on the degree of hypotension acceptable in the individual case. Some decrease in systolic blood pressure, often accompanied by a reduction in heart rate, is usual after epidural block and a low rate-pressure product results. Since this is associated with low myocardial oxygen demands, there is a beneficial effect on the normal myocardium. In the patient with ischaemic heart disease though, perfusion pressure is more important than flow in forcing oxygenated blood past atheromatous obstructions, so systolic pressure (and heart rate) should be kept within 20% of normal, angina-free limits (Merin 1981).

If serious hypotension develops, the patient should be tilted head-down and increments of ephedrine 3–7.5 mg given intravenously up to 30 mg. If this fails to restore the blood pressure, other causes for the hypotension, such as undetected surgical haemorrhage, should be sought, and the central venous pressure measured.

Retention of urine

This is a recognized complication of epidural block. In many cases, such as major gynaecological and arterial procedures and operations on the lower abdomen, a catheter will in any case be required for urinary output measurements. In other major procedures, catheterization may be required solely to deal with urinary retention resulting from the epidural, particularly when the block is continued into the postoperative period. However, it is in these cases that an epidural has the most to offer and it may be argued that catheterization of the bladder is an acceptable price to pay.

Catheter problems

Transections and *kinking* of epidural catheters, and the methods for avoiding these complications, have been discussed. Studies in which radiopaque dye has been injected down epidural catheters have shown that a catheter inserted by the midline approach may loop if excessive length is introduced, and a *knot* may form when an attempt is made to remove it and the loop is drawn tight (Nash & Openshaw 1968). This complication can be avoided by inserting a short length of catheter.

Unfortunately, although a length such as 2.5 cm may be satisfactory for the operative period when the patient is lying still, it tends to be displaced when he becomes more mobile. Not less than 5 cm should be inserted if this is to be avoided postoperatively. The risk of knotting is reduced if the catheter is introduced through a needle inserted by the paramedian approach. A knotted catheter, or one which for any reason is *difficult to remove*, may be freed by flexing the patient to the position in which it was originally inserted and exerting traction. If this is ineffective, extension of the back may allow it to be withdrawn. If this also fails or if the catheter breaks, surgical removal may be considered, but it is worth bearing in mind that Dawkins (1969), faced with this problem, left the broken end in situ. No symptoms had occurred 2 years later when he reported the case.

Infection

It is unlikely that every case is reported, but infection of the epidural space is nevertheless very rare. When it does occur, it is generally secondary to sources in the respiratory or urinary tracts, or the skin. A review of 39 cases of epidural abscess, collected over 27 years (Baker et al 1975) revealed only one case in which the infection could have been due to an epidural catheter, although this review extended over a period when epidural anaesthesia was not so widely practised as it is today. More recently, Saady (1976) has reported an abscess attributable to epidural anaesthesia, the probable cause being the development of infection in the haematoma produced, presumably, when the catheter was inserted. Epidural abscess has also been described after a *single-shot* epidural injection in a diabetic patient (Goucke & Graziotti 1990) and after spinal anaesthesia (Loarie et al 1978, Beaudoin & Klein 1984).

Two of the invariable signs of an epidural abscess – pyrexia and leukocytosis – first appear 3 or 4 days after the block. They may easily be attributed to surgical causes or respiratory infection, but local tenderness and back pain are also always present, CSF protein levels are raised and myelography reveals narrowing or obstruction of the theca at the level of the abscess. Antibiotics, surgical decompression and drainage are required before irreversible neurological damage has occurred. *Staphylococcus aureus* is usually the causative organism.

Neurological sequelae

Permanent neurological disability following an epidural often attracts publicity, so it is not surprising that the occasional patient is unhappy about having a block. Such complications are very rare, but the anaesthetist must be able to quote the risk for the patient. Kane (1981) found that three out of a total of 50 000 patients had persistent paralysis of the lower limbs, but pointed out that the incidence in any specific survey is lower than the sum total of individual case reports. In a review of the literature, Dawkins (1969) estimated an incidence of 1 in 5000 for permanent paralysis and 1 in 1000 for transient paralysis.

More recently, Scott & Hibbard (1990) undertook a retrospective study of complications associated with epidural block in obstetric practice. The total number of epidurals given during the review period was over half a million and 38 mothers suffered damage to a single spinal nerve or nerve root. In one case, the neuropathy appeared to be permanent, but symptoms resolved within 3 months in the other 37. A further two patients developed irreversible lesions of the spinal cord, but the contribution, if any, of the epidural to their symptoms is uncertain. One developed thrombosis in a congenital cervical haemangioma 10 days after delivery, and the other probably developed the anterior spinal artery syndrome 12 hours after delivery when she had apparently recovered from the effects of the epidural. Permanent neurological damage has occurred when the treatment of complications such as hypotension, haematoma, abscess and accidental subarachnoid injection was inadequate or was commenced too late. It has also followed the accidental epidural injection of a highly irritant solution such as potassium chloride.

Sequelae of uneventful blocks

Nerve damage has apparently followed the otherwise uncomplicated administration of a local anaesthetic solution. Preservatives, such as metabisulphite and methylparaben, and vasoconstrictors have been suspected of contributing to this. Metabisulphite added to chloroprocaine was almost certainly responsible for permanent paralysis after the accidental intrathecal injection of an epidural dose (Covino 1984). Solutions containing preservative should be avoided when epidural and spinal block is to be performed.

Many of the affected patients had received adrenaline, but this may simply reflect the frequency of its use. However, the dose given has often been unacceptably high and it is unwise to exceed the optimal concentration of 1:200 000. Commercial solutions which contain a vasoconstrictor are more acidic than those which do not, so it is better practice to add the adrenaline just before use.

Latent neurological disease

Occasionally, some previously symptomless pathology may be unmasked by an epidural block. During epidural injection, pressure up to 60 cm H_2O may be generated. This rapidly dissipates, but it could serve to hasten the onset of symptoms in a patient who would in any case develop them later. One patient who developed paraplegia after an epidural was cured when a laminectomy relieved her spinal stenosis (Chaudhari et al 1978). The only case of permanent paralysis in Dawkins' personal series of 4000 patients (Dawkins 1969) was a man who was found to have secondary spinal deposits from a carcinoma of the prostate.

REFERENCES

Abouleish E, Wadhwa R K, de la Vega S, Tan R N, Uy N T L 1975 Regional analgesia following epidural blood patch. Anesthesia and Analgesia (Current Researches) 54: 634–636

Aitkenhead A R, Hothersall A P, Gilmour D G, Ledingham I Mc A 1979 Dural dimpling in the dog. Anaesthesia 34: 14–19

Apostolou G A, Zarmakoupis P K, Mastrokostopoulos G T 1981 Spread of epidural anesthesia and the lateral position. Anesthesia and Analgesia (Current Researches) 60: 584–586

Armitage E N 1989 Postoperative pain – prevention or relief? British Journal of Anaesthesia 63: 136–137

Bach S, Noreng M F, Tjellden N U 1988 Phantom limb pain in amputees during the first 12 months following limb amputation after preoperative lumbar epidural blockade. Pain 33: 297–301

Baker A S, Ojemann R G, Swartz M N, Richardson E P 1975 Spinal epidural abscess. New England Journal of Medicine 293: 463–468

Beaudoin M G, Klein L 1984 Epidural abscess following multiple spinal anaesthetics. Anaesthesia and Intensive Care 12: 163–164

Blomberg R G 1988 Technical advantages of the paramedian approach for lumbar epidural puncture and catheter introduction. A study using epiduroscopy in autopsy subjects. Anaesthesia 43: 837–843

Bromage P R 1969 Ageing and epidural dose requirements. Segmental spread and predictability of epidural analgesia in youth and extreme age. British Journal of Anaesthesia 41: 1016–1022

Bromage P R 1981 The price of intraspinal narcotic analgesia: basic constraints. Anesthesia and Analgesia (Current Researches) 60: 461–463

Brown D T, Morison D H, Covino B G, Scott D B 1980 Comparison of carbonated bupivacaine and bupivacaine hydrochloride for extradural anaesthesia. British Journal of Anaesthesia 52: 419–422

Burn J M, Guyer P B, Langdon L 1973 The spread of solutions injected into the epidural space. A study using epidurograms in patients with the lumbosciatic syndrome. British Journal of Anaesthesia 45: 338–345

Chambers W A, Sinclair C J, Scott D B 1981 Extradural morphine for pain after surgery. British Journal of Anaesthesia 53: 921–925

Chaudhari L S, Kop B R, Dhruva A J 1978 Paraplegia and epidural analgesia. Anaesthesia 33: 722–725

Covino B G 1984 Current controversies in local anaesthetics. In: Scott D B, McClure J H, Wildsmith J A W (eds) Regional anaesthesia 1884–1984, p 74–81. ICM, Sodertalje

Covino B G, Marx G F, Finster M, Zsigmond E K 1980 Prolonged sensory/motor deficits following inadvertent spinal anesthesia. Anesthesia and Analgesia (Current Researches) 59: 399–400

Cowen M J, Bullingham R E S, Paterson G M C, McQuay H J, Turner M, Allen M C, Moore A 1982 A controlled comparison of the effects of extradural diamorphine and bupivacaine on plasma glucose and plasma cortisol in postoperative patients. Anesthesia and Analgesia (Current Researches) 61: 15–18

Crawford J S 1972 The prevention of headache consequent upon dural puncture. British Journal of Anaesthesia 44: 598–600

Crawford J S 1980 Experiences with epidural blood patch. Anaesthesia 35: 513–515

Dahl J B, Kehlet H 1991 Non-steroidal anti-inflammatory drugs: rationale for use in postoperative pain. British Journal of Anaesthesia 66: 703–712

Dahl J B, Rosenberg J, Dirkes W E, Mogensen T, Kehlet H 1990 Prevention of postoperative pain by balanced analgesia. British Journal of Anaesthesia 64: 518–520

Dawkins C J M 1966 Postoperative pain relief by means of continuous drip epidural block. Acta Anaesthesiologica Scandinavica 23(supplement): 438–441

Dawkins C J M 1969 An analysis of the complications of extradural and caudal block. Anaesthesia 24: 554–563

Dripps R D, Eckenhoff J E, Vandam L D 1961 Introduction to anesthesia. The principles of safe practice, 2nd edn, p 155. W B Saunders, Philadelphia

Goodman L S, Gilman A 1975 The pharamacological basis of therapeutics, 5th edn, p 483. Macmillan, New York

Goucke C R, Graziotti P 1990 Extradural abscess following local anaesthetic and steroid injection for chronic low back pain. British Journal of Anaesthesia 65: 427–429

Griffiths D P G, Diamond A W, Cameron J D 1975 Postoperative extradural analgesia following thoracic surgery. A feasibility study. British Journal of Anaesthesia 47: 48–55

Grundy E M, Ramamurthy S, Patel K P, Mani M, Winnie A P 1978a Extradural re-visited. A statistical study. British Journal of Anaesthesia 50: 805–809

Grundy E M, Rao L N, Winnie A P 1978b Epidural anesthesia and the lateral position. Anesthesia and Analgesia (Current Researches) 57: 95–97

Hodgkinson R, Husain F J 1981 Obesity, gravity and spread of epidural anesthesia. Anesthesia and Analgesia (Current Researches) 60: 421–424

Holmdahl M H, Sjogren S, Strom G, Wright B 1972 Clinical aspects of continuous epidural blockade for postoperative pain relief. Uppsala Journal of Medical Science 77: 47–56

Husemeyer R P, White D C 1980 Topography of the lumbar epidural space. A study in cadavers using injected polyester resin. Anaesthesia 35: 7–11

Jacobson L, Phillips P D, Hull C J, Conacher I D 1983 Extradural versus intramuscular diamorphine. A controlled study of analgesic and adverse effects in the postoperative period. Anaesthesia 38: 10–18

Kane R E 1981 Neurologic deficits following epidural and spinal anesthesia. Anesthesia and Analgesia (Current Researches) 60: 150–161

Lee A, Simpson D, Whitfield A, Scott D B 1988 Postoperative analgesia by continuous extradural infusion of bupivacaine and diamorphine. British Journal of Anaesthesia 60: 845–850

Loarie D S, Fairlie H B 1978 Epidural abscess following spinal anesthesia. Anesthesia and Analgesia 57: 351–353

Macintosh R R 1950 New inventions 2: extradural space indicator. Anaesthesia 5: 98

Macintosh R R, Mushin W W 1947 Observation on the epidural space. Anaesthesia 2: 100–104

Merin R G 1981 Local and regional anaesthetic techniques for the patient with ischemic heart disease. Cleveland Clinic Quarterly 48: 72–74

Michael S, Richmond N M, Birks R J S 1989 A comparison between open-end (single hole) and closed-end (three lateral holes) epidural catheters. Complications and quality of sensory blockade. Anaesthesia 44: 578–580

Murphy D F, MacGrath P, Stritch M 1984 Postoperative analgesia in hip surgery. A controlled comparison of epidural buprenorphine with intramuscular morphine. Anaesthesia 39: 181–183

Nash T G, Openshaw D J 1968 Unusual complication of epidural anaesthesia. British Medical Journal i: 700

Park W Y, Hagins F M, Rivat E L, MacNamara T E 1982a Age and epidural dose response in adult men. Anesthesiology 56: 318–320

Park W Y, Poon K C, Massengale M D, MacNamara T E 1982b Direction of needle bevel and epidural anesthetic spread. Anesthesiology 57: 327–328

Ready L B, Oden R, Chadwick H S, Benedetti C, Rooke G A, Caplan R, Wild L M 1988 Development of an anesthesiology-based postoperative pain management service. Anesthesiology 68: 100–106

Report 1990 Pain After Surgery. Commission on the provision of surgical services. The Royal College of Surgeons of England and The College of Anaesthetists, London

Report 1991 High dependency care – acute care in the future. Association of Anaesthetists of Great Britain and Ireland, London

Ross R A, Clarke J E, Armitage E N 1980 Postoperative pain prevention by continuous epidural infusion. A study of the clinical effects and the plasma concentrations obtained. Anaesthesia 35: 663–668

Saady A 1976 Epidural abscess complicating thoracic epidural analgesia. Anesthesiology 45: 244–246

Schweitzer S A, Morgan D J 1987 Plasma bupivacaine concentrations during postoperative continuous analgesia. Anaesthesia and Intensive Care 15: 425–430

Scott D B 1975a Management of epidural block during surgery. British Journal of Anaesthesia 47: 271–272

Scott D B 1975b Evaluation of the clinical tolerance of local anaesthetic agents. British Journal of Anaesthesia 47: 328–331

Scott D B 1983 Abdominal and perineal surgery. In: Henderson J J, Nimmo W S (eds) Practical regional anaesthesia. Blackwell. Oxford

Scott D B, Hibbard B M 1990 Serious non-fatal complications associated with extradural block in obstetric patients. British Journal of Anaesthesia 64: 537–541

Scott D B, Schweitzer S, Thorn J 1982 Epidural block in postoperative pain relief. Regional Anesthesia 7: 135–139

Sharrock N E 1978 Epidural anesthetic dose responses in patients 20 to 80 years old. Anesthesiology 47: 425–428

Sinclair C J, Scott D B 1984 Comparison of bupivacaine and etidocaine in extradural blockade. British Journal of Anaesthesia 56: 147–153

Soresi A L 1932 Peridural anesthesia: a preliminary report. Medical Record (New York) 35: 165–166

Torda T A, Pybus D A 1984 Extradural administration of morphine and bupivacaine. A controlled comparison. British Journal of Anaesthesia 56: 141–146

Valentine S J, Jarvis A P, Shutt L E 1991 Comparative study of the effects of air or saline to identify the extradural space. British Journal of Anaesthesia 66: 224–227

Verniquet A J W 1980 Vessel puncture with epidural catheters. Experience in obstetric patients. Anaesthesia 35: 660–662

Weddell S J, Ritter R R 1980 Epidural morphine: serum levels and pain relief. Anesthesiology 53: 419

Welchew E A 1983 The optimum concentration for epidural fentanyl. A randomised double-blind comparison with and without 1:200 000 adrenaline. Anaesthesia 38: 1037–1041

Wheatley R G, Madej T H, Jackson I J B, Hunter D 1991 The first year's experience of an acute pain service. British Journal of Anaesthesia 67: 353–359

Woolf C J 1989 Recent advances in the pathophysiology of acute pain. British Journal of Anaesthesia 63: 139–146

9. Sacral epidural (caudal) block

L. V. H. Martin

The sacral approach to the epidural space produces a more reliable and effective block of the sacral nerves than does the lumbar route and is therefore to be preferred for operations on the anus and rectum, the perineum, the penis and urethra, and the vagina and cervix.

The technique of caudal block depends upon the accurate localization of the sacral hiatus through which access to the sacral epidural space is gained. Unfortunately, there are considerable anatomical variations in this area resulting in differences in the size and shape of the hiatus which may make its identification difficult, and in some cases the insertion of a needle into the sacral canal may be impossible.

Anatomical variations (Fig. 9.1)

Interest in the anatomy of the sacrum was aroused in the 1940s in the USA and was associated with the development of continuous caudal anaesthesia for the relief of pain in childbirth (Edwards & Hingson 1942, Hingson 1947a,b). Reviews of large collections of skeletons delineated the wide range of normal measurements and recorded the variations that may occur (Trotter and Lanier 1945). The important variations relate to the dorsal wall of the sacral canal and are due to differing degrees of fusion between the component sacral vertebrae (Trotter 1947).

The sacral hiatus, which is roughly triangular in shape, results from failure of fusion of the laminae of the fifth sacral vertebra, and its apex is commonly accepted as being at the level of the lower third of the body of S_4. However, this was found to be the case in only 35% of bones studied and it was at a higher level in 45% and lower in the

remaining 20%. Consequently, there is variation in the distance from the apex to a line joining the two sacral cornua. The mean of this measurement was found to be 20 mm with a range of 0–66 mm, but in some instances there was complete failure of fusion of the sacral arches and in other cases the hiatus was completely obliterated by bone. Failure of fusion of the upper sacral vertebrae may also occur and result in separate defects through which solution may escape during injection. The base of the hiatus (the line joining the sacral cornua) is subject to some variation, having a mean length of 16 mm and a range of 7–28 mm.

In Trotter's study the anteroposterior diameter of the sacral canal had a mean of 5.3 mm (range 0–16 mm), but was less than 2 mm in 5.5% of cases. Complete obliteration of the canal was found in a small number of bones. This was caused either by a tranverse fold in the posterior wall of the canal with a corresponding projection from the anterior wall, or by the dorsal projection of a sacral body into the canal.

Studies of cadavers (Lanier et al 1944) have shown similar variations in the position of the inferior extremity of the dura, which was found to have a mean position at the middle third of the body of S_2, being caudad to this in 46% of cases and cephalad in 38%. The mean distance from the dura to the apex of the sacral hiatus was 47 mm with a range of 19–75 mm.

Technique of sacral epidural block

Position of patient

Caudal injections are usually carried out either with the patient prone or in the lateral position.

127

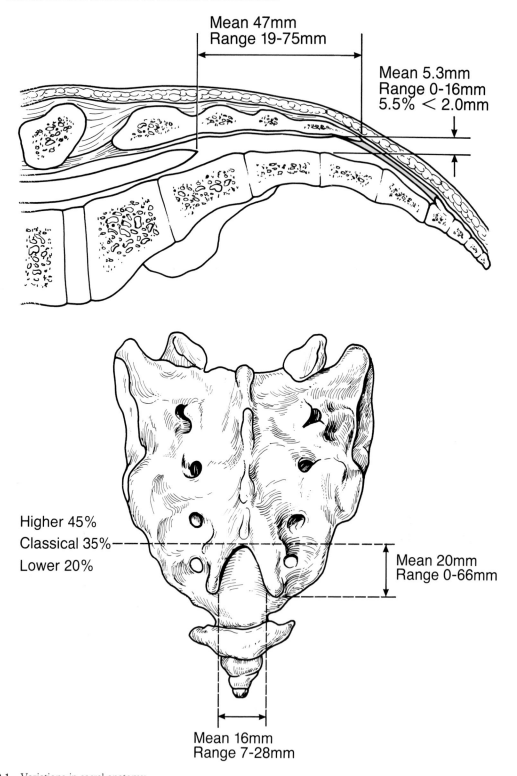

Fig. 9.1 Variations in sacral anatomy.

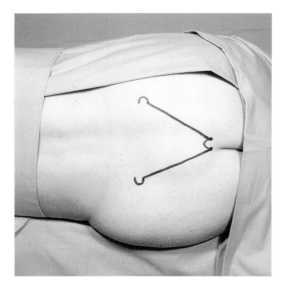

Fig. 9.2 Patient in lateral position. Note how the natal cleft does not correspond to midline bony structures.

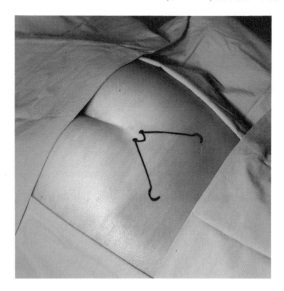

Fig. 9.3 Triangular relationship of bony landmarks for caudal block.

The *prone position* is easier for the operator, but is less comfortable for the patient, particularly if there is any respiratory embarrassment. The patient's head and shoulders should be supported by a suitable pillow or padding and another pillow should be placed under the pelvis to tilt it and bring the sacral hiatus into greater prominence. The ankles should also be supported on a pillow with the lower limbs slightly abducted and the heels encouraged to flop outwards. This prevents tightening of the gluteal muscles which can make identification of the landmarks more difficult.

In the *lateral position* the patient should arch the back and draw up the knees in front of the abdomen and the sacral region should be brought to the edge of the table to allow the operator greater freedom of movement. The anaesthetist should sit or crouch and, if the anaesthetist is right handed, the patient should be placed in the left lateral position so that the natural movement of the anaesthetist's wrist facilitates the insertion of the needle. In this position the patient's buttock may fall over the sacral region and obscure the region of the hiatus (Fig. 9.2).

Caudal injection with the patient in the lithotomy position has been described (Berstock 1979).

Location of the sacral hiatus

The approximate position of the sacral hiatus can be located in two ways. Firstly, an equilateral triangle with its base on the line joining the two posterior superior iliac spines will have its apex over the sacral hiatus (Fig. 9.3). Secondly, if the anaesthetist's finger is laid in the natal cleft with

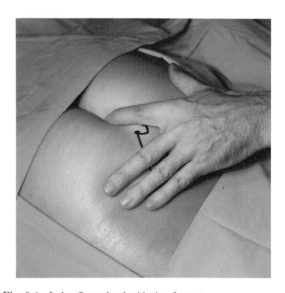

Fig. 9.4 Index finger level with tip of coccyx.

the distal end at the tip of the coccyx, the sacral hiatus will be level with the proximal interphalangeal joint (Fig. 9.4). When the approximate position has been indicated, the sacral spines are palpated with gradual movement in a caudad direction until a depression is felt. Identification of the sacral cornua laterally will then confirm the exact location.

Choice of needle

Ordinary disposable hypodermic needles can be used for injection, but their length may be inadequate, particularly in obese subjects, and breakage is always a possibility. It is more satisfactory to use a longer, more substantial needle, preferably with a trocar in situ. Spinal needles of 18 g or 19 g can be used, as can epidural needles with a straight point. Huber-pointed needles, although recommended by some, are less satisfactory and are more difficult to insert through the sacrococcygeal ligament.

Malleable stainless steel needles as described by Hingson (Fig. 9.5) are now difficult to obtain, but were originally intended for continuous caudal anaesthesia before the development of suitable catheters. They have a side opening near the distal end to allow injection in case the point becomes embedded in periosteum or otherwise occluded. A small expansion at the proximal end prevents the needle being lost in the sacral canal in the event of breakage at the hub – a recognized hazard with the early needles.

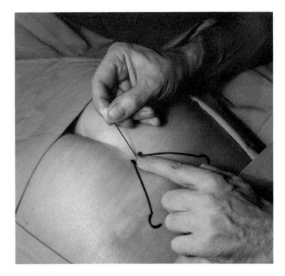

Fig. 9.6 Needle alignment for initial insertion.

Needle insertion

During preparation of the skin, care should be taken to avoid antiseptic solutions irritating the perineum. A skin wheal should be raised over the hiatus and the subcutaneous tissue infiltrated with a small quantity of local anaesthetic. Infiltration of the sacrococcygeal ligament and the adjacent periosteum should also be carried out, but large amounts of anaesthetic should be avoided since the landmarks, which may already be difficult to palpate, are easily obscured.

The caudal needle should then be inserted (Fig. 9.6) through the skin wheal at right angles to the

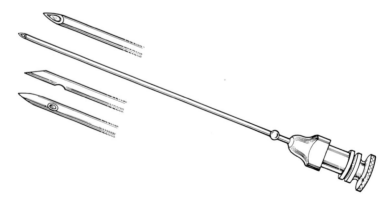

Fig. 9.5 Hingson needle.

sacrococcygeal ligament until the ligament is penetrated and the bone of the underlying sacral body is reached. The needle should be withdrawn slightly to disengage the point from the periosteum, and the hub of the needle depressed until it is estimated that the shaft of the needle is in the plane of the sacral canal (Fig. 9.7). The needle is then advanced along the canal. There is often a sensation of 'give' and the needle is then firmly held by bone and ligament. The needle should be maintained in the midline and sufficient length inserted to establish its position, but without penetration of the dura. The measurements and variations detailed earlier must be borne in mind.

Incorrect insertion

It is easy to place the needle incorrectly and a number of possibilities exist. The needle may be inserted superficial to the canal (Fig. 9.8A) and injection made into the subcutaneous tissue. It is usually possible to see or palpate a swelling if this occurs, but in cases of doubt the injection of a few millilitres of air will produce localized surgical emphysema which will confirm the misplacement. The needle may enter the canal, but become embedded in the periosteal lining. Injection will then meet with considerable resistance.

The needle may enter the canal, but may leave it through a superior defect and subcutaneous injection will then occur. A more serious malposition may occur if the needle is inserted too vigorously and too far. It may then pass through the sacrococcygeal joint, or lateral to the coccyx, into the pelvic cavity beyond (Fig. 9.8B) and in this case both the rectum and birth canal may be entered. The needle will then be contaminated and subsequent withdrawal and insertion into the sacral canal will carry with it the danger of infection. If this malposition is suspected the

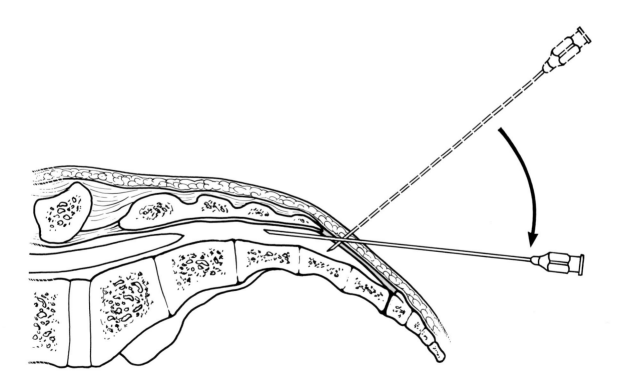

Fig. 9.7 Change of alignment needed to advance needle along sacral canal.

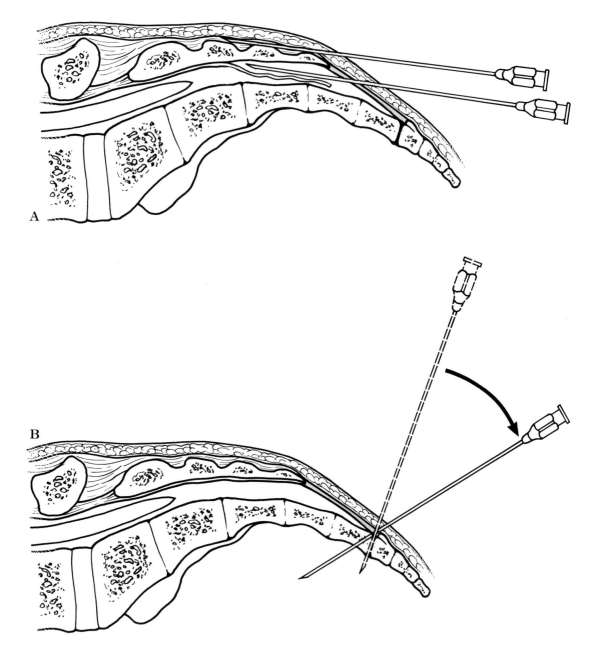

Fig. 9.8 Some possible misplacements of needle during caudal block.

procedure should be abandoned. Failure to recognize incorrect needle placement during labour has resulted in the injection of local anaesthetic into the fetal skull (Sinclair et al 1965). It is also possible to force the point of the needle into the marrow cavity of a sacral vertebra and any local anaesthetic injected will be rapidly absorbed (DiGiovanni 1971, McGown 1972).

Injection

When the needle is satisfactorily positioned, the syringe with local anaesthetic should be attached and an aspiration test carried out for both cerebrospinal fluid and blood. A dural tap is, in fact, very rare, but should it occur it is wise to abandon the procedure and proceed to a low spinal injection through the lumbar region. The aspiration of blood is more common and is usually due to damage to veins during insertion with bleeding into the sacral canal, rather than to intravenous placement of the needle tip. Slight withdrawal of the needle and the injection of a small quantity of local anaesthetic can be carried out and the patient questioned and observed for signs of toxicity. If none appear the full dose of anaesthetic can then be injected.

If the needle is correctly placed in the sacral canal there will be only slight resistance to injection, similar to an epidural or intravenous injection. If any force is required to inject the solution a malposition of the needle should be suspected. Rotation of the needle should be tried before it is repositioned. If there is doubt about the position of the needle tip, the anaesthetist may inject 2–5 ml of air while listening with a stethoscope placed over the lumbar vertebrae. If the needle is within the sacral canal a loud bruit will be heard (Lee 1988).

Volume of solution

The spread of solution in the sacral canal is dependent on the volume injected. The early anatomical studies suggested that the volume of the sacral canal in adults was slightly more than 30 ml (with a range of 12–65 ml) and that this was the volume of solution required to block the sacral nerves. However, this was the volume of dry bones and in life the canal is filled with dura, nerves, blood vessels and connective tissue so that smaller volumes are required. Spread up the epidural space occurs on injection and there is also leakage through the foramina to a variable and unpredictable extent.

Cousins & Bromage (1971), using a standard dose of 20 ml of 2% lignocaine, found wide variations in the upper level of analgesia, there

being no correlation with age, height or weight of the patient. However, 20 ml of solution can be relied upon to produce analgesia of the sacral nerves and although spread into the lower thoracic region takes place on occasion, this seldom causes clinical problems and 20 ml is recommended as a standard dose irrespective of the drug used.

Agent

Any standard agent is suitable. When a single-injection technique is used a longer-acting drug such as 0.5% bupivacaine is preferable. Maximum analgesia is established after approximately 20 minutes and, in the case of bupivacaine, lasts several hours. The addition of adrenaline will prolong the action of the drug, but there is wide and unpredictable variation in its effect. This is particularly noticeable after haemorrhoidectomy when analgesia may last many hours and outlast the recovery of other sensations. It may be that the prevention of initial muscle spasm prevents the initiation of a pain–spasm–pain cycle. For out-patient surgery in adults bupivacaine should be avoided, since prolonged weakness of the leg muscles may delay discharge. Lignocaine is to be preferred.

The rate of absorption of the drug from the sacral canal into the bloodstream is intermediate between that from intercostal and lumbar epidural injections and this, together with the known characteristics of the drug used, will enable a safe dose to be calculated. The caudal route has also been used for epidural opioid administration, with morphine being given alone and in combination with local anaesthetics. The results have been variable (Jensen et al 1982, Farad & Naguib 1985).

Continuous caudal analgesia

When this was originally developed for use in obstetrics, catheters of suitable size were not available and the technique had to be carried out using semi-rigid needles. With the development of epidural catheters it is now possible to insert a catheter in the sacral region. Because the size of the canal may limit the diameter of the needle, the smallest available catheter should be to hand. It is inserted through the caudal needle and, provided that the needle point is lying freely in the canal, no difficulty should be experienced in threading the catheter through it. About 5 cm should be threaded beyond the needle tip. After the needle is withdrawn, the entry point of the catheter through the skin should be dressed and the catheter held firmly in place by Sleek.

A standard top-up dose of 10 ml of local anaesthetic is recommended.

REFERENCES

Berstock D A 1979 Haemorrhiodectomy without tears. Annals of the Royal College of Surgeons of England 61: 51–54

Cousins M J, Bromage P R 1971 A comparison of the hydrochloride and carbonated salts of lignocaine for caudal analgesia in out-patients. British Journal of Anaesthesia 43: 1149–1155

DiGiovanni A J 1971 Inadvertent interosseous injection – a hazard of caudal anesthesia. Anesthesiology 34: 92–94

Edwards W B, Hingson R A 1942 Continuous caudal anesthesia in obstetrics. American Journal of Surgery 57: 459–464

Farad H, Naguib M 1985 Caudal morphine for pain relief following anal surgery. Annals of the Royal College of Surgeons of England 67: 257–258

Hingson R A 1947a Continuous caudal analgesia in obstetrics, surgery and therapeutics. Current Researches in Anesthesia and Analgesia 26: 177–191

Hingson R A 1947b Continuous caudal analgesia in obstetrics, surgery and therapeutics – conclusion. Current Researches in Anesthesia and Analgesia 26: 238–247

Jensen P J, Siem-Jorgensen P, Nielsen B N, Wichmand-Nielsen H, Wintherreich E 1982 Epidural morphine by the caudal route for postoperative pain relief. Acta Anaesthesiologica Scandinavica 26: 511–513

Lanier V A, McKnight H E, Trotter M 1944 Caudal analgesia: an experimental and anatomical study. American Journal of Obstetrics and Gynecology 47: 633–641

Lee M G 1988 Identification of the caudal epidural space. Anaesthesia 43: 705–706

McGown R G 1972 Accidental marrow sampling during caudal anaesthesia. British Journal of Anaesthesia 44: 613–614

Sinclair J C, Fox H A, Lenty J F, Fuld G L, Murphy J 1965 Intoxication of the fetus by a local anesthetic. New England Journal of Medicine 273: 1173–1177

Trotter M 1947 Variations of the sacral canal: their significance in the administration of caudal analgesia. Current Researches in Anesthesia and Analgesia 26: 192–202

Trotter M, Lanier P F 1945 Hiatus canalis sacralis in American whites and negroes. Human Biology 17: 368–381

10. Regional techniques in obstetrics

L. E. S. Carrie

General considerations

Regional analgesia in obstetrics is an art based on a science. The science involves knowledge of the anatomy of the nervous system and reproductive tract, of the physiology of pregnancy and of the pharmacology of local anaesthesia. The anaesthetist learns the art by long experience in the labour ward, performing regional techniques, assessing their results and learning how to modify them in the best interests of the mother and her baby. There is no short cut to this experience and it is in large measure the justification for having specialists in obstetric anaesthesia.

There are several reasons for the popularity of regional analgesia in labour. Firstly, the main alternative methods of analgesia – parenteral and inhalational – have the potential for producing maternal and fetal central nervous system depression. In the mother this can range from amnesia for the birth of her child, to confusion and disorientation such that she loses the ability to cooperate with attendant staff. In the neonate the effect can extend from mild neurobehavioural abnormalities, detectable only by sophisticated testing, to severe respiratory depression with failure to initiate normal respiration at birth. The use of regional analgesia in obstetrics offers the possibility of maternal pain relief without clouding of consciousness or neonatal depression.

A second reason for the popularity of regional techniques is that parenteral and inhalational methods may fail, even when carefully applied, to provide satisfactory analgesia in as many as 40% of women (Beazley et al 1967). Regional analgesia, when expertly performed and carefully timed, provides much better results.

In recent years, regional anaesthesia has become increasingly preferred for operative obstetrics, especially for Caesarean section. The main impetus for this change has come from the mothers themselves, the majority of whom would rather remain conscious with husband present at the time of delivery. This produces a feeling of well-being which is continued into the puerperium. Other benefits include less postoperative pain, fewer chest complications and earlier establishment of breast feeding (Morgan et al 1984). Most obstetric anaesthetists encourage this trend towards regional anaesthesia because the preservation of the protective respiratory reflexes considerably decreases the risks of failed endotracheal intubation and inhalational pneumonitis.

Innervation of birth canal (Fig. 10.1)

The pain associated with uterine contraction is transmitted in visceral afferent fibres which traverse the uterine, cervical and hypogastric plexuses to reach the sympathetic chains. The fibres then pass through the white rami communicantes and the posterior nerve roots of the 11th and 12th thoracic and first lumbar segments of the spinal cord. Pain is therefore felt mainly in the lower abdomen and in the back in the area innervated by the corresponding posterior primary rami. Bonica (1979) pointed out that this area may extend down as far as the sacrum. Back pain in the first stage of labour, especially that associated with persistent occipitoposterior positions, may be due to pressure of the presenting part on the lumbosacral plexus or other pelvic structures and is referred to the lower lumbar and sacral segments.

135

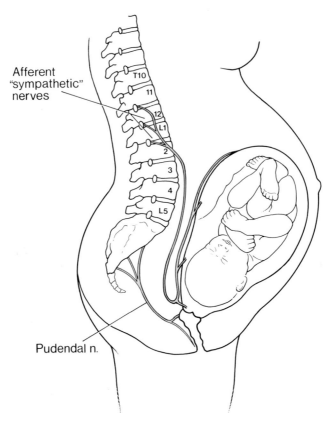

Afferent
"sympathetic"
nerves

Pudendal n.

Fig. 10.1   Innervation of the birth canal.

Pain during the second stage of labour caused by distension of, or surgical manipulations upon, the vagina, vulva and perineum, is transmitted in somatic nerves – mainly the pudendal nerves and perineal branches of the posterior cutaneous nerve of the thigh – to the second, third and fourth sacral segments of the spinal cord. Other afferent fibres run in the cutaneous branches of the ilio-inguinal and genital branches of the genitofemoral nerves. Thus the pain of the first stage of labour can usually be relieved by block of the 11th and 12th thoracic and first lumbar segments; the pain of the second stage requires additional block of the second to fourth sacral segments.

Aorto-caval occlusion

There is conclusive evidence that all pregnant women in the supine position near term have complete or nearly complete occlusion of the inferior vena cava (and sometimes the aorta) due to compression between the gravid uterus and the vertebral column. Flow through the vena cava may not always be normal even in the full lateral position and the extent to which venous return is compromised depends entirely on the adequacy of the collateral circulation through the paravertebral and azygos systems of veins. Severe occlusion is 'revealed' (Crawford 1972) to the patient and her medical attendants by faintness or nausea and hypotension. Less severe cases may be 'concealed' if blood pressure is maintained by peripheral vasoconstriction. Unfortunately this vasoconstriction affects the uteroplacental circulation and may cause varying degrees of birth asphyxia.

The importance of aorto-caval occlusion to regional analgesia in obstetrics is that it renders the pregnant woman much more susceptible to hypotension from sympathetic block. Preloading and avoidance of the full supine position improve cardiovascular status, but venous return is never quite normal until the infant is delivered.

Local anaesthetic drugs

The two drugs most commonly used at present for obstetric analgesia in the UK are lignocaine and bupivacaine. Both agents are used for epidural and spinal block, although bupivacaine is usually chosen for the latter. Lignocaine is also used for local infiltration and peripheral blocks. Their pharmacology has been considered in Chapter 4. The large doses of local anaesthetic sometimes used both for epidural anaesthesia for Caesarean section and for continuous epidural techniques in labour run the theoretical risk of producing cumulative toxicity. Reynolds and colleagues (1973) calculated that a dose rate of 0.4 mg min^{-1} of plain bupivacaine (about 10 ml of the 0.5% solution every 2 hours) would produce potentially toxic blood concentrations in 5% of patients after 320 mg (more than 60 ml of the 0.5% solution).

Recently, sensitive neurobehavioural tests have been developed which detect more subtle degrees of neonatal depression than are measured by methods such as fetal acid–base status and Apgar testing (Scanlon et al 1974, Amiel-Tison et al 1982). The tests assess motor behaviour, habituation to stimuli and attentiveness and have been used to detect the less obvious effects of local anaesthetic drugs in the neonate. Early studies indicated that there may be diminished muscle tone without central nervous system (CNS) depression ('floppy but alert') after lignocaine (Scanlon et al 1974, Hollmen et al 1978), but more recent work (Abboud et al 1983a,b, Kuhnert et al 1984, Kileff et al 1984) has failed to demonstrate this. Wiener and colleagues (1977) found neurobehavioural abnormalities for 48 hours after epidural bupivacaine, but this has not been confirmed (Scanlon et al 1976, Corke 1977, Hodgkinson et al 1977, McGuinness et al 1978). Useful though these tests may be in comparing local anaesthetic drugs and techniques, the long-term significance of the results, if any, is unknown.

LUMBAR EPIDURAL BLOCK

Lumbar epidural block is now the sheet-anchor of obstetric regional anaesthesia, being applicable as a method of pain relief throughout labour, as well as for all types of operative obstetrics and for postoperative pain control.

Effect on placental blood flow

Information of great interest to obstetric anaesthetists has been produced by the measurement of intervillous placental blood flow using Xenon-133 clearance (Rekonen et al 1976). The method has been used in several investigations of the effect of regional techniques on placental blood flow (Jouppila et al 1978a,b, Hollmen et al 1982). Hollmen and colleagues (1982) showed that, during established labour, epidural block produced by 10 ml doses of 0.25% plain bupivacaine or 2% 2-chloroprocaine caused an increase in placental blood flow of about 35%, whereas it decreased by 19% in controls. Other workers have shown that this beneficial effect also occurs in patients with pre-eclamptic toxaemia (Jouppila et al 1982). These studies are important because they show that epidural analgesia can be of positive benefit to the fetus.

Epidural analgesia in labour

Methods of identifying the epidural space have been discussed in Chapter 8. The second or third lumbar interspace is usually chosen and the procedure performed with the patient in the left lateral or sitting position. An epidural catheter should almost *always* be inserted because, even when delivery seems imminent, labour has a contrary way of lingering on when a single-shot technique has been used. It is important to perform the epidural as expeditiously as possible because it is seldom easy for the labouring patient to lie in the flexed position.

Practical problems

The more general problems associated with epidural block have also been discussed in Chapter

8. However, obstetric practice presents anaesthetists with the rare challenge of maintaining analgesia for many hours over several spinal segments. The skill of the obstetric anaesthetist lies not so much in inserting the epidural catheter into the right place as in making the block effective.

Unilateral and patchy block. For an epidural block to be effective from T_{11} to S_4, 11 nerve roots must be blocked on each side. Although this might seem easy to achieve by using a large enough volume of drug, it does not always happen in practice and recent research provides an explanation. Several workers have demonstrated varying degrees of posteromedian folding of the dura mater, which may be attached to the ligamentum flavum by a connective tissue band or septum. These structures tend to divide the posterior epidural space into two or more compartments (see Ch. 6) and may be the cause of patchy or asymmetrical blocks. If the septum is complete, a unilateral block will result (Singh 1967).

The upper limit of the block is usually determined by pinching the skin between the nails of the thumb and index finger or by using a blunt needle. Alternatively, the level of loss of temperature discrimination may be used. The lower limit of block is adequately (and more aesthetically) assessed by enquiring about numbness or paraesthesiae over the buttocks. If dermatome charts are provided in every delivery room, midwives become very adept at assessing the extent of the block.

Hypotension. Hypotension during epidural analgesia in the pregnant patient results from the combination of sympathetic block and aorto-caval occlusion. The lateral or wedged position encourages uterine displacement and limits the adverse effects of aorto-caval occlusion, but the latter cannot always be overcome entirely by posture (see p.136), and it is customary to 'preload' the circulation with 500 ml of crystalloid solution. Persistent hypotension is better treated with a small dose of a vasopressor (e.g. ephedrine 5–10 mg intravenously) rather than administering large volumes of fluid. It is obviously important to avoid giving a dose of local anaesthetic which produces a block higher than that required for effective analgesia because this will increase the possibility of hypotension.

Motor block and instrumental delivery. Motor block in the lower limbs and an increased incidence of instrumental delivery are the two commonest side-effects of epidural local anaesthetics. Epidural opioids do not produce these complications, but, used alone, they are neither fully effective nor free from serious side-effects. However, the *combination* of opioids with local anaesthetics allows effective analgesia to be obtained with smaller amounts of both types of drug. At present the most popular combination is bupivacaine with fentanyl. Although this mixture still produces some impairment of motor function, it is claimed that the combination of bupivacaine with sufentanil will produce effective pain relief while maintaining the ability to walk (Naulty et al 1989). Unfortunately, this does not seem to be accompanied by a significant reduction in the need for instrumental delivery (Chestnut et al 1988).

Technique

Pain relief in labour can be achieved by giving either bolus injections or infusions.

Bolus injections. For the first injection 5–10 ml is administered, smaller volumes being used in short or obese patients in whom spread tends to be more extensive. Larger volumes are more appropriate for taller patients, possibly combined with head-up tilt for those in whom sacral analgesia is required from the outset. The latter group includes patients who are expected to deliver within the duration of the first dose of local anaesthetic. The initial dose must take into account the test dose (if used) and the volume required to prime the filter and catheter. Analgesia will last from 1 to 2 hours, after which a *top-up* will be required if the block is to be maintained. The volume given will be influenced by the effect and duration of the initial dose, but it will also depend on the stage of labour and the likelihood of instrumental delivery.

Recently, opioids have been added to bolus injections of local anaesthetic and almost every drug has been tried. A typical mixture would be 0.125% bupivacaine with fentanyl 20 µg in each

10 ml. In general, the use of a mixture allows the local anaesthetic concentration to be approximately halved, with consequently less reduction in motor power.

Infusions. While bolus injections are still commonly used for the relief of pain in labour, epidural infusions have become increasingly popular because they eliminate the problem of pain developing between injections and make fewer demands on the anaesthetist's time. However, regular assessment is still essential because analgesic requirements alter as labour progresses. There is no ideal concentration of local anaesthetic for infusion because of individual variation. If too strong a solution is used, motor block becomes intense; if the solution is too weak, additional boluses may be required too frequently. A typical regime, after a test dose and the establishment of analgesia with a bolus injection of 0.125 or 0.25% bupivacaine, is an infusion of 0.125% bupivacaine at a rate of 8–12 ml h^{-1}.

Combinations of local anaesthetics and opioids can also be given by infusion and, again, numerous combinations have been tried, bupivacaine with fentanyl being the most popular. An effective regime is the infusion, at 10–12 ml h^{-1}, of 0.0625% bupivacaine with fentanyl 20 μg in each 10 ml (Chestnut et al 1988).

Imperfect blocks. Several adjustments can be made to try and improve an imperfect block:

1. The catheter may be partially withdrawn so that the tip lies more posteriorly in the epidural space. This manoeuvre may also withdraw the tip from one of the subcompartments of the space. When making this adjustment it is important to remember that the proximal hole in many catheters is more than 1 cm from the tip.
2. The patient's posture may be changed before the next dose is administered. Gravity has some effect on the spread of solution in the epidural space and the patient should be positioned so that the missed segments are dependent.
3. A higher concentration of local anaesthetic can be used or a different drug may be tried.

4. A larger volume of a more dilute solution may be effective. For example, 14 ml of 0.25% bupivacaine may be injected instead of 7 ml of 0.5% solution.
5. If an opioid has not already been used, it may be given alone or added to the local anaesthetic. This is particularly effective for pain in the sacral segments during the first stage of labour (Reynolds & O'Sullivan 1989).

Because it takes 15–20 minutes to establish whether any of the above adjustments has been effective, it is often wise to carry out more than one at a time.

During an infusion, it may be necessary to alter either the extent of the block *or* its quality. The extent of the block may be influenced by changing the patient's position or increasing the volume infused. The quality of the block depends on the dose of drug given.

If the block remains ineffective, the best remedy is to remove the catheter and reinsert it in an adjacent interspace. This is particularly appropriate when a previously effective block becomes ineffective, because it is more than likely that, despite careful fixation, the catheter has become displaced.

Timing

Provided vena caval occlusion is avoided, epidural analgesia has little effect on the strength or frequency of uterine contractions (Schellenberg 1979). In spontaneous, unaugmented labour, Studd and colleagues (1980) found the first stage lasted 1 hour longer in epidural than in non-epidural patients. In induced, augmented labour there was no statistical difference in the length of the first stage. Epidural analgesia is not usually commenced in either primiparous or multiparous patients until labour is well established. An exception may be the group of patients who find surgical induction of labour painful. Caseby (1974) found 22% of women in this category and, if they can be identified beforehand, it is reasonable to offer them an epidural block before induction. Thereafter it is quite possible, if the patient so wishes, to let the analgesia wear off until labour becomes established.

Some women who have an effective epidural throughout labour may feel 'deprived' of part of the experience of labour. This is less likely in units where epidural analgesia is not commenced until labour is well established and becoming painful. This 'on demand' arrangement, which is only possible in a unit well-staffed with experienced anaesthetists, may nevertheless miss a few multiparous patients who, once they are in strong, established labour, spend little time in the first stage. As few epidurals are effective in less than 20 minutes from the time the anaesthetist is called to the patient's room, the request may come too late. If a multiparous patient wishes to have an epidural, the catheter should be inserted as soon as possible after the start of labour.

Management of the second stage

If an epidural or spinal block is fully effective in the sacral segments, then the bearing-down reflex will be obtunded. The actual ability to bear down is virtually unimpaired as this effort is produced by the diaphragm and abdominal muscles, but the effectiveness is undoubtedly reduced in many cases in the absence of the afferent side of the reflex. If the woman is exhorted to push as soon as full dilatation is diagnosed, no matter how high the head, then mid-cavity or rotational forceps will frequently be required to deliver an exhausted mother of her distressed infant.

Pearson & Davies (1974) have shown that progressive maternal and fetal metabolic acidosis develop in the second stage and this is probably the basis for the commonly accepted maximum time limit for the length of the second stage – 'One hour in a primigravid patient – half an hour in a multiparous'. However, they also showed that an effective epidural, with suppression of the bearing-down reflex, prevented the metabolic acidosis in the mother. There was still a tendency towards acidosis in the fetus, but this may have been due to the fact that the dorsal lithotomy position was maintained throughout.

Many obstetricians and obstetric anaesthetists now feel that it is acceptable to let the second stage continue for much longer than the above limits and that in these circumstances the fetal head will be brought down into the pelvis by uterine action. This assumes that the mother does not bear down, that she is properly positioned in the full lateral or supine wedged position and that the fetus is being carefully monitored. Spontaneous delivery or outlet forceps can then be carried out easily. Adherence to this regime greatly reduces the need for mid-cavity or rotation forceps, but if they should still be necessary, an effective epidural allows them to be applied painlessly and delivery to be facilitated through a relaxed pelvic floor. The incidence of forceps delivery can also be reduced by using lower concentrations of local anaesthetic agents, but this benefit results in a lower proportion of patients obtaining satisfactory pain relief (Thorburn & Moir 1981).

Indications

Pain relief. The primary indication for lumbar epidural analgesia in labour is the relief of pain and for this it is unsurpassed. Barely 60% of women are satisfied with the pain relief afforded by carefully given parenteral and inhalational methods (Beazley et al 1967), but most centres which have established epidural services claim satisfactory analgesia in about 80% of cases. This figure can be improved on if labour does not progress too fast to allow the anaesthetist to make adjustments to the epidural block.

Pre-eclamptic toxaemia. The blood pressure of toxaemic patients is particularly sensitive to circulating catecholamines. Thus patients with mild, untreated pre-eclampsia may show abrupt increases in blood pressure, particularly during uterine contractions. Patients with more severe pre-eclampsia will be controlled with antihypertensive drugs in the antenatal period, but the blood pressure may 'break through' this control during labour. In both groups an epidural block is often the only treatment required because it relieves pain and produces a mild degree of sympathetic block. However, it is a mistake to try and extend the block higher if the blood pressure does not return to an acceptable level. In such patients further antihypertensive therapy is necessary.

Vaginal breech delivery. Although obstetricians are increasingly favouring elective Caesarean section for the delivery of women with breech presentations, some are still delivered vaginally. These patients sometimes have an uncontrollable urge to bear down before the cervix is fully dilated. This can cause severe oedema and bruising of the cervix, making delivery difficult. The main risk to the infant is damage to the after-coming head, which may be delivered precipitously through a tight pelvic floor, and this may result in intracranial haemorrhage if the infant is premature. Both these problems are admirably managed with epidural analgesia because the bearing-down reflex is eliminated and the obstetrician has gentle control of the head. Earlier fears that epidural analgesia would increase the incidence of breech extraction, with its high incidence of morbidity and mortality, have proved to be unfounded.

Multiple pregnancy. During vaginal delivery the second twin may be at risk from uterine inertia, cord compression or partial separation of the placenta, and modern obstetric opinion favours expediting its delivery. Oxytocin can be used to stimulate the flagging uterus, but if spontaneous delivery does not take place soon, forceps, an assisted breech delivery or even internal version and breech extraction may be required. An effective epidural allows the obstetrician to proceed immediately with the method of his choice without the risks associated with general anaesthesia in these circumstances. If uterine tone is too high to permit version and breech extraction, it has been suggested that inhalation of salbutamol is an effective, but safer, method of producing uterine relaxation than inducing general anaesthesia with halothane.

Premature infants. Many of the above remarks about breech deliveries also apply to premature infants presenting by the vertex. Delivery tends to be precipitate and this increases the risk of intracranial haemorrhage. Epidural analgesia, by abolishing the bearing-down reflex, permits a slow, controlled delivery and avoids the need to give the mother systemic analgesics which may depress the premature infant.

Diabetes mellitus. Diabetic mothers have reduced placental function and their babies consequently have a high perinatal mortality rate. If elective Caesarean section is not planned, labour is usually induced at 37–38 weeks and babies of diabetic mothers benefit from epidural anaesthesia for the same reasons as premature babies.

Cardiovascular disease. It is impossible to generalize about heart disease because of the wide variety of congenital and acquired conditions and all cases should be discussed with a cardiologist. However, if a patient is to have a vaginal delivery, most of the adverse factors are best treated by a carefully given lumbar epidural block. As hypotension is more likely in these patients, the first dose of local anaesthetic should err on the small side. The block allows the use of syntocinon to augment labour without maternal distress and it can then be extended to the sacral segments to avoid the Valsalva manoeuvres which result from uncontrolled bearing-down in the second stage. Furthermore, vasodilatation resulting from epidural block helps to accommodate the increase in venous return in the third stage which occurs as caval occlusion is released and the uterus retracts after delivery. Because of its vasoconstrictor effect, ergometrine should be avoided in these patients. Oxytocin is a safer alternative.

The obstetric anaesthetist is now seeing an increasing number of women who have artificial heart valves. Their cardiac function is often extremely good, but they are usually receiving long-term anticoagulant therapy. The decision as to whether this therapy can be stopped and normal coagulation restored for an epidural to be performed can only be made in close consultation with a cardiologist.

The use of regional anaesthesia for Caesarean section in the rare patient with severe cardiac disease is debatable. Hypotension is much more likely with the high block required for this operation, and there is considerable difficulty in knowing how to react when faced with the sudden changes in cardiovascular haemodynamics which occur during these operations. Many anaesthetists would consider light, muscle relaxant anaesthesia the technique of choice for these patients.

Respiratory disease. Few patients now come to the labour ward with severe disease of the lower respiratory tract. The most likely exceptions are those with asthma or an acute upper respiratory infection which has spread downwards. These patients are likely to be very distressed during hyperventilation and Valsalva manoeuvres and they find lumbar epidural analgesia very helpful.

For Caesarean section, mild respiratory disease has little effect on the choice between general and regional anaesthesia. In more severe cases, the choice depends largely on the degree of productive cough suffered by the patient. Although some might advocate regional block, general anaesthesia prevents repeated coughing (which may make conditions difficult for the surgeon) and also allows the anaesthetist to perform careful tracheo-bronchial toilet before extubation. While these are not sufficient reasons for making general anaesthesia mandatory, it must be remembered that epidural block high enough to allow Caesarean section decreases peak expiratory flow rate and impairs the ability to cough, particularly while the abdomen is open (Gamil 1989). However, an epidural sufficient to produce wound analgesia, started at the end of the operation, does much to help the patient cough effectively thereafter.

Incoordinate uterine action. This is a condition in which painful, but ineffective, uterine contractions produce slow dilatation of the cervix and, eventually, an exhausted patient. It is often associated with maternal vomiting, dehydration, ketosis and indications of fetal distress. Epidural analgesia alone in these cases produces a more normal type of uterine contraction (Moir & Willocks 1967) although oxytocin is administered as well. An intravenous infusion to correct the dehydration and electrolyte imbalance, along with the removal of fear and pain by the epidural, may save the patient an emergency Caesarean section (Moir & Willocks 1967, Maltau & Anderson 1975). Severe examples of this condition are now seldom seen in well-run obstetric units.

Contraindications

It is customary to classify certain conditions as 'absolute' contraindications to epidural anaesthesia in obstetrics. These include a bleeding diathesis, whether iatrogenic or due to disease,

refusal by the patient to accept the technique, skin sepsis near the needle entry site, and inadequate facilities for caring for the patient after the epidural has been performed.

Other conditions are often referred to as 'relative' contraindications. This may be misleading since some of the conditions formerly classified in this way (e.g. vaginal breech delivery) are now considered to be indications. There are, however, certain circumstances where particular care or caution is required.

Hypotension and hypovolaemia. These conditions must always be treated before an epidural is performed, since any sympathetic block reduces the patient's ability to compensate for them. In addition, it is important to establish the underlying cause, because hypotension due to conditions such as pre-eclamptic toxaemia or placental abruption can be associated with coagulation defects.

Neurological disease. Diseases such as multiple sclerosis and myasthenia gravis are sometimes said to be contraindications to epidural block but there seems no obvious reason why the epidural injection of local anaesthetic should worsen these conditions and there is no good evidence that it does so. The quality of life for these patients is already less than perfect, so it seems unreasonable to deprive them of the benefits of an epidural if it is indicated. However, a full explanation should be given to the patient and her agreement obtained.

Previous back trouble or spinal surgery. There is no reason why epidural anaesthesia per se should make this worse. The removal of bony landmarks during previous spinal surgery, and subsequent skin scarring, may make identification of the epidural space difficult. Access to operation notes and radiographs may be helpful in such cases. After spinal surgery — especially some types of spinal fusion — adhesions may form in the epidural space, making access by local anaesthetic to the nerve roots unpredictable. However, Daley and colleagues (1990) have shown that epidural block is almost as effective in patients who have undergone lumbar spinal surgery as in those who have not. If the epidural block is inadequate or the epidural space cannot be found, a spinal may be successful.

Uterine scar. A uterine scar following hysterotomy or previous Caesarean section may rupture during labour. The use of epidural block in these cases is controversial because the pain associated with the impending rupture may be concealed. However, pain is a relatively rare warning of scar rupture and other clinical features, such as fetal distress and vaginal bleeding, are more common. All such patients require meticulous maternal and fetal monitoring whether an epidural is used or not.

Crawford (1976) states that if pain occurs with uterine rupture it 'breaks through' an effective epidural. He calls this effect the epidural 'sieve'. Whether it is always seen in the presence of an effective block with high concentrations of local anaesthetic solution is uncertain and it may be wiser to use a lower concentration of drug (e.g. 0.25% bupivacaine) in these patients.

Complications

The complications of epidural block in general have been discussed in Chapter 8. All of those mentioned may occur in the obstetric patient, but one problem which causes particular concern is the late occurrence of *backache* in patients who have no previous history of it. A recent study has suggested that there may be an increased incidence of symptoms after an obstetric epidural, probably due to the patient adopting spine-stressing postures during labour. Extreme flexion of the lumbar spine is said to be particularly dangerous (MacArthur et al 1990).

Establishment of an epidural service

The setting up of an obstetric epidural service has implications for obstetricians and midwives, as well as for anaesthetists and patients. The first requirement is that all staff should be enthusiastic and understand the part which regional analgesia can play in obstetric practice. Acceptance of the advantages does not always come easily as it may require fundamental changes in obstetric management and in attitudes towards pain in labour. A regular obstetric department meeting is an ideal setting for liaison, discussion and education when an epidural service is being planned. Once the service has been established it serves as a forum at which problems can be ironed out.

It is important that obstetricians and midwives appreciate the effect of epidural analgesia on the clinical features of labour and it is particularly important that everyone concerned has a clear understanding of the aorto-caval syndrome and how its effects may be exacerbated by epidural block. Because of the possible complications associated with epidural analgesia (see Ch. 8), it is vital that a doctor should be available who is competent to pass an endotracheal tube and ventilate the patient, treat hypotension and provide full cardiopulmonary resuscitation in the event of cardiac arrest. An anaesthetist is the most suitable person to provide this service. Ideally he should be resident in the maternity hospital with no other commitment but, if he is required to undertake other duties, they should not be arduous and should not take him far from the obstetric department. The safety of an epidural service depends to a large extent on the anaesthetist's availability. In some units epidurals have been performed by an obstetrician. Although this arrangement has apparently proved satisfactory, there is little justification for it in present day practice. The obstetrician becomes an 'operator–anaesthetist' and on the occasions when he has to decide between epidural and obstetric considerations, he will quite naturally tend to favour the latter. Most obstetricians will admit that, should an emergency arise, they cannot intubate as quickly or carry out cardiopulmonary resuscitation as effectively as an anaesthetist.

Epidural anaesthesia for Caesarean section

Caesarean section is by far the most common major operation regularly performed under unsupplemented regional anaesthesia, and use of the latter in preference to general anaesthesia is increasing for two reasons. More women are requesting it because it enables them to be conscious of, and to enjoy, the birth of the baby. Anaesthetists recognize that the risks of failed tracheal intubation and inhalation of gastric contents are greatly reduced.

Abdominal cavity innervation

The innervation of the abdomen is considered in detail in Chapter 11, but a few points are relevant here. Caesarean section is performed through a lower abdominal incision and while a block to the level of the umbilicus (T_{10}) should be adequate for the skin incision, visceral afferents from intra-abdominal structures reach the spinal cord at levels at least as high as T_5. Even a block to that level will still leave vagal fibres and those from the dia-phragm (C_3–C_5) unaffected, and the obstetrician should therefore prevent blood or liquor from running up under the diaphragm and should handle the bowel gently. Postpartum delivery of the uterus through the incision to facilitate sutur-ing is a potent cause of discomfort and should be avoided whenever possible.

Preoperative visit

Before *elective* Caesarean section no premedication is given, but the anaesthetic technique should be discussed fully with the patient. The anaesthetist should warn her that some sensations may arise from the abdomen even with a good block. The possibility of complete or partial failure can be mentioned and the available remedies outlined. Symptoms and signs of caval occlusion should be sought with care. There is considerable variation in the administration of antacids and H_2 antago-nists prior to Caesarean section. Every obstetric unit should have a clear policy in regard to the use of these drugs. If the epidural is inadequate and a general anaesthetic becomes necessary, an antacid should be given in theatre.

In the *emergency* situation the same principles are followed, although the time for discussion will obviously be short.

Epidural technique

When regional anaesthesia – especially epidural block – is used for Caesarean section, it is fundamental that the surgeon is flexible about the starting time. It is not always possible to predict when the block will be fully effective, but the surgeon must be ready to start as soon as it is. A few patients develop hypotension which is resis-tant to therapy and it is important that the baby is delivered as expeditiously as possible.

Several detailed descriptions of epidural tech-niques for Caesarean section have been published (Milne & Murray Lawson 1973, Thorburn & Moir 1980, Crawford 1980, Laishley & Morgan 1988). The differences between them represent, in part at least, various views on the best way of avoiding problems due either to excessive height of block or to inadequate spread. Most obstetric anaesthetists insert the catheter at the second or third lumbar interspace and inject 0.5% bupiva-caine (or 2% lignocaine with adrenaline).

Mode of injection. In essence, there are two approaches to injection and dosage once the test dose has been administered. The first is to give the full dose (15–20 ml depending on the patient's size) as one bolus. This may be injected through the needle (Laishley & Morgan 1988) or the catheter but, whichever route is chosen, it is essential that it is injected slowly, and that constant verbal contact is maintained with the patient. This ensures that an intravascular injection is detected before a large mass of drug has been given. The single-bolus technique is simple and has the advantage of rapid onset. However, the block may be patchy (Thorburn & Moir 1980, Laishley & Morgan 1988). In addition, hypotension may be marked if the block spreads higher than needed, and maternal plasma concentrations of local anaesthetic are greater than after an incremental technique (Thompson et al 1985).

The second approach is to give two smaller increments (8–10 ml) separated by an interval of 5–10 minutes. This repeated application of drug aims to reduce the incidence of patchy blocks. If after a third or fourth increment the block is still inadequate, or is spreading slowly, a physical obstruction to the flow of solution is probably present within the epidural space. Whichever technique is used – single bolus or incremental – analgesia from T_4 to the lowest sacral segment is necessary.

Posture. Traditionally, obstetric epidural block is induced with the patient in the 'wedged' lateral position to minimize aorto-caval occlusion, although there is no reason for preferring this to alternate full lateral positions (Carrie 1989). In order to avoid unilateral block, the patient is turned from one side to the other, usually when a second increment is injected. Thorburn & Moir (1980) recommend that the patient should sit for the first 10 minutes after injection to improve anaesthesia in the sacral segments, but it is doubtful whether this produces a significantly better block.

Inadequate block. There are four remedies to this problem (Carrie 1986). A general anaesthetic may be given, especially if time is short, but this is a disappointment for all concerned. The use of yet more local anaesthetic has been advocated but carries the risk of severe systemic toxicity. Thorburn & Moir (1984) reported convulsions in two patients given large volumes of local anaesthetic in an attempt to extend recalcitrant lumbar epidural blocks. Those skilled in thoracic epidural analgesia might perform such a block above the level of any obstruction. A small volume (5–6 ml) is almost invariably effective since it is deposited precisely at the required segment. Lastly, a spinal anaesthetic may be induced. This is the method of choice where the epidural block has developed in such a patchy or asymmetrical way that a small volume of local anaesthetic in the thoracic region is unlikely to complete the required spread of analgesia.

"Other factors". 'Fractionated' techniques, as outlined above, are used widely and successfully, but they have the disadvantage of being very time-consuming and the surgeon has to be very flexible about the starting time. These adverse factors may account for the increasing popularity of spinal anaesthesia in busy obstetric units.

It is also important to consider the systemic concentrations of local anaesthetic produced by the various techniques. Thompson and colleagues (1985) measured venous bupivacaine concentrations in several groups of patients. In the elective groups, the bolus technique resulted in greater concentrations than with the incremental method, but the highest concentrations were found in patients who were having emergency Caesarean section after a block had been in use during labour and toxic convulsions have been reported in these circumstances (Thorburn & Moir 1984). Obstetric anaesthetists must beware that, in avoiding the

hazards associated with general anaesthesia, they do not subject their patients to overdosage of local anaesthetic.

Hypotension is related to speed of onset of the block, and also to aorto-caval occlusion. All the methods produce an incidence of hypotension, but this is less if the patient is turned from one full lateral position to the other until the block is effective. The author uses this technique and turns the patient into the supine 'wedged' position just before surgery. Hypotension severe enough to require ephedrine is unusual.

Bupivacaine and lignocaine in various formulations are the local anaesthetic agents used in the UK for obstetric epidural anaesthesia. The former, in 0.5% concentration, has been the preferred solution for many years, but dissatisfaction with its ability to provide effective analgesia in awake patients has led to a reappraisal of 2% lignocaine with 1:200 000 adrenaline. Despite the enthusiasm for this solution, there has been little controlled work comparing it with other solutions. Although one investigation suggested that it is quicker in onset and gives a more effective block than 0.5% bupivacaine, the same study found it to be inferior in both these respects to 0.5% bupivacaine with adrenaline (Howell et al 1990). However, the adrenaline was added 'fresh' to the plain solutions, resulting in a solution of bupivacaine with adrenaline having a higher pH than that commercially available, a factor which might enhance its rate of onset.

Patient management

Every attempt should be made to prevent caval compression, and an inflatable wedge (Carrie 1982) will allow the degree of lateral tilt to be varied during the procedure. Full-length elastic stockings will help decrease venous pooling in the lower limbs. A large-bore intravenous cannula is essential so that blood volume can be maintained if much bleeding occurs. The author infuses 1–1.5 litres of crystalloid immediately before and during onset of the block, the timing being more important than the volume since the crystalloid passes rapidly out of the circulation. Because of this, some have recommended colloid for preloading, but this has been shown to be no more effective than crystalloid (Ramanathan et al 1983) and all colloids carry a small risk of severe anaphylactoid reactions. If a vasopressor is required, the drug usually recommended is ephedrine (which has a predominantly β-adrenergic action) because investigation in animals has shown that drugs with a predominanttly α-adrenergic effect may cause fetal asphyxia by producing vasoconstriction in the uteroplacental circulation. However, Ramanathan & Grant (1988), in a careful comparison of ephedrine and phenylephrine, found that both drugs were equally effective and without adverse affect on the fetus, but that phenylephrine produced less tachycardia. Furthermore, they concluded that both drugs act by an α-adrenergic effect on capacitance vessels, resulting in an increase in the preload. The circulation should be monitored closely during the establishment of the block and, in the interests of the baby, oxygen should be administered to the mother until after delivery.

In the conscious patient, syntocinon is the oxytocic of choice. After delivery 5 IU is given as a bolus and another 15–20 IU should be infused over the next hour because the effect is transient.

There is little point in sedating a pain-free, relaxed patient after the baby is born. The company of her new baby and her husband, if present, is all the distraction that is required. Minor discomforts during the operation are managed by reassurance and the inhalation of a low concentration (e.g. 30%) of nitrous oxide. Potent intravenous sedatives (e.g. diazepam) are ineffective or unsafe in this situation, but small increments of an opioid (e.g. 1–2 mg of diamorphine), although seldom necessary, may be used after delivery. Proper assessment of the block prior to surgery should ensure that it is never necessary to administer a general anaesthetic during the procedure because of pain.

Both local anaesthetic and opioids may be injected epidurally to control postoperative pain. Most women resent the numbness which even dilute solutions of local anaesthetic produce because the immobility enforced by the continuation of the block interferes with their ability to care for their newborn babies. Epidural opioids allow greater mobility, and fentanyl 50 μg plus 0.5% bupivacaine 2 ml, in 6 ml of normal saline usually gives excellent pain control, without numbness, for 2–5 hours. However, the risk of respiratory depression must be kept in mind and an appropriate level of nursing supervision provided.

SPINAL ANAESTHESIA

Varieties of block

Both from a practical point of view and for the purposes of discussion, it is useful to identify three levels of spinal block in obstetrics. Techniques for producing these have been described in Chapter 7 and they may be applied to the obstetric patient, but there is some evidence that intrathecal drugs spread further in the pregnant patient and this should be taken into account. Hyperbaric solutions are perhaps more predictable than plain ones in this situation.

Low, or saddle, block

This was first used by Burton of Stoke on Trent (Burton 1943), who coined the term 'saddle back' anaesthesia and later by Resnick of Salford (Resnick 1945). Adriani popularized the term 'saddle block' (Adriani & Roma Vega 1946). It anaesthetizes the vagina, vulva and perineum, so the extent of analgesia is limited, being adequate for a low forceps delivery or an episiotomy repair, but not much else. It has no effect on the pain of uterine contractions, nor is there any analgesia for intrauterine manipulation.

Mid-spinal block

In obstetric practice the aim of this block is to produce analgesia of the whole birth canal so that the pain of uterine contraction is abolished, and intrauterine manipulation and operative vaginal delivery can be carried out painlessly. The block is therefore suitable for all types of forceps delivery, for breech delivery and for manual removal of a retained placenta. Rather than use the technique described in Chapter 7, the author injects a hyperbaric solution with the patient on her left side and tilts the table about 10° head-up. The L_2–L_3 interspace is preferred so that the solution has not far to spread to reach T_{11}, the upper level required. After injection the patient is immediately turned supine, but 'wedged' to the right.

High spinal block

Anaesthesia to the mid-thoracic level permits the performance of Caesarean section, although a profound block of reasonably long duration is needed. In most circumstances this can be ensured by injecting a slightly larger than usual dose of local anaesthetic, but in the pregnant patient the risk of excessive spread must be countered. With 0.5% hyperbaric bupivacaine, the following technique produces excellent results and maintains the full lateral position (to minimize caval occlusion) for as long as possible.

The operating table is tilted 5–10° head-down and the patient is placed on her left side with an inflatable wedge under her shoulder and three pillows under her head. This produces a gradient between the mid-thoracic and cervical sections of the spine and should result in a high concentration of local anaesthetic restricted to mid-thoracic level. After the injection of 2.5–3.0 ml of hyperbaric bupivacaine the patient is turned into an identical position on her right side. The onset of the block is noted at 2 minute intervals and postural adjustments are made if necessary. Just before the start of surgery the supine 'wedged' position is assumed and one of the three pillows is removed.

Advantages

A major advantage of spinal anaesthesia over epidural block is its *speed of onset*. Often the patient, if in labour, does not feel the first uterine contraction after injection of local anaesthetic, and surgical anaesthesia is excellent within minutes. This means that a skilled anaesthetist can block the whole birth canal about 10 minutes after approaching the patient, whereas nearer 30 minutes would be required with an epidural technique. Another advantage of spinal anaesthesia is its *reliability*. Unblocked segments, which are some-

times a problem during epidural block, are rarely if ever encountered. A third advantage is the almost complete *lack of systemic drug toxicity*. No other technique, be it general or regional, can provide such extensive anaesthesia with such a small amount of drug.

Disadvantages

Unfortunately, *post-lumbar puncture headache* has its highest incidence in women of child-bearing age and it may be that the pregnant woman is especially prone to this complication. A severe headache, which is worse when the patient is sitting or standing, is particularly distressing because it interferes with the mother's attempts to feed and care for her new baby. The incidence is related to needle size and is 3–10% even with 26 g needles, so 29 g and 30 g sizes have been tried (Carrie & Collins 1991, Lesser et at 1990). However, they are more difficult to use (Flaatten et al 1989, Dahl et al 1990, Lesser et al 1990) and there are manufacturing problems in bonding transparent hubs to such fine shafts. These disadvantages have led to the reassessment of needles with atraumatic or 'pencil-point' tips first described over 40 years ago (Haraldson 1951, Hart & Whitacre 1951). Fine-gauge versions (24 g and 27 g) are now available, and the early results are encouraging, the incidence of headache being reduced to less than 2% (Cesarini et al 1990, Carrie & Donald 1991). This suggests that needles of this design should be used whenever possible in obstetrics. Although the need for treatment with an epidural blood patch should be infrequent, it is reassuring to know that this almost certain cure is available if required.

As already mentioned, aorto-caval occlusion makes *hypotension* more likely in the pregnant patient when the sympathetic outflow is blocked. Hypotension should not be produced by a saddle block, but it is a possibility with mid-spinal and quite likely with high spinal block. Spinals tend to produce a higher incidence of, and more profound, hypotension than epidural blocks of similar extent, probably because of the faster onset which allows less time for compensatory vasoconstriction to occur in unaffected sympathetic segments.

Prophylaxis in the case of saddle and mid-spinal block consists only of avoiding the supine position until after the baby is born and preloading with up to 1 litre of crystalloid. During high spinal block for Caesarean section prophylaxis is as for epidural block, but many consider that a vasopressor should also be given routinely (Moya & Smith 1962, Shnider 1970, Gutsche 1976). Ephedrine 50 mg in 500 ml titrated against blood pressure is particularly effective (Kang et al 1982). As for epidural block, it may be that phenylephrine or other vasopressors will gain in popularity.

A third potential disadvantage of spinal anaesthesia is the possibility of *respiratory depression* with a high block. In the non-pregnant patient, even a block which produces paralysis of all the intercostal muscles leaves the innervation of the diaphragm (C_3–C_5) unaffected, and consequently the patient has adequate respiratory reserve. However, in the recumbent, pregnant patient the gravid uterus may hinder diaphragmatic respiration, so in theory a motor block extending into the upper thoracic region might produce respiratory embarrassment. In practice, most patients tolerate a high spinal or epidural block perfectly well, possibly because the differential nature of the block at its upper limit leaves motor function intact.

The remaining disadvantage of spinals is that they are usually used as *single-shot techniques* in the UK because most anaesthetists are reluctant to insert catheters into the subarachnoid space. Two of the benefits of an epidural are therefore lost – the ability to extend the analgesia produced by the initial dose of local anaesthetic, and the provision of postoperative pain control.

It was hoped that the development of extremely fine (32 g) polyimide catheters, which will pass through 26 g spinal needles, might make continuous spinal block a more feasible proposition, even in obstetric patients. However, case reports of cauda equina syndrome following the use of hyperbaric solutions for continuous spinal block in the USA have cast doubt on the safety of the technique (Rigler et al 1991).

The advantages of both spinal and epidural blocks can be obtained by use of the *combined spinal–epidural technique*. The spinal provides speed of onset, reliability and low toxicity, while the epidural catheter allows modification of the block and provision of postoperative analgesia. The most popular version of the technique involves locating the epidural space with a Tuohy needle and passing a longer needle through it into the subarachnoid space. After the spinal anaesthetic has been injected, the spinal needle is withdrawn and an epidural catheter passed through the Tuohy needle (Carrie & O'Sullivan 1984). The epidural needle is a useful guide for the fine-gauge spinal needle and excellent results have been obtained using both 26 g and 29 g Quincke and 26 g pencil-point needles (Carrie & Collins 1991, Carrie & Donald 1991). If a hyperbaric solution is used, it may be 'trapped' in an appropriate region of the subarachnoid space (usually mid- to upper thoracic) while the epidural catheter is being introduced (Carrie 1990). This is achieved by placing the patient in the lateral position, with a support under the dependent shoulder and three or four pillows under the head to produce additional lateral flexion of the cervical and upper thoracic spines. After the catheter has been inserted, the patient is turned to the identical position on the other side.

An alternative method is that described by Brownridge (1981), who inserts the epidural catheter first and then performs the spinal block at a different interspace.

Indications

Increasingly, spinal anaesthesia is being used as an alternative to epidural block for Caesarean section and, as stated above, there are good reasons for making this part of a combined spinal–epidural technique. The other group of indications for its use comprises vaginal procedures where *quick, reliable analgesia* is required in cases where an epidural catheter is not already in situ. This includes rotational forceps delivery, breech presentation and twin deliveries where urgent surgical intervention may be required in the interests of the second twin. The sudden return of the mother's comfort and self-control in these cases, without incurring the dangers of emergency general anaesthesia, is most impressive and it should be the technique of choice in these situations.

Other indications for spinal anaesthesia are insertion of a *cervical circumsuture*, or any situation in which *epidural anaesthesia has failed*, especially for Caesarean section (see under 'Epidural anaesthesia for Caesarean section', above).

OTHER TECHNIQUES

Spinal and lumbar epidural blocks can be used not only to provide analgesia for labour, but also for most types of obstetric surgery. However, other more peripheral techniques are also useful in obstetrics and these will be described briefly.

Local infiltration

Local infiltration with solution such as 0.5% lignocaine with 1:200 000 adrenaline provides good analgesia for outlet forceps delivery or an episiotomy and its repair, but a severe tear requires a more extensive block. It is possible to perform Caesarean section under local infiltration alone. Essentially, the technique consists of liberal infiltration with dilute local anaesthetic solution by the surgeon, each layer being infiltrated prior to incision. The analgesia can leave much to be desired, but may be acceptable in the most primitive or desperate circumstances. Large volumes of solution are required, so 0.25% lignocaine with 1:400 000 adrenaline or 1% plain procaine (Ranney & Stanage 1975) are the agents of choice.

Pudendal block

This requires bilateral injection of the pudendal nerves in the region of the ischial spines (Eriksson 1969). Usually a transvaginal approach is used with a guarded needle, but a transperineal approach, using a 10 cm needle, has the advantage that the perineal branches of the posterior cutaneous nerve of the thigh can be blocked through the same injection site. Either method should be accompanied by infiltration of the labia to block the perineal branches of the ilio-inguinal and genitofemoral nerves. The technique gives good analgesia for low and some mid-cavity forceps deliveries, but if much traction or intrauterine manipulation is required pain relief will be inade-

quate. Being a purely somatic block, it has no effect on the pain of uterine contraction. In a carefully performed trial, Scudamore & Yates (1966) found that only 36% of pudendal blocks gave effective, bilateral analgesia of the perineum and vulva, and concluded that much of the apparent efficacy of pudendal blocks was due to the associated local infiltration of the labia and perineum. This low success rate may seem surprising, but the study was carried out by experienced operators in ideal conditions.

Paracervical block

This is a purely visceral afferent block, so it relieves the pain of uterine contractions, but not that transmitted in somatic fibres during the second stage. Bilateral injections of local anaesthetic solution are made into the parametrium at the base of the broad ligament lateral to the cervix, so that the sensory nerves are blocked as they leave the uterus. The technique enjoyed considerable popularity in some countries – particularly the USA – but not in the UK. Suspicions that the method could have adverse effects on the fetus were confirmed by the more widespread use of continuous fetal heart monitoring, which showed a high incidence of bradycardia. The technique is associated with an increased incidence of depressed neonates and occasionally even intrauterine death. Initially it was concluded that the absorption of the local anaesthetic from the intervillous space produced a toxic effect on the fetal myocardium. More recent work has shown that the application of local anaesthetic to a section of uterine artery from a pregnant human or ewe caused marked vasoconstriction (Cibils 1976, Greiss et al 1976). This occurred at a concentration of local anaesthetic likely to be obtained during paracervical block.

If they are to provide complete pain relief in the second stage of labour, bilateral paracervical blocks have to be supplemented with bilateral pudendal blocks. Since up to 10 ml of solution is required for each block, there is a real risk of a toxic reaction in the mother, especially if previous doses of anaesthetic have been given. In the face of the clinical and experimental evidence, there seems little justification for the continued use of paracervical blocks in obstetrics.

Lumbar sympathetic chain and paravertebral blocks

These two blocks have been used to relieve the pain of the first stage of labour. They have the disadvantage of requiring bilateral, multiple injections and are of historical interest only, paravertebral block being the method by which Cleland (1933) originally identified the spinal segments involved in the pain of the first stage of labour.

Sacral epidural (caudal) block

Caudal blocks (usually performed by the obstetrician) were popular in a few centres in the UK before lumbar epidural analgesia provided by anaesthetists became more freely available. Even in units with well-established caudal services the method soon disappeared in competition with the lumbar route because of several major disadvantages: greater pain on insertion of the needle; a

higher failure rate because of anatomical variations in the sacral hiatus; the necessity for much larger (and potentially more toxic) volumes of local anaesthetic; unnecessarily early analgesia in the sacral segments, usually with motor block of the lower limbs; a theoretically greater risk of infection; and the possibility of piercing the fetal skull and injecting a lethal dose of local anaesthetic if the block is performed late in labour (Finster et al 1965).

There are two claimed advantages for the caudal over the lumbar epidural route. Firstly there is said to be less risk of dural puncture, though since Trotter (1947) found that the distance from the sacral hiatus to the lower end of the dural sac could be as little as 1.6 cm this is debatable. It is also alleged that there is a more rapid onset of analgesia in the sacral segments, but if speed is necessary a spinal block has an even more rapid onset. Few obstetric anaesthetists would disagree that lumbar epidural and spinal block will suit most situations and that the caudal approach should be reserved for situations when there are technical difficulties with the lumbar route.

REFERENCES

Abboud T K, Sarkis F, Blikian A, Varakian L, Earl S, Henriksen E 1983a Lack of adverse neonatal neurobehavioral effects of lidocaine. Anesthesia and Analgesia (Current Researches) 62: 473–475

Abboud T K, Kyung C K, Noueihed R, Kuhnert B K, DerMardirossian N, Moumdjian J, Sarkis F, Nagappala S 1983b Epidural bupivacaine, chloroprocaine, or lidocaine for Cesarean section – maternal and neonatal effects. Anesthesia and Analgesia (Current Researches) 62: 914–919

Adriani J, Roma Vega D 1946 Saddle block anesthesia. American Journal of Surgery 71: 12–18

Amiel-Tison C, Barrier G, Shnider S M, Levinson G, Hughes S C, Stefani S J 1982 A new neurologic and adaptive capacity scoring system for evaluating obstetric medications in full-term newborns. Anesthesiology 56: 340–350

Beazley J M, Leaver E P, Morewood J H M, Bircumshaw J 1967 Relief of pain in labour. Lancet i: 1033–1035

Bonica J J 1979 Peripheral mechanisms and pathways of parturition pain. British Journal of Anaesthesia 51(Supplement 1): 3–9

Brownridge P 1981 Epidural and subarachnoid analgesia for elective Caesarean section. Anaesthesia 36: 70

Burton H 1943 Low spinal anaesthesia during labour in cases of cardiac failure. British Medical Journal ii: 389–390

Carrie L E S 1982 An inflatable obstetric anaesthetic 'wedge'. Anaesthesia 37: 745–747

Carrie L E S 1986 Local analgesic convulsions and epidural analgesia for Caesarean section. Anaesthesia 41: 87

Carrie L E S 1989 A plea for lateral thinking by obstetric anaesthetists. Anaesthesia 44: 145–146

Carrie L E S 1990 Spinal and/or epidural blockade for Caesarean section. In: Reynolds F (ed) Epidural and spinal blockade in obstetrics, pp 146–148. Baillière Tindall, London

Carrie L E S, Collins P D 1991 29-gauge spinal needles. British Journal of Anaesthesia 66: 145–146

Carrie L E S, Donald F 1991 A 26-gauge pencil-point needle for combined-epidural anaesthesia for Caesarean section. Anaesthesia 46: 230–231

Carrie L E S, O'Sullivan G M 1984 Subarachnoid bupivacaine 0.5% for Caesarean section. European Journal of Anaesthesia 1: 275–283

Caseby N G 1974 Epidural analgesia for the surgical induction of labour. British Journal of Anaesthesia 46: 747–751

Cesarini M, Torrielli R, Lahaye F, Mene J M, Cabiro C 1990 Sprotte needle for intrathecal anaesthesia for Caesarean section: incidence of postdural puncture headache. Anaesthesia 45: 656–658

Chestnut D H, Owen C L, Bates J N, Ostman L G, Choi W W, Geiger M W 1988 Continuous infusion epidural analgesia during labor: a randomized, double-blind comparison of 0.0625% bupivacaine/0.0002% fentanyl versus 0.125% bupivacaine. Anesthesiology 68: 754–759

Cibils L A 1976 Response of human uterine arteries to local anesthetics. American Journal of Obstetrics and Gynecology 126: 202–210

Cleland J G P 1933 Paravertebral anesthesia in obstetrics, experimental and clinical basis. Surgery, Gynecology and Obstetrics 57: 51–54

Corke B C 1977 Neurobehavioural responses of the newborn. Anaesthesia 32: 539–543

Crawford J S 1972 The second thousand epidural blocks in an obstetric hospital practice. British Journal of Anaesthesia 44: 1277–1287

Crawford J S 1976 The epidural sieve and MBC (minimum blocking concentration): an hypothesis. Anaesthesia 31: 1277–1280

Crawford J S 1980 Experiences with lumbar extradural analgesia for Caesarean section. British Journal of Anaesthesia 52: 821–825

Dahl J B, Schultz P, Anker-Moller E, Christensen E F, Staunstrup H G, Carlsson P 1990 Spinal anaesthesia in young patients using a 29-gauge needle: technical considerations and an evaluation of postoperative complaints compared with general anaesthesia. British Journal of Anaesthesia 64: 178–182

Daley M D, Rolbin S H, Hew E M, Morningstar B A, Stewart J A 1990 Epidural anesthesia for obstetrics after spinal surgery. Regional Anesthesia 15: 280–284

Eriksson E 1969 (ed) Illustrated handbook in local anaesthesia, pp 94–96. Munksgaard, Copenhagen

Finster M, Poppers P J, Sinclair J C, Morishima H O, Daniel S S 1965 Accidental intoxication of the fetus with local anesthetic drug during caudal anesthesia. American Journal of Obstetrics and Gynecology 92: 922–924

Flaatten H, Rodt S A, Vamnes J, Rosland J, Koller M E 1989 Postdural puncture headache. A comparison between 26- and 29- gauge needles in young patients. Anaesthesia 44: 147–149

Gamil M 1989 Serial peak expiratory flow rates in mothers during Caesarean section under extradural anaesthesia. British Journal of Anaesthesia 62: 415–418

Greiss F C, Still J G, Anderson S G 1976 Effects of local anesthetic agents on the uterine vasculature and myometrium. American Journal of Obstetrics and Gynecology 124: 889–898

Gutsche B 1976 Prophylactic ephedrine preceding spinal analgesia for Cesarean section. Anesthesiology 45: 462–465

Haraldson S 1951 Headache after spinal anesthesia: experiments with a new spinal needle. Anesthesiology 12: 321–327

Hart J R, Whitacre R J 1951 Pencil-point needle in prevention of postspinal headache. Journal of the American Medical Association 147: 657–658

Hodgkinson R, Marx G F, Kim S S, Miclat N M 1977 Neonatal neurobehavioral tests following vaginal delivery under ketamine, thiopental and extradural anesthesia. Anesthesia and Analgesia (Current Researches) 56: 548–552

Hollmen A I, Jouppila R, Koivisto M, Maatta L, Pihlajaniemi R, Puuka M, Rantakyla P 1978 Neurological activity of infants following anesthesia for Caesarean section. Anesthesiology 48: 350–356

Hollmen A I, Jouppila R, Jouppila P, Koivula A, Vierola H 1982 Effect of extradural analgesia using bupivacaine and 2-chloroprocaine on intervillous blood flow during normal labour. British Journal of Anaesthesia 54: 837–842

Howell P, Davies W, Wrigley M, Tan P, Moran B 1990 Comparison of four local extradural anaesthetic solutions for elective Caesarean section. British Journal of Anaesthesia 65: 648–653

Jouppila R, Jouppila P, Kuikka J, Hollmen A 1978a Placental blood flow during Caesarean section under lumbar extradural analgesia. British Journal of Anaesthesia 50: 275–279

Jouppila R, Jouppila P, Hollmen A, Kuikka J, 1978b Effect of segmental extradural analgesia on placental blood flow during normal labour. British Journal of Anaesthesia 50: 563–567

Jouppila P, Jouppila R, Hollmen A, Koivula A 1982 Lumbar epidural analgesia to improve intervillous blood flow during labor in severe pre-eclampsia. Obstetrics and Gynecology 59: 158–161

Kang Y G, Abouleish E, Caritis S 1982 Prophylactic intravenous ephedrine infusion during spinal anesthesia for Cesarean section. Anesthesia and Analgesia (Current Researches) 61: 839–842

Kileff M E, James F M, Dewan D M, Floyd H M 1984 Neonatal neurobehavioral responses after epidural anesthesia for Cesarean section using lidocaine and bupivacaine. Anesthesia and Analgesia (Current Researches) 63: 413–417

Kuhnert B K, Harrison M J, Linn P L, Kuhbert P M 1984 Effects of maternal epidural anesthesia on neonatal behavior. Anesthesia and Analgesia (Current Researches) 63: 301–308

Laishley R S, Morgan B M 1988 A single dose epidural technique for Caesarean section. A comparison between 0.5% bupivacaine plain and 0.5% bupivacaine with adrenaline. Anaesthesia 43: 100–103

Lesser P, Bembridge M, Lyons G, MacDonald R 1990 An evaluation of a 30-gauge needle for spinal anaesthesia for Caesarean section. Anaesthesia 45: 767–768

MacArthur C, Lewis M, Knox E G, Crawford J S 1990 Epidural anaesthesia and long term backache after childbirth. British Medical Journal 301: 9–12

McGuinness G A, Merkow A J, Kennedy R L, Erenberg A 1978 Epidural anesthesia with bupivacaine for Cesarean section. Anesthesiology 49: 270–273

Maltau J M, Anderson H T 1975 Epidural anaesthesia as an alternative to Caesarean section in the treatment of prolonged exhaustive labour. Acta Anaesthesiologica Scandinavica 19: 349–354

Milne M K, Murray Lawson J I 1973 Epidural analgesia for Caesarean section. British Journal of Anaesthesia 45: 1206–1210

Moir D D, Willocks J 1967 Management of inco-ordinate uterine action under continuous epidural analgesia. British Medical Journal iii: 396–400

Morgan B M, Aulakh J M, Barker J P, Reginald P W, Goroszeniuk T, Trojanowski A 1984 Anaesthetic morbidity following Caesarean section under epidural or general anaesthesia. Lancet i: 328–330

Moya F, Smith B 1962 Spinal anesthesia for Caesarean

section. Journal of the American Medical Association 179: 609–614

Naulty J S, Ross R, Bergen W 1989 Epidural sufentanil–bupivacaine for analgesia during labor and delivery. Anesthesiology 71: A842

Pearson J F, Davies P 1974 The effect of continuous lumbar epidural analgesia upon foetal acid–base status during the second stage of labour. British Journal of Obstetrics and Gynaecology 81: 957–979

Ramanathan S, Grant G J 1988 Vasopressor therapy for hypotension due to epidural anesthesia Caesarean section. Acta Anaesthesiologica Scandinavica 32: 559–565

Ramanathan S, Masih A, Rock I, Chalon J, Turndorf H 1983 Maternal and fetal effects of prophylactic hydration with crystalloids or colloids before epidural anesthesia. Anesthesia and Analgesia 62: 673–678

Ranney B, Stanage W F 1975 Advantages of local anesthesia for Cesarean section. Obstetrics and Gynecology 45: 163–167

Rekonen A, Luotola H, Pitkanen M, Kuikka J, Pyorala T 1976 Measurement of intervillous and myometrial blood flow by an intravenous ^{133}Xe method. British Journal of Obstetrics and Gynaecology 83: 723–728

Resnick I 1945 Heavy Nupercaine spinal analgesia in operative obstetrics with report on 394 cases. British Medical Journal 2: 722–723

Reynolds F, O'Sullivan G 1989 Epidural fentanyl and perineal pain in labour. Anaesthesia 44: 341–344

Reynolds F, Hargrove R L, Wyman J B 1973 Maternal and foetal concentrations of bupivacaine after epidural block. British Journal of Anaesthesia 45: 1049–1053

Rigler M L, Drasner K, Krejcie T C, Yelick S J, Schohuck F T, DeFontes J, Bohner D 1991 Cauda equina syndrome after continuous spinal anesthesia. Anesthesia and Analgesia 72: 275–281

Scanlon J W, Brown W U, Weiss J B, Alper M H 1974 Neurobehavioral responses of newborn infants after maternal epidural anesthesia. Anesthesiology 40: 121–128

Scanlon J W, Ostheimer G W, Lurie A C, Brown W U, Weiss J B 1976 Neurobehavioral responses and drug concentrations in newborns after maternal epidural anesthesia and bupivacaine. Anesthesiology 45: 400–405

Schellenberg J C 1979 Uterine activity during lumbar epidural analgesia with bupivacaine. American Journal of Obstetrics and Gynecology 127: 26–31

Scudamore J H, Yates M J 1966 Pudendal block – a misnomer? Lancet i: 23–24

Shnider S M 1970 Obstetrical anesthesia. Current concepts and practice, pp 94–106. Williams and Wilkins, Baltimore

Singh A 1967 Unilateral epidural analgesia. Anaesthesia 22: 147–149

Studd J W W, Crawford J S, Duignan N M, Rowbotham C J F, Hughes A O 1980 The effect of lumbar epidural analgesia on the rate of cervical dilation and the outcome of labour of spontaneous onset. British Journal of Obstetrics and Gynaecology 87: 1015–1021

Thompson E M, Wilson C M, Moore J, McClean E 1985 Plasma bupivacaine levels associated with extradural anaesthesia for Caesarean section. Anaesthesia 40: 427–432

Thorburn J, Moir D D 1980 Epidural analgesia for elective Caesarean section. Anaesthesia 35: 3–6

Thorburn J, Moir D D 1981 Extradural analgesia: the influence of volume and concentration of bupivacaine on the mode of delivery, analgesic efficacy and motor block. British Journal of Anaesthesia 53: 933–939

Thorburn J, Moir D D 1984 Bupivacaine toxicity in association with extradural analgesia for Caesarean section. British Journal of Anaesthesia 56: 551–553

Trotter M 1947 Variations of the sacral canal: their significance in the administration of caudal analgesia. Current Researches in Anesthesia and Analgesia 26: 192–202

Wiener P C, Hogg M I, Rosen M 1977 Neurobehavioural changes in neonates following maternal pethidine and bupivacaine administration and the effect of naloxone hydrochloride. Anaesthesia 32: 99

11. Regional anaesthesia of the trunk

D. G. Littlewood   A. Lee

The somatic innervation

The thoracic and first lumbar spinal cord segments supply the major part of the innervation of the trunk (see Fig. 3.6). The course, branches and relations of the first 11 thoracic nerves are sufficiently similar to allow them to be described as 'typical' segmental nerves (Fig. 11.1). Each has a ventral and a dorsal ramus, the latter passing posteriorly to supply the muscles and skin of the paravertebral region. Close to its origin the ventral ramus communicates with the associated sympathetic ganglion through the white and grey rami communicantes. It then continues as the intercostal nerve which has three main branches:

1. *The lateral cutaneous branch* arises approximately in the mid-axillary line and pierces the internal and external intercostal muscles obliquely before dividing into anterior and posterior branches. The anterior branch runs forward to supply skin over the pectoral region (T_1–T_6) or that of the anterior abdominal wall (T_7–T_{12}). The posterior supplies skin over the scapula and latissimus dorsi.
2. *The anterior terminal branch* pierces the external intercostal and pectoralis major muscles to supply the skin of the anterior part of the thorax near the midline (T_1–T_6) or pierces the posterior rectus sheath to supply the rectus muscle and the overlying skin (T_7–T_{12}).
3. *A collateral branch* arises from most nerves in the posterior intercostal space and runs forward in the inferior part of the space. It

lies parallel to the main nerve and may rejoin it anteriorly or end as a separate anterior cutaneous nerve.

Other branches exist, but are less easily defined. Numerous slender filaments supply the intercostal muscles and parietal pleura and these branches may cross to adjoining intercostal spaces.

Exceptions to this typical pattern occur at either end of the thoracic outflow. Most of the fibres from T_1 join those from C_8 to form the inferior trunk of the brachial plexus. Some fibres from T_2 and T_3 join to form the intercostobrachial nerve which supplies the medial aspect of the upper arm. The nerve from T_{12} is subcostal and most of its ventral ramus joins that of L_1 to form the iliohypogastric, ilio-inguinal and genitofemoral nerves (Fig. 11.2).

The course and relations of an intercostal nerve (Fig. 11.1) must be understood if safe, effective blocks are to be produced. In its most posterior course, medial to the angle of the rib, the nerve lies deep to the posterior intercostal membrane with very little tissue separating it from the pleura. At the angle of the rib it comes to lie in the subcostal groove, inferior to the intercostal artery and between the subcostal and internal intercostal muscles. The nerve continues in the subcostal groove until it reaches the anterior end of the space. It is apparent that any solution placed in the same tissue plane as the nerve may track centrally and gain access to the paravertebral space, the sympathetic ganglion and even the epidural space. Posteriorly, at least, there are communications with the adjacent spaces.

153

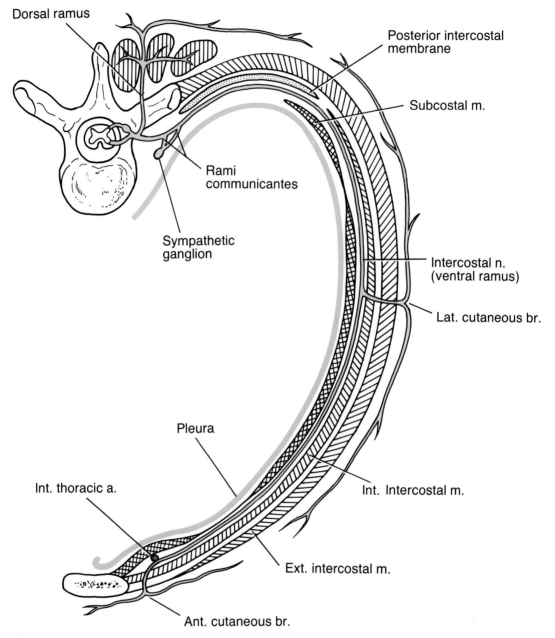

Fig. 11.1 Anatomy of a typical intercostal nerve. The recurrent and smaller muscular branches have been omitted.

These nerves may be blocked at several 'central' sites, that is, in the subarachnoid, epidural and paravertebral spaces. More peripherally the intercostal nerves and even their cutaneous branches may be blocked.

The autonomic innervation (Fig. 11.3)

The 12 thoracic, together with the first and occasionally the second lumbar, segments give rise to the entire sympathetic innervation of the trunk.

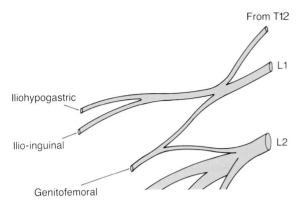

Fig. 11.2 Formation of the nerves supplying the inguinal region.

The parasympathetic supply is primarily through the vagus, which runs a completely separate anatomical course. The pelvic viscera receive their parasympathetic supply through the second to fourth sacral nerves. Preganglionic sympathetic fibres from each segment run forward from the intervertebral foramen in white rami communicantes to the paravertebral sympathetic ganglia where they either synapse diffusely or pass uninterrupted to peripheral sites such as the coeliac plexus and adrenal glands. In the thoracic region the sympathetic chain and ganglia are located immediately anterior to the heads or necks of the ribs and from there postsynaptic fibres travel to segmental nerves in the grey rami communicantes (Fig. 11.3).

The sympathetic outflow from T_1 to T_3 forms the stellate ganglion which lies in the thoracic inlet, anterior to the neck of the first rib in close proximity to the vertebral artery and the pleura (see Fig. 17.1). The sympathetic rami from T_3 to T_5 form a diffuse network of cardiac sympathetic nerves. From T_5 to T_{12} the rami are more discrete, running caudally and somewhat anteriorly as the great, lesser and least splanchnic nerves. At first these are closely applied to the vertebral bodies of T_{11} and T_{12} but, after piercing the crus of the

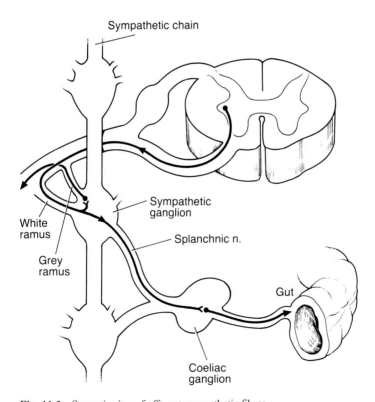

Fig. 11.3 Synaptic sites of efferent sympathetic fibres.

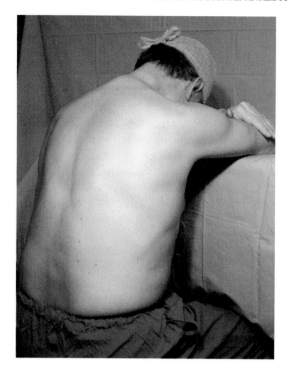

Fig. 11.4 Position for intercostal nerve block in ambulant patient.

diaphragm, they coalesce to form the diffuse coeliac plexus overlying the aorta and the coeliac axis at the level of the first lumbar vertebral body (see Fig. 17.7). From there sympathetic fibres accompany blood vessels to supply the abdominal viscera. The sympathetic supply to the pelvis and urogenital tract is derived from T_{10} to L_1 and runs in the lumbar sympathetic chain and the ill-defined hypogastric plexus.

The sympathetic and somatic innervation are thus closely related near the neuraxis, but become separated peripherally. It follows that spinal or paravertebral block will cause significant sympathetic block, which may result in major cardiovascular changes and other physiological effects. Conversely, peripheral nerve blocks only affect somatic innervation and leave sympathetic efferents intact. It is also apparent that, if complete denervation of the viscera is required, vagal afferents have to be obtunded by a separate procedure such as coeliac plexus block.

INTERCOSTAL NERVE BLOCK

The intercostal nerve may be blocked at any point in its course, but for the best analgesia and muscle relaxation the injection should be made proximal to the origin of the lateral branch (i.e. posterior to the mid-axillary line).

Positioning and preparation

In the premedicated patient the prone or lateral decubitus position is recommended, whereas the ambulant subject can be seated leaning forwards over the edge of the bed or operating table, head on hands (Fig. 11.4). A pillow should be placed under the chest of the prone patient. In either position the shoulders should be abducted and the arms forward so that the scapulae move laterally and allow access to the posterior rib angles where the rib is usually easily palpated. At this point the intercostal space is relatively deep and the nerve is separated from the pleura by the subcostal muscle. In very obese or muscular individuals the ribs and spaces may be more easily defined in the posterior axillary line, anterior to latissimus dorsi.

Surface markings can greatly help accurate needle placement. A line is drawn in the coronal plane along the edge of the paraspinous muscles, approximately 8–10 cm from the midline, and the point at which it crosses the lower border of each rib is marked.

Injection technique (Fig. 11.5)

The skin is drawn cephalad with the 'palpating hand' and a 23 g or 25 g short bevelled needle is introduced over the rib and advanced perpendicular to the skin until bony contact is made. A small quantity of local anaesthetic may be injected on to the periosteum as this is the most painful part of the procedure. The 'palpating hand' then holds the hub of the needle firmly between thumb and index finger with the hypothenar eminence pressed firmly on to the patient's back. The 'injecting hand' then gently walks the needle caudally while the skin is allowed to move back over the rib until the tip just passes under its lower edge. If the needle becomes barbed by repeated bony contact, it should be changed.

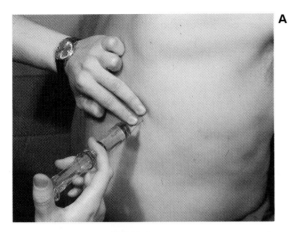

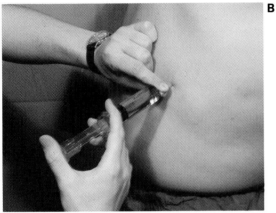

Fig. 11.5 Technique of intercostal nerve block. **A** The fingers of the left hand have pushed the skin that normally lies over the rib headwards. The needle tip has been advanced down to the rib. **B** The left hand then grips the needle hub and the needle is 'walked' down until it slides under the rib.

Occasionally a slight 'pop' is felt as the needle is advanced through the external intercostal muscle and the posterior intercostal membrane. The patient is asked to hold his breath as the needle is passed under the rib and while the injection is made. This minimizes lung movement over the needle point so that if it has accidentally penetrated the pleura the risk of serious pneumothorax is decreased. If a careful aspiration test is negative for air and blood, up to 5 ml of local anaesthetic solution is injected.

For upper abdominal midline surgery, 12 nerves have to be blocked (T_6–T_{11} bilaterally) and up to 60 ml of solution may be required. Systemic

absorption of local anaesthetic is very rapid due to the vascularity of the area and this technique may produce high blood concentrations (Moore et al 1976, Scott et al 1972), particularly after liver transplantation (Bodenham & Park 1990). The concentrations produced are surpassed only by those which may follow inadvertent intravascular injection or endotracheal instillation (Braid & Scott 1965). These factors mean that the drug and its concentration have to be chosen with care. From the point of view of toxicity prilocaine would have much to offer, but if the block is to be of real benefit to the patient, a longer-acting agent is needed. Bupivacaine 0.25% with 1:200 000 adrenaline is recommended. The addition of adrenaline decreases the rate of absorption and the peak blood concentration, but there is little evidence that it significantly prolongs the duration of this block. A significant dose of adrenaline may be administered so it is important to bear in mind the contraindications to this drug and to use solutions without vasoconstrictor when indicated. Intercostal blocks are by no means painless and they involve multiple injections, so additional systemic analgesia or sedation may be needed.

The anatomical distribution of solution deposited in the intercostal space is of relevance to both the resultant analgesia and the likely complications, but remains subject to debate. A claim that it is anatomically possible for a single large volume injection to spread to several adjacent spaces (Nunn & Slavin, 1980) resulted in further studies suggesting that medial spread to the paravertebral space might be responsible for this effect (Mowbray et al 1987, Crossley 1988, Moore 1985). Moore (1985) suggested that the posterior intercostal membrane has to be pierced before solution will spread to adjacent spaces, and this requires that the needle be placed posteriorly and close to the pleura, with concomitant risk of pneumothorax. It is debatable (Moore 1981) whether this is useful in practice, recent evidence suggesting that multiple injections are more effective and reliable than the single-injection technique (Renck et al 1984, Mowbray & Wong 1988). However, repeat injection through an indwelling catheter has been used to extend the duration of analgesia by eliminating the need for further painful injections and the increased risk of pneumothorax (Ablondi et al 1966, Murphy 1983, Kolvenbach et al 1989).

Indications

For unilateral thoracic procedures, intercostal block produces rather better postoperative analgesia than conventional opioid therapy. It may be performed by the anaesthetist before or immediately after surgery, or by the surgeon from inside the chest. When the chest is open, the intercostal nerves can be injected under direct vision, a catheter inserted (Sabanathan et al 1988, Sabanathan et al 1990) or a cryoprobe used to freeze the nerves (Glynn et al 1980). Intercostal block has no effect on visceral structures so by itself it is inadequate for surgery. The duration of its analgesic effect, even with the longer-acting amide drugs such as bupivacaine, is only 4–8 hours, although pinprick analgesia may be demonstrable for 12–18 hours.

Unilateral intercostal block (T_6–T_{11}) provides good somatic analgesia for a subcostal incision, but muscle relaxation is usually inadequate for the surgical procedure and neuromuscular blocking drugs are required. Better relaxation is produced by bilateral block, but again this may not be sufficient for upper abdominal surgery.

Complications

The *physiological effects* of intercostal block are usually slight. Minimal cardiovascular changes are seen unless either large quantities of adrenaline have been used or the injected solution has tracked posteriorly to involve the sympathetic chain. As well as upper limb sympathetic block (Purcell-Jones et al 1987), dramatic hypotension (Benumof & Semenza 1975, Cottrell 1978, Brodsky 1979, Skretting 1981) and total spinal anaesthesia (Friesen & Robinson 1987) have been recorded, so the anaesthetist must be ready to deal with such rare, but potentially serious, complications. With regard to the respiratory system, intercostal block offers some slight advantages in the postoperative period when compared with conventional analgesia, but the results of different studies are not always comparable or conclusive. This block tends to reduce the impairment of respiratory function which occurs after thoracic and upper abdominal procedures. It improves the result of effort-dependent tests such as vital capacity, forced expiratory volume and peak expiratory flow rate and reduces to some extent the degree and duration of postoperative hypoxaemia (Engeberg 1975, Kaplan et al 1975). There is some evidence to suggest that postoperative chest infection is slightly less common than with opioid analgesia (Engeberg 1983).

The incidence of *pneumothorax* depends on the skill of the operator and the zeal with which this complication is sought. Published series quote an incidence of between 0.075 and 19% (Moore 1975, Cronin & Davies 1976). If a pneumothorax occurs, it is usually small and resolves spontaneously, but occasionally an intercostal drain is required, particularly if the patient is being artificially ventilated since tension pneumothorax is then a real danger. Significant haemorrhage may occur after intercostal nerve block if coagulation is impaired (Nielsen 1989), so, as with all regional techniques, the coagulation status of the patient must be taken into account.

OTHER NERVE BLOCKS IN THE TRUNK

Interpleural block

Interpleural analgesia was first described by Kvalheim & Reiestad in 1984. After some initial scepticism the analgesic action of interpleural injection of local anaesthetic was confirmed, but the duration of effect of a single injection is less than originally reported (VadeBoncouer et al 1989). The technique has proved useful after rib fractures and unilateral trunk operations (Reiestad & Stromskag 1986, Rocco et al 1987), but it does not appear that respiratory function is better maintained with this technique than with systemically administered opioid (Oxorn & Whatlet 1989, Scott et al 1989, Lee et al 1990b). The place of interpleural analgesia in anaesthetic practice remains to be established, particularly with the advent of laparoscopic cholecystectomy.

Mechanism of block

Radiographic studies have demonstrated that 20 ml of solution spreads posteriorly in the pleural cavity from the diaphragm to the apex of the lung in the supine subject (Brismar et al 1987). It is probable that the local anaesthetic diffuses through the parietal pleura to produce multiple intercostal nerve block and this is supported by the finding of diminished sensitivity to cold in the same dermatomes (Lee et al 1990b). Both sympathetic and splanchnic nerve block may also be produced. Horner's syndrome and upper limb vasodilatation have been described in association with the technique (Parkinson et al 1989) and the sympathetic block may contribute to the analgesia. Splanchnic nerve block may alleviate visceral pain and account for the profound analgesia described after left-sided interpleural block in a patient with severe pancreatic pain (Durrani et al 1988).

Technique

Local anaesthetic may be injected through a previously inserted chest drain which is then clamped for up to 30 minutes, or through a catheter placed in the pleural cavity at thoracotomy. More commonly, a catheter is inserted percutaneously into the closed chest. Great care must be taken to avoid producing a pneumothorax secondary to either lung puncture or accidental air entry during catheter insertion.

The catheter is usually inserted through an intercostal space in the posterior axillary line with the patient in the lateral position, although a more anterior puncture site may be used in supine patients. Full aseptic precautions and a no-touch technique are essential. The skin is first punctured with a sharp hypodermic needle and then a Tuohy epidural needle is advanced until a rib is contacted. The needle is then 'walked' superiorly off the rib into the intercostal space, where its passage through the external intercostal muscle is easily appreciated. Methods of insertion vary from this

stage and may be described as either 'open' or 'closed'.

Open techniques

During open techniques the pleural space is in direct communication with the atmosphere at some stage, but the methods are technically straightfoward.

1. The original technique for identifying the subatmospheric pressure in the pleural cavity involves attachment of an air-filled syringe to the Tuohy needle and observing the plunger of the syringe moving down the barrel once the needle tip enters the space (Reiestad & Stromskag 1986). The syringe is then removed and the catheter threaded through the needle.
2. A 'hanging-drop' technique, similar to that used for epidural catheter insertion may also be employed (Squier et al 1989). A drop of saline suspended from the hub of the Tuohy needle is drawn inwards when a subatmospheric pressure is detected.
3. Alternatively, the catheter may be placed in the needle while its tip is in the intercostal muscles. One hand advances the needle and the other tries to thread the catheter. When the pleural space is entered it is possible to advance the catheter without resistance (Gin et al 1990).
4. The pleural space may be identified using loss of resistance to the injection of air or saline as in epidural anaesthesia (Seltzer et al 1987).

With the first two methods it is necessary to have the patient breathing spontaneously, but even with the latter two methods the patient should be disconnected from positive-pressure ventilation to minimize the risk of lung puncture.

Closed techniques

Systems which allow the catheter to be fed through a silicone or rubber seal will prevent air entry during catheter insertion. The pleural space is identified by the collapse of a small balloon on a side arm or by the ability to run in saline rapidly from a bag connected to that side arm (Scott 1991). The ability to thread 10 cm of catheter easily confirms placement. Extrapleural placement may occur in error because the pressure in this space is subatmospheric at some points of the respiratory cycle, although analgesia may still be effective (Lee et al 1990b).

Dosage

A dose of 20 ml of 0.5% bupivacaine with 1:200 000 adrenaline will last 4–5 hours (Vade-Boncouer et al 1989). Infusions of 10 ml of 0.2–0.25% bupivacaine have been used by the authors in adults and smaller volumes have proved effective in children (McIlvaine et al 1988).

Indications

Interpleural block has been used successfully after a variety of trunk operations such as mastectomy, cholecystectomy and nephrectomy (Reiestad & Stromskag 1986, Lee et al 1980a). Results after thoracotomy are more variable (Rosenberg et al 1987, McIlvaine et al 1988) and this may be related to loss of bupivacaine through the chest drain in some circumstances. Bilateral blocks have been used after midline abdominal operations, but large doses of bupivacaine are required and there is some risk of producing bilateral pneumothoraces (El-Naggar et al 1988). Interpleural analgesia may be useful after chest trauma or in the management of some chronic pain states (Rocco et al 1987, Durrani et al 1988).

Complications

Small pneumothoraces secondary to air entry through the needle when using an open system have been described, but are of little consequence and resolve spontaneously (Brismar et al 1987). Pneumothorax secondary to lung puncture is more serious and may require insertion of an underwater seal chest drain until it is certain there is no further leak of air from the lung.

Local anaesthetic toxicity because of rapid drug absorption has followed injection of bupivacaine into an inflamed pleural cavity (Seltzer et al 1987). Peak plasma concentrations of bupivacaine are reduced when adrenaline-containing solutions are used (Kambam et al 1989, Gin et al 1990).

Hemidiaphragmatic paralysis has been reported with a catheter placed next to the diaphragm, but this is probably not a common complication (Landesberg et al 1990, Lee et al 1990b). Sympathetic block of the upper extremity and head may occur, but hypotension is not a feature (Parkinson et al 1989). Catheter breakage has been described (Rosenberg et al 1987), but not empyema, which would be a serious complication.

Contraindications are relative, but a past or present history of pleurisy, pneumonia, pulmonary embolus, severe chronic obstructive airways disease or other major lung or pleural pathology should probably rule out the use of this technique.

Paravertebral block

This may be carried out with the patient in the prone, lateral or sitting position, and at any appropriate level from high thoracic to mid-lumbar regions (Moore 1979). It may be used for postoperative pain control after thoracotomy, cholecystectomy or nephrectomy and both single-injection and catheter techniques may be used. In chronic pain conditions, both local anaesthetics and neurolytic solutions can be injected. Anatomical studies, using radiopaque contrast media or computerized tomography (CT) scanning in patients, or injections of dyes and latex in cadavers, have shown considerable variation in the dimensions of the paravertebral space. Highly variable patterns of spread may be seen with injected solutions tracking over several segments in either cephalad or caudad directions, into the pleural space and, by no means infrequently, into the epidural space (Conacher & Kokri 1987, Conacher 1988, Purcell-Jones et al 1989). In concept, this technique is attractive because it would produce relatively localized unilateral analgesia with less hypotension or urinary retention than epidural block (Matthews & Govenden 1989). However, it is not an easy block to perform, the degree of spread is variable and there is in fact considerable potential for hypotension, bilateral block, pneumothorax or even a total spinal (Gilbert & Hultman 1989). In chronic pain practice the use of an image intensifier is mandatory if reliable diagnostic results from low-volume local anaesthetic injections are to be obtained, or if neurolytic procedures are to be undertaken safely.

Peripheral blocks

Due to the branching of segmental nerves, there is considerable overlap in their distribution. The more peripheral the block, therefore, the more widespread must be the infiltration of local anaesthetic drug. This necessitates multiple injections of large volumes of dilute solution and brings with it the problems of overdosage. Historically, such blocks have been used for abdominal surgery and involve infiltration of the skin incision, multiple injections into the rectus sheath on each side, infiltration of the parietal peritoneum and either coeliac plexus block or intraperitoneal local anaesthetic lavage. Two important peripheral blocks are used, with apparently increasing frequency, for inguinal herniorrhaphy and for operations on the penis.

Field block for herniorrhaphy

This technique can be used alone for day case surgery or poor-risk patients. When combined with light general anaesthesia, it gives good operating conditions and postoperative pain control. The musculocutaneous innervation of the inguinal region is through the ventral rami of T_{11} and T_{12} and two upper branches of the lumbar plexus, the iliohypogastric and ilio-inguinal nerves (Fig.11.2).

Anatomy (Fig. 11.6)

The ventral ramus of the 12th thoracic or *subcostal nerve* is larger than the other thoracic roots and sends a large branch to join the first lumbar root. The anterior branch follows the lower border of the 12th rib, continues between the transversus and internal oblique muscles, becomes superficial at the lower end of the rectus sheath and supplies skin over the lower anterior abdominal wall.

The anterior cutaneous branch of the *iliohypogastric nerve* lies first between the internal oblique and transversus muscles. About 2 cm medial to the anterior iliac spine it passes through the internal oblique to lie between it and the external oblique. About 3 cm above the superficial ring it pierces the external oblique aponeurosis to supply the skin above the pubis and medial end of the inguinal ligament.

The *ilio-inguinal* nerve pierces the internal oblique muscle a little lower and further forward than does the iliohypogastric nerve. It then enters the inguinal canal and lies below the spermatic cord. It accompanies the cord through the superficial ring and supplies skin over the root of the penis and scrotum. Throughout its course it supplies branches to the cord and cremaster muscle.

The genital branch of the *genitofemoral nerve* also runs in the inguinal canal and may supply skin in the medial part of the groin.

Autonomic fibres supply the spermatic cord throughout its length, originating from the lower thoracic segments and travelling with the testicular blood vessels and somatic nerves.

Technique

Because the subcostal, iliohypogastric and ilio-inguinal nerves lie close together anteromedial to the anterior superior iliac spine (Fig. 11.6) and between the abdominal muscle layers, they may be conveniently blocked here. With the patient supine, a point 2.5 cm anterior and inferior to the iliac spine is marked and infiltrated with local anaesthetic. A short-bevel 20 g 10 cm spinal needle is inserted at this point and directed laterally to contact the inner surface of the ilium. Approximately 10 ml of local anaesthetic is infiltrated through the full thickness of the abdominal wall to ensure spread of solution between all muscle layers. From the same point, the needle is directed inferomedially, parallel to the inguinal ligament,

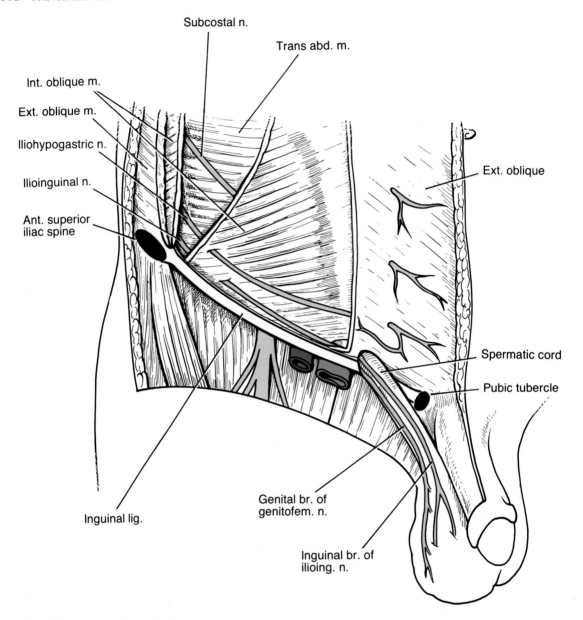

Fig. 11.6   Nerves in the inguinal region.

and more solution (10 ml) is injected both deep and superficial to the external oblique aponeurosis.

The pubic tubercle is now palpated and the overlying skin infiltrated. The spinal needle is inserted to the tubercle and angled superolaterally so that it just clears its superior border. A further injection (10 ml) is made at this point and in a 'fan' pattern from it. This will block any fibres of the genitofemoral or the lower intercostal nerves which extend to this area. Once the cord has been exposed during surgery, it and the neck of the peritoneal sac should receive separate injections (5 ml) at the level of the deep inguinal ring to block impulses transmitted in the visceral nerves.

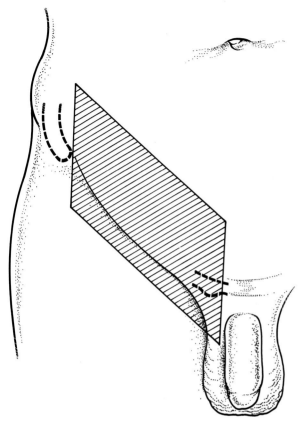

Fig. 11.7   The shaded area should be infiltrated once the primary injections near the anterior superior iliac spine and pubic tubercle have been made.

The area of the skin incision will also need to be infiltrated. It is wise to ask the surgeon to outline the area within which he will make his incision (Fig.11.7). Infiltration of this zone should ensure effective analgesia even if the incision has to be extended, so it is more satisfactory than linear infiltration. It is performed with the 10 cm spinal needle inserted through the upper skin wheal. In almost every case, the needle is long enough for the infiltration to be completed without the need for repeated skin puncture.

At least 40 ml of solution is needed for this procedure. In the poor-risk patient 0.5–1% plain prilocaine should be used. For the healthy out-patient 0.5% bupivacaine may be used for the deep injections and 0.25% bupivacaine with adrenaline for the skin infiltration.

Patience, understanding and gentle tissue handling on the part of the surgeon do a great deal to improve the success rate in conscious patients. Small intravenous doses of short-acting agents such as midazolam and alfentanil may also be helpful. If a long-acting local anaesthetic such as bupivacaine is used, at least 20 minutes must be allowed for the block to become effective, but postoperative analgesia may last for up to 6 hours (Glasgow 1976) and may be prolonged further by adding high molecular weight dextran to the local anaesthetic solution (Navaratnarajah & Davenport 1985).

Indications

When herniorrhaphy is to be carried out under regional anaesthesia alone, this technique has some advantages over spinal and epidural block in poor-risk cases and out-patients, even though a large dose of local anaesthetic is required. There is little sympathetic block, so significant pulse and blood pressure changes are rare. There is also less disturbance of bladder function, and early ambulation is possible because there is no block of the lower limb muscles. It may be the method of choice for the severe respiratory cripple in whom general anaesthesia is inadvisable and in whom the respiratory muscle paralysis caused by spinal or epidural anaesthesia may be sufficient to precipitate respiratory failure.

Penile block

Anatomy

Most of the somatic supply of the penis is supplied by the second, third and fourth sacral nerve roots. The fibres run in the dorsal nerve of the penis, which is the terminal branch of the pudendal nerve. The dorsal nerve runs with the artery along the inferior ramus of the pubis, through the suspensory ligament of the penis and under the pubic arch where it lies in the floor of the suprapubic space, before entering Buck's fascia, the fibrous tissue which invests the corpus cavernosum (Dalens et al 1989) (Fig.11.8). It supplies the skin and glans. The autonomic supply arises

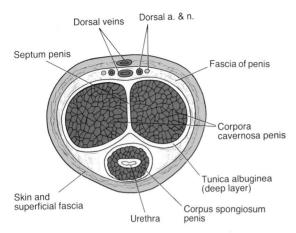

Fig. 11.8   Cross-section of penis to show the position of the dorsal nerves (n).

from the inferior hypogastric plexus in the pelvis. Some fibres run with the pudendal nerves, but others accompany the blood vessels to the corpus spongeosum and corpus cavernosum. The base of the penis and scrotum are innervated by cutaneous branches of the genitofemoral nerve through its genital branch (Fig. 11.6).

Technique

Spinal, epidural or caudal techniques may be used for penile surgery, but block of the dorsal nerves and terminal branches of the genitofemoral nerve produces more localized anaesthesia. With the patient supine a finger is placed under the pubic symphysis in the midline. A skin wheal is raised before a 5 cm 23 g needle is inserted in the midline vertical to the skin to pass under the pubis into the subpubic space. Then, 5 ml of local anaesthetic (0.25–0.5% *plain* bupivacaine) should be injected without resistance, first to one side of the midline, and then to the other. Alternatively the needle may be directed in a more caudal direction on to the tough dorsal fascia of the penis and, after careful aspiration, 2–5 ml of solution should be injected without resistance. Forced injection of large volumes of solution, especially in children, within the non-elastic tissues of Buck's fascia may cause arterial compression and penile gangrene even if no adrenaline has been used (Sara & Lowry 1984).

Frequent aspiration is required to avoid intravascular injection in this highly vascular area. *It is imperative that adrenaline is not used.* For complete anaesthesia another 5–10 ml of solution should be placed subcutaneously in a 'ring' around the base of the penis.

Indications

This is a useful, simple procedure for reduction of paraphymosis, and for dorsal slit, circumcision or meatotomy. It gives excellent postoperative pain control, but erection can occur as some of the autonomic supply is unaffected. It is an excellent adjunct to general anaesthesia, is easier and quicker than spinal or caudal anaesthesia and avoids motor block, bladder disturbance and central sympathetic block.

CHOICE OF BLOCK FOR SURGERY TO THE TRUNK

There is no doubt that regional anaesthesia for surgery on the trunk offers many advantages both during and after operation. Several techniques are available, each with advantages and disadvantages so the anaesthetist must decide which is the most appropriate. Consideration must be given to several factors, including the skills and experience of the anaesthetist, the availability of adequate monitoring and supervision during and after the procedure, anatomical and physiological features of the individual patient, and the amount of time available. If there are major reasons for avoiding general anaesthesia, even mastectomy may be performed under a field block (Dennison et al 1985).

For *thoracic surgery* the practical choice lies between intercostal, interpleural, paravertebral and thoracic epidural block. Apart from simple procedures on the chest wall, thoracic surgery requires general anaesthesia, with intermittent positive-pressure ventilation, to allow adequate control of respiration and manipulation of the diaphragm. The latter is innervated from the cervical region, so it is unaffected by either technique. Regional anaesthesia is therefore used as a supplement to general anaesthesia, particularly to provide post-operative pain control. Intercostal block by the surgeon or anaesthetist is the easiest technique and has a relatively low incidence of serious side-effects, but it is limited in efficacy and duration of effect. Cryoanalgesia, applied from within the chest, may be used, or placement of a paraverte-bral or interpleural catheter considered, but close monitoring of infusions and injections is vital, particularly in the first few postoperative hours because the effects are so variable. The best pain control is probably obtained with an epidural infusion, but meticulous monitoring and control of hydration is required.

For *abdominal surgery* the choice lies between subarachnoid, epidural or intercostal block. During upper abdominal procedures, conscious patients will not tolerate large packs or stimulation of the diaphragm, so general anaesthesia with controlled ventilation is required. Regional techniques may be used as supplements to, but virtually never as replacements for, general anaesthesia. For lower abdominal and pelvic procedures, however, excellent anaesthesia and relaxation is obtained with spinal or epidural techniques, and if any sedation or light general anaesthesia is required, it may be considered to be the supplement. Given adequate postoperative facilities and expertise, epidural anaesthesia is superior to other methods since it is suitable for long surgical procedures and excellent postoperative pain control can be obtained with top-ups or continuous infusion of local anaesthetic, or with the epidural injection of opioid. If this form of postoperative analgesia is not to be used and if the surgery is sure to be completed in the available time, spinal anaesthesia is preferable because it is quicker to perform, has a more rapid onset and is more effective than epidural anaesthesia.

Intercostal block is useful in abdominal surgery in three situations: firstly, where spinal or epidural techniques are not possible, because of a major spinal deformity such as spina bifida or ankylosing spondylitis; secondly, for subcostal incisions (for surgery of the gallbladder) when it is quick and easy to apply at the end of surgery and gives reasonable postoperative analgesia; thirdly, and most important, where sympathetic block may result in dangerous hypotension due to the relative hypovolaemia associated with many acute conditions, such as haematemesis, peritonitis and intestinal obstruction. Spinal and epidural anaesthesia are contraindicated in these conditions, but it should also be remembered that sympathetic block, although rare, is also possible after posteriorly placed intercostal injections.

The type of regional anaesthesia applicable to *renal surgery* depends to a large extent on the patients's position during surgery. The 'renal position', with the patient on his side and with maximum operating table 'break', may impair venous return regardless of the anaesthetic technique employed, but the use of epidural or spinal anaesthesia considerably magnifies the problem. This is a situation where low unilateral intercostal injections have advantages.

Low spinal, lumbar or caudal epidural blocks are all useful in a variety of *gynaecological, urological, perineal* and *anal* procedures. After some of these, for example transurethral prostatectomy, profound postoperative analgesia is not necessary and spinal anaesthesia with an agent of suitable duration is the technique of choice. For anal procedures (but only those in which sphincter relaxation is surgically acceptable or desirable) low spinal or caudal block may be employed. If the patient is to remain conscious, the spinal technique is less painful, quicker in onset and considerably more effective than caudal block, which has a significant failure rate even in expert hands. The main advantage of the caudal approach is that it avoids postspinal headache, which may be a serious disability in younger patients who would normally mobilize quickly after surgery. For this reason spinal anaesthesia should not be used routinely in day case surgery.

Regional anaesthesia is commonly used for *inguinal hernia repair*. Peripheral nerve block has gained popularity particularly in day case surgery and for the very frail patient. The obvious advantages include lack of sympathetic block and resulting hypotension, lack of accessory respiratory muscle involvement, no risk of spinal headache and no muscle paralysis of the lower limbs, the patient being able to walk from the table. However, the technique requires careful patient counselling and the co-operation of both patient and surgeon. It involves several rather uncomfortable injections, but if the block is performed after induction of general anaesthesia this discomfort is avoided. Minimal general anaesthesia is required thereafter, and the advantage of good postoperative pain control is retained. Spinal anaesthesia is a perfectly acceptable technique for inpatients and, rarely, a lumbar epidural catheter is desirable especially after bilateral hernia repair when continuous analgesia techniques allow excellent management of a patient with respiratory disability.

FURTHER READING

McClure J H, Wildsmith J A W 1991 Conduction blockade for postoperative analgesia. Edward Arnold, London

REFERENCES

Ablondi M A, Ryan J F, O'Connell C T, Harley R W 1966 Continuous intercostal nerve blocks for postoperative pain relief. Anesthesia and Analgesia 45: 185–190

Benumof J L, Semenza J 1975 Total spinal anesthesia following intercostal nerve blocks. Anesthesiology 43: 124–125

Bodenham A, Park G R 1990 Plasma concentrations of bupivacaine after intercostal nerve block in patients after orthotopic liver transplantation. British Journal of Anaesthesia 64: 436–441

Braid D P, Scott D B 1965 The systemic absorption of local anaesthetic drugs. British Journal of Anaesthesia 37: 394–404

Brismar B, Pettersson N, Tokics L, Standberg A, Hedenstierna G 1987 Postoperative analgesia with intrapleural administration of bupivacaine–adrenaline. Acta Anaesthesiologica Scandinavica 31: 515–520

Brodsky J B 1979 Hypotension from intraoperative intercostal nerve blocks. Regional Anaesthesia 4/3: 17–18

Conacher I D 1988 Resin injection of thoracic paravertebral spaces. British Journal of Anaesthesia 61: 657–661

Conacher I D, Kokri M 1987 Postoperative paravertebral blocks for thoracic surgery. A radiological appraisal. British Journal of Anaesthesia 59: 155–161

Cottrell W M 1978 Hemodynamic changes after intercostal nerve blocks with bupivacaine-epinephrine solution. Anesthesia and Analgesia 57: 492–495

Cronin K D, Davis M J 1976 Intercostal block for postoperative pain relief. Anaesthesia and Intensive Care 4: 259–261

Crossley A W A 1988 Intercostal catheterisation: an alternative approach to the paravertebral space? Anaesthesia 43: 163–164

Dalens B, Vanneuville G, Dechelotte P 1989 Penile block via the subpubic space in 100 children. Anesthesia and Analgesia 69: 41–45

Dennison A R, Walkins R M, Ward M E, Lee E C G 1985 Simple mastectomy under local anaesthesia. Annals of the Royal College of Surgeons of England 67: 243–244

Durrani Z, Winnie A P, Ikuta P 1988 Interpleural catheter analgesia for pancreatic pain. Anesthesia and Analgesia 67: 479–481

El-Naggar M A, Bennett B, Raad C, Yogaratnam G 1988 Bilateral intrapleural intercostal nerve block. Anesthesia and Analgesia 67: S57

Engeberg G 1975 Single dose intercostal block for pain relief after upper abdominal surgery. Acta Anaesthesiologica Scandinavica 60(supplement): 43–49

Engeberg G 1983 Intercostal block for prevention of pulmonary complications after upper abdominal surgery. Acta Anaesthesiologica Scandinavica 78(supplement): 73

Friesen D, Robinson R H 1987 Total spinal anesthesia – a complication of intercostal nerve block. Kansas Medicine 88: 84–96

Gilbert J, Hultman J 1989 Thoracic paravertebral block: a method of pain control. Acta Anaesthesiologica Scandinavica 33: 142–145

Gin T, Chan K, Kan A F, Gregory M A, Wong Y C, Oh T E 1990 Effect of adrenaline on venous plasma concentrations of bupivacaine after interpleural administration. British Journal of Anaesthesia 64: 662–666

Glasgow F 1976 Short stay surgery for repair of inguinal hernia. Annals of the Royal College of Surgeons of England 58: 133–139

Glynn C J, Lloyd J W, Barnard J G W 1980 Cryoanalgesia in the management of pain after thoracotomy. Thorax 35: 325–327

Kambam J R, Hammon J, Parris W C V, Lupinetti F M 1989 Intrapleural analgesia for postthoracotomy pain and blood levels of bupivacaine following intrapleural injection. Canadian Journal of Anaesthesia 36: 106–109

Kaplan J A, Miller E D, Gallagher E G 1975 Post operative analgesia for thoracotomy patients. Anesthesia and Analgesia 54: 773–777

Kolvenbach H, Lauven P M, Schneider B, Kunath U 1989 Repetitive intercostal nerve block via catheter for postoperative pain relief after thoracotomy. Thoracic and Cardiovascular Surgeon 37: 273–276

Kvalheim L, Reiestad F 1984 Interpleural catheter in the management of postoperative pain. Anesthesiology 61: A231

Landesberg G, Meretyk S, Lankovsky Z, Shapiro A 1990 Intra-operative intrapleural catheter placement for continuous bupivacaine administration. European Journal of Anaesthesiology 7: 149–152

Lee A, Boon D, Bagshaw P, Kempthorne P A 1990a Randomised double-blind study of interpleural analgesia after cholecystectomy. Anaesthesia 46:1028–1031

Lee T L, Boey W K, Tan W C 1990b Analgesia and respiratory function following intrapleural bupivacaine after cholecystectomy. Journal of Anesthesiology 4: 20–28

McIlvaine W B, Knox R F, Fennessey P V, Goldstein M 1988 Continuous infusion of bupivacaine via intrapleural catheter for analgesia after thoracotomy in children. Anesthesiology 69: 261–264

Matthews P J, Govenden V 1989 Comparison of continuous paravertebral and extradural infusions of bupivacaine for pain relief after thoracotomy. British Journal of Anaesthesia 62: 204–205

Moore D C 1975 Intercostal nerve block for postoperative somatic pain following surgery of the thorax and upper abdomen. British Journal of Anaesthesia 47: 284–286

Moore D C 1979 Regional block, 4th edn, pp 200–220. Thomas, Springfield

Moore D C 1981 Intercostal nerve block: spread of india ink injected to the rib's costal groove. British Journal of Anaesthesia 53: 325–329

Moore D C 1985 Intercostal blockade. British Journal of Anaesthesia 57: 543–544

Moore D C, Mather L E, Bridenbaugh P O 1976 Arterial and venous plasma levels of bupivacaine following epidural and intercostal nerve blocks. Anesthesiology 45: 39–45

Mowbray A, Wong K K S 1988 Low volume intercostal injection. A comparative study in patients and cadavers. Anaesthesia 43: 633–634

Mowbray A, Wong K K S, Murray J M 1987 Intercostal catheterisation. An alternative approach to the paravertebral space. Anaesthesia 42: 958–961

Murphy D F 1983 Continuous intercostal nerve blockade for pain relief following cholecystectomy. British Journal of Anaesthesia 55: 521–524

Navaratnarajah M, Davenport H T 1985 The prolongation of local anaesthetic action with dextran. The effect of molecular weight. Anaesthesia 40: 259–262

Nielsen C H 1989 Bleeding after intercostal nerve block in a patient anticoagulated with heparin. Anesthesiology 71: 162–164

Nunn J F, Slavin G 1980 Posterior intercostal nerve block for pain relief after cholecystectomy. British Journal of Anaesthesia 52: 253–260

Oxorn D C, Whatlet G S 1989 Post-cholecystectomy pulmonary function following interpleural bupivacaine and intramuscular pethidine. Anaesthesia and Intensive Care 17: 440–443

Parkinson S K, Mueller J B, Rich T J, Little W L 1989 Unilateral Horner's syndrome associated with interpleural catheter injection of local anesthetic. Anesthesia and Analgesia 68: 61–62

Purcell-Jones G, Speedy H M, Justins D M 1987 Upper limb sympathetic blockade following intercostal nerve blocks. Anaesthesia 42: 984–986

Purcell-Jones G, Pither C E, Justins D M 1989 Paravertebral somatic nerve block: a clinical, radiographic, and computed tomographic study in chronic pain patients. Anesthesia and Analgesia 68: 32–39

Reiestad F, Stromskag K E 1986 Interpleural catheter in the management of postoperative pain. A preliminary report. Regional Anesthesia 11: 89–91

Renck H, Johansson A, Aspellin P, Jacobsen H 1984 Multiple intercostal nerve blocks by a single injection – a clinical and radiological investigation. In: Van Kleef J, Burns T, Spierdijk J (eds) Current concepts in regional anaesthesia, pp 1–7. Martinus Nijhoff, Amsterdam

Rocco A, Reiestad F, Gudman J, McKay W 1987 Interpleural administration of local anaesthetics for pain relief in patients with multiple rib fractures. Preliminary report. Regional Anesthesia 12: 10–14

Rosenberg P H, Scheinin B M A, Lepantalo M J A, Lindfors O 1987 Continuous intrapleural infusion of bupivacaine for analgesia after thoracotomy. Anesthesiology 67: 811–813

Sabanathan S, Smith P J B, Pradhan G N, Hashimi H, Eng J, Mearns A J 1988 Continuous intercostal nerve block for pain relief after thoracotomy. Annals of Thoracic Surgery 46: 425–426

Sabanathan S, Mearns A J, Smith P J B et al 1990 Efficacy of continuous extrapleural intercostal nerve block on post-thoracotomy pain and pulmonary mechanics. British Journal of Surgery 77: 221–225

Sara C A, Lowry C J 1984 A complication of circumcision and dorsal nerve block of the penis. Anaesthesia and Intensive Care 13: 79–85

Scott D B, Jebson P J R, Braid D P, Ostengren B, Frisch P 1972 Factors affecting plasma levels of lignocaine and prilocaine. British Journal of Anaesthesia 44: 1040–1049

Scott N B, Mogensen T, Bigler D, Kehlet H 1989 Comparison of the effects of continuous intrapleural vs epidural administration of 0.5% bupivacaine on pain, metabolic response and pulmonary function following cholecystectomy. Acta Anaesthesiologica Scandinavica 33: 535–539

Scott P V 1991 Interpleural regional analgesia: detection of the interpleural space by saline infusion. British Journal of Anaesthesia 66: 131–133.

Seltzer J L, Larijani G E, Goldberg M E, Marr A T 1987 Intrapleural bupivacaine – a kinetic and dynamic evaluation. Anesthesiology 67: 798–800

Skretting P 1981 Hypotension after intercostal nerve block during thoracotomy under general anaesthesia. British Journal of Anaesthesia 53: 527–529

Squier R C, Morrow J S, Roman R 1989 Hanging-drop technique for intrapleural analgesia. Anesthesiology 70: 882

VadeBoncouer T R, Riegler F X, Gautt R S, Weinberg G L 1989 A randomized, double-blind comparison of the effects of interpleural bupivacaine and saline on morphine requirements and pulmonary function after cholecystectomy. Anesthesiology 71: 339–343

12. Upper limb blocks

T. J. Hughes   D. A. Desgrand

With the exception of epidural and spinal techniques, blocks of the upper limb have the greatest potential for wide application in anaesthetic practice. Virtually all operations on this limb may be performed under local anaesthesia, but the anaesthetist must have realistic expectations of the available methods since each has its own limitations, particularly in regard to the extent of block produced. Occasionally, local infiltration, sedation or light general anaesthesia will be needed to supplement the block. The planned combination of a brachial plexus technique with general anaesthesia has many advantages, not the least of which is profound analgesia extending into the postoperative period. The clinical features of each block differ and Table 12.1 provides a guide to the selection of the most appropriate technique.

BRACHIAL PLEXUS ANAESTHESIA

Anatomy

Formation and distribution of plexus (Fig. 12.1)

The nerve supply of the upper limb is derived mainly from the brachial plexus, which is formed from the anterior primary rami of the fifth cervical to the first thoracic roots. Contributions may also be received from C_4 and T_2. The roots form three trunks, each of which divides into an anterior and a posterior division. The six divisions then unite to form three cords. Each cord has two terminal branches and these are the nerves which supply the greater part of the arm. The branches of the proximal parts of the plexus supply the deep structures of the shoulder girdle. The skin over the shoulder is innervated by the supraclavicular

Table 12.1 Techniques for brachial plexus block

Technique	Area blocked	Advantages	Disadvantages
Intravenous regional	Hand, forearm	Simple to do; very low failure rate; suitable for out-patients	Tourniquet discomfort; tourniquet must be reliable
Interscalene	Shoulder, humerus, elbow, lateral aspect of forearm and hand	Good for shoulder injury	Lower dermatomes (C_8T_1) and skin over shoulder (C_4) may be missed
Subclavian perivascular	Whole arm except shoulder skin	Widest distribution of block	Slight risk of pneumothorax; difficult in the obese
Axillary	Hand, ulnar aspect of forearm	Pulsatile landmark; simple	Painful arm must be positioned; radial and musculocutaneous nerves may be missed

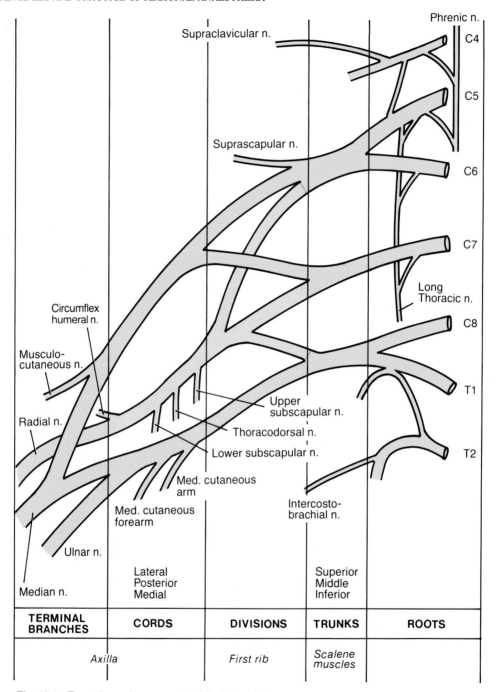

Fig. 12.1 Formation and components of the brachial plexus.

branches of the cervical plexus (Fig. 12.2). The lateral cutaneous branch of the second thoracic nerve – the intercostobrachial nerve – supplies the skin of the inner aspect of the upper arm and, with a branch from the third thoracic nerve, the skin of the axilla.

As a result of interbranching within the plexus, most of the peripheral nerves carry fibres from

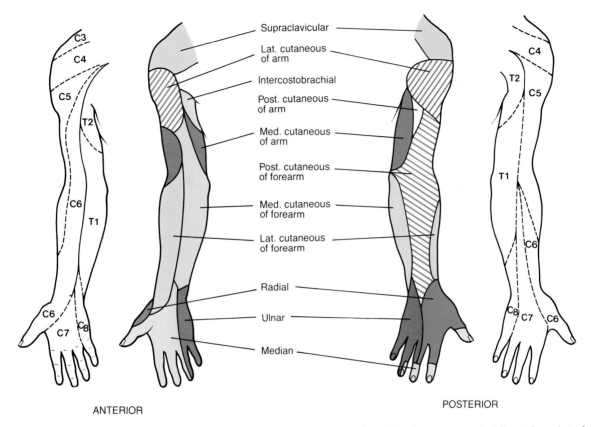

Fig. 12.2 Cutaneous innervation of the upper limb. The dermatomal innervation of the deep structures is different from that of the skin. C_5 supplies the shoulder, C_7 the elbow and T_1 the hand.

several roots. Each nerve supplies a recognized area, as does each segmental root, but the segmental innervation of deep and cutaneous structures is different (Fig. 12.2).

Position and relations (Figs 12.3 and 12.4)

After emerging from the intervertebral foramina, the plexus *roots* lie between the scalene muscles, which arise from the tubercles of the transverse processes of the cervical vertebrae and are inserted into the first rib. At this level the vertebral artery, the stellate ganglion and the contents of the cervical spinal canal are close relations. The phrenic nerve (C_3–C_5) lies on the anterior surface of the scalenus anterior, posterior to the carotid sheath. The recurrent laryngeal nerve, lying in the groove between oesophagus and trachea, is also close to the plexus. Laterally the external jugular

vein crosses the interscalene groove, classically at the level of the sixth cervical vertebra and the cricoid cartilage.

As the *trunks* approach the first rib they are arranged vertically and are named 'superior', 'middle' and 'inferior'. They are grouped closely together. The subclavian artery comes to lie between the plexus and the scalenus anterior muscle, with the dome of the pleura as a major inferomedial relation. At the lateral edge of the rib each trunk divides into two *divisions* and these pass behind and under the clavicle where the *cords* are formed. In the axilla, the components of the plexus completely surround the artery. As they pass behind the lateral border of the pectoralis minor muscle, the three cords divide into the *terminal branches*. The axillary vein lies medial to the artery and the surrounding plexus, and partially overlaps them. High in the axilla the musculocutaneous

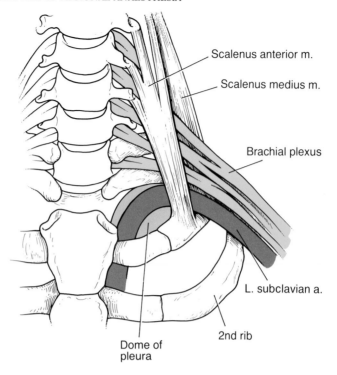

Fig. 12.3   Major relationships of the brachial plexus.

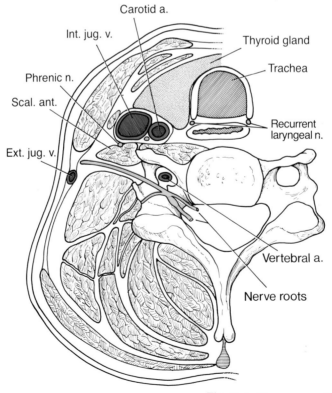

Fig. 12.4   Transverse section of neck.

nerve (from the lateral cord) leaves the plexus and enters the substance of the coracobrachialis muscle (Fig. 12.5). This may be several centimetres proximal to the point of needle entry for axillary block.

The sheath concept

Over its entire length, from the cervical vertebrae to the distal axilla, the plexus lies within a tube of fibrous tissue continuous with the prevertebral fascia. The clinical importance of this sheath has been discussed in detail by Winnie (1970) and an appreciation of its existence greatly simplifies our understanding and application of brachial plexus anaesthesia. Solution injected into the sheath at any point will tend to spread in both directions. Superiorly the sheath is continuous with that surrounding the cervical plexus, and this explains why block of the cervical nerves is sometimes seen after interscalene block. Distally the major axillary vessels are also enclosed by the sheath.

Studies with cadavers (Thompson & Rorie 1983) and observations on patients during surgery in the axilla have demonstrated the presence of septa inside the axillary sheath which separate one nerve from another. The septa may provide an explanation for incomplete blocks, although they do not prevent the spread of methylene blue injected inside the sheath in cadavers (Partridge et al 1987).

Potential sites for block

Numerous techniques for injecting local anaesthetic into the brachial plexus have been described. Starting with the most proximal they are:

1. Interscalene (Winnie 1970)
2. Parascalene (Vongvises & Panijayanond 1979)
3. Subclavian perivascular (Winnie & Collins 1964)
4. Supraclavicular (Macintosh & Mushin 1967)
5. Infraclavicular (Raj et al 1973)
6. Axillary (de Jong 1961).

Each of these approaches has its advocates, but it is doubtful whether any one anaesthetist could master them all, even if there were definite indications for each. The supraclavicular is the classical approach and the others have been introduced in attempts to produce easier methods with clearer landmarks and less risk of pneumothorax. The supraclavicular and subclavian perivascular methods produce the most complete limb block (Lanz et al 1983), whereas the axillary technique does not block the shoulder and the interscalene often misses the ulnar aspect of the hand and forearm. Although the infraclavicular approach has a satisfactory distribution of block, its application is complicated by the need for a nerve stimulator. Neither the parascalene nor the infraclavicular approach has achieved widespread popularity and their usefulness is difficult to assess. The interscalene and axillary methods are somewhat easier to learn and perform than the others, and are therefore more suitable for the occasional user who can choose between them according to the distribution of block required. With its wide distribution of block and lower risk of pneumothorax, the subclavian perivascular technique is probably the optimum method. The interscalene, subclavian and axillary approaches will therefore be described in detail.

General remarks on technique

Equipment

The use of *short-bevel* regional block needles is preferable (see Ch. 5) because they reduce the risk of nerve injury (Selander et al 1977, 1979) and sheath penetration is more easily appreciated. Standard hypodermic needles are less satisfactory alternatives.

It is advantageous to use an *immobile needle* technique (Winnie 1969) in which an extension set joins the needle to the syringe. The system is primed with local anaesthetic to prevent air embolism. This method allows the operator to hold the needle while the assistant aspirates and injects, thus minimizing movements of the needle. Although an aseptic technique should always be employed, gloves are unnecessary and make the palpation of landmarks more difficult. Although a nerve stimulator is not necessary for successful brachial plexus block (Smith 1990), many anaes-

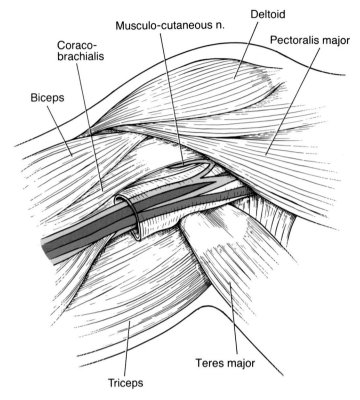

Fig. 12.5   Position of neurovascular bundle in the upper arm. Both vessels and nerves are within the sheath.

thetists find it a useful alternative to eliciting paraesthesiae.

Drugs and dosage

Prilocaine 1–2%, bupivacaine 0.25–0.5% and lignocaine 1–2% are all suitable and are available in the UK. Due to the plasma concentrations which follow brachial plexus block, *prilocaine* is the drug of choice, although the 1% solution may not provide adequate muscle relaxation. To minimize the risk of systemic toxicity, bupivacaine and lignocaine should be used with adrenaline, particularly when the higher concentrations are used (Wildsmith et al 1977).

Generally speaking, the lower concentrations of drug will give satisfactory depth of block and allow the use of the larger volumes which greatly increase the chance of successful brachial plexus block. In adults, between 30 and 40 ml of solution is recommended for the subclavian perivascular and interscalene approaches, while up to 50 ml is advocated for axillary block. The use of 1% prilocaine or 0.25% bupivacaine allows supplementary nerve block to be performed without risk of systemic toxicity. Higher concentrations of drug, while restricting volume, can provide more profound muscle relaxation and a more rapid onset of action.

An approximate guide to maximum dosage is given in Table 12.2. These doses are for the average adult and may need to be reduced in elderly patients, those with severe systemic disease and in children.

Latency and duration of block

Although onset of anaesthesia may be slow with any brachial plexus technique, most blocks should be well established within 20 minutes, but up to

Table 12.2 Maximum dosage of local anaesthetics for the average adult

Drug	Plain solution	With adrenaline
Prilocaine	600 mg (60 ml of 1%)	—
Bupivacaine	125 mg (50 ml of 0.25%)	200 mg (40 ml of 0.5%)
Lignocaine	300 mg (30 ml of 1%)	500 mg (50 ml of 1%)

40 minutes may have to be allowed on occasion. To some extent this variation is related to the drug and concentration used. Motor block often becomes apparent before sensory block, so it is possible to predict whether the injection has been successful by testing for muscle weakness after a few minutes. The earliest sign of a successful axillary block is inability to extend the elbow, but it is movement at the shoulder which is first affected by the interscalene and subclavian perivascular blocks. If there is no evidence of motor weakness within 10 minutes of injection, success is unlikely. Testing for sensory loss too early may undermine the patient's confidence so at least 15 minutes should elapse before this is done.

Duration is also variable and bupivacaine may be associated with anaesthesia that lasts for up to 24 hours (Brockway et al 1989). Plain prilocaine and lignocaine (with adrenaline) will provide at least 90 minutes, and bupivacaine 3 hours, of reliable surgical anaesthesia. If longer durations are required, a continuous catheter technique should be considered. Such techniques have been used successfully for postoperative analgesia (Gauman et al 1988) and the management of pain due to advanced malignancy (Clarke et al 1990), although the risk of cumulative toxicity from repeated injections must not be forgotten.

Paraesthesiae and nerve damage

Before the injection the patient should be told to expect paraesthesiae and to describe, rather than point to, their location because movement may disturb the position of the needle. Once paraesthesiae have been elicited, the needle should be withdrawn slightly to minimize needle damage. Severe pain on starting the injection indicates that the needle is intraneural, so it should be withdrawn further. Discomfort on injection may be due to 'pressure paraesthesiae', a sensation caused by over-rapid distension of the plexus sheath. Nerve damage has been associated with brachial plexus block (Plevak et al 1982) and can vary from mild paraesthesiae lasting a few weeks to more serious motor and sensory disturbances lasting months or years. Symptoms may appear almost immediately the block has worn off or take one week or more to develop. It may be difficult to determine the aetiology of nerve damage after brachial plexus anaesthesia because a variety of possible factors other than needle and injection trauma have to be considered. Many of these are unrelated to the local anaesthetic technique and may also be associated with general anaesthesia. There may be pre-existing nerve damage or the nerve may be injured as a result of the surgical procedure. Excessive tourniquet pressure, prolonged tourniquet application and malposition of the arm can all damage nerves.

Interscalene block

The interscalene technique is the most proximal approach to the brachial plexus. Local anaesthetic is injected into the plexus sheath at the level of the sixth cervical vertebra.

Clinical application

The main advantage of this approach is that pneumothorax is avoided, but the price paid is inconsistent blocking of the lower roots of the plexus. Structures innervated by C_5–C_7, the deep tissues of the shoulder, elbow joint, and the superficial areas of the radial aspect of the forearm and hand will be blocked reliably (Fig. 12.6). Supplementary blocks may be required for surgery involving other parts of the limb.

Position

The patient lies supine with the head resting on one pillow. The head is turned a little to the

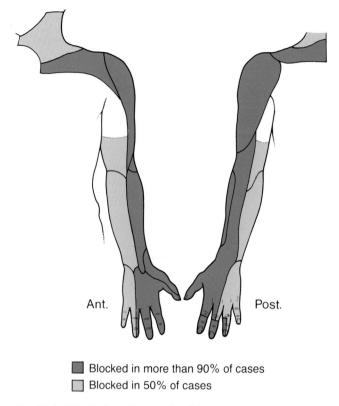

Ant.   Post.

■ Blocked in more than 90% of cases
□ Blocked in 50% of cases

Fig. 12.6   Distribution of interscalene block.

opposite side and the shoulder gently depressed. If the head is turned too far, the scalene muscles will be stretched and more difficult to palpate.

Landmarks

Interscalene block is performed by inserting a needle at the point where the cricoid line crosses the interscalene groove. The cricoid cartilage is palpated and a line is drawn laterally from it around the neck (Fig. 12.7). This line should run parallel to the clavicle rather than follow the skin creases which slope upwards. The lateral border of the sternomastoid is found next. If this is not obvious, the patient is asked to lift the head just off the pillow. A finger is then placed on the line from the cricoid and immediately lateral to the edge of the sternomastoid. The patient should relax completely. The finger now lies on the belly of the scalenus anterior muscle and is moved laterally until the groove between the scalene muscles is

felt. The groove can be accentuated by asking the patient to sniff several times. A fairly constant additional landmark is the external jugular vein which crosses the point of injection. To avoid a haematoma the needle is inserted so as to miss the vein.

Technique

The index finger is placed in the interscalene groove just below the point of injection. The needle is inserted level with the cricoid line and at right angles to the skin in all planes (Fig. 12.7) so that its direction is medial, slightly caudal and a little dorsal. If it is directed horizontally, it may pass between the transverse processes of two cervical vertebrae and could pierce the vertebral artery or enter the intervertebral foramen.

The needle is advanced slowly until paraesthesiae are obtained. These should radiate to the arm rather than the shoulder tip or scapula. Paraesthe-

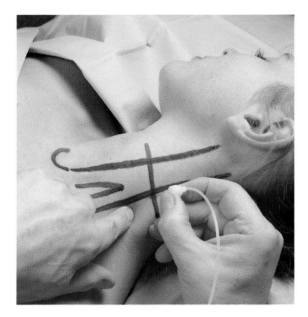

Fig. 12.7 Needle insertion for interscalene block. The left index finger is palpating the groove.

siae of the latter areas are often caused by stimulation of the suprascapular or supraclavicular nerves. Since these lie outside the sheath subsequent injection will be ineffective. The sensation described as a 'click', when the needle pierces the fascial sheath, is a useful guide to its correct placement, but is not always felt. If paraesthesiae are not evoked, or a response to nerve stimulation is not obtained, the needle is withdrawn to the skin and redirected a little more dorsally or caudally. It is important to stress that the plexus is rarely more than 2.5 cm from the skin (Yasuda et al 1980).

Once paraesthesiae have been elicited, the neck is compressed firmly by a finger placed above the needle to promote caudal spread. After aspiration the local anaesthetic solution is injected slowly with repeated aspiration.

Complications

Phrenic nerve block. Radiographic evidence of diaphragmatic paralysis has been reported in 36% of patients with interscalene and subclavian perivascular blocks (Farrar et al 1981). Although this rarely causes symptoms unless the patient has severe respiratory disease, significant alterations in

measurements of respiratory function have been reported (Urmey & McDonald 1990). The anaesthetist should take this into account when selecting a block for such patients.

Recurrent laryngeal nerve block. Both the interscalene and subclavian perivascular techniques are associated with a low incidence of recurrent laryngeal nerve block. The hoarseness is of no significance and the patient should be reassured. Bilateral blocks may result in laryngeal incompetence, and should be avoided.

Horner's syndrome. At least half the patients with interscalene or subclavian perivascular blocks develop Horner's syndrome. Some occasionally complain of flushing of the face. In a patient with both upper limb and head injuries unequal pupils may be misleading.

Vertebral artery injection. The injection of even a small dose of local anaesthetic into a vertebral artery will cause severe cerebral toxicity. Avoidance of this complication by accurate needle placement and careful aspiration is vital.

Epidural and subarachnoid injection. Injections into the epidural and subarachnoid spaces are possible and both have been reported. These complications can be avoided by correct needle angulation and by bearing in mind the superficial position of the plexus (i.e. 2.5 cm from the skin).

Subclavian perivascular block

This technique involves injection into the subclavian perivascular space which lies between the scalene muscles and above the first rib. It differs from the supraclavicular approach in that the needle is directed caudally from a more posteromedial position and strikes the plexus where the trunks lie one on top of the other behind the subclavian artery (Fig. 12.3).

Clinical application

The subclavian perivascular technique consistently blocks the arm, forearm and hand (Fig. 12.8) and can be used for most upper limb surgery. The lower trunk of the plexus (C_8T_1) may be missed if it lies below the subclavian artery, but the use of a generous volume of solution (see above) should

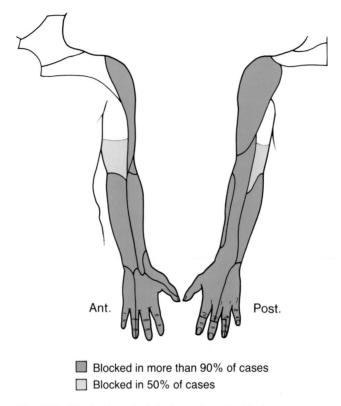

Ant.   Post.

■ Blocked in more than 90% of cases
□ Blocked in 50% of cases

Fig. 12.8   Distribution of subclavian perivascular block.

avoid this problem. The risk of pneumothorax is less than with the supraclavicular approach, but is sufficient to contraindicate this block in day case surgery, obese patients with poorly defined landmarks and those with severe chest disease.

Position

The patient lies supine with the head on a pillow and the arm by his side. The head is turned slightly to the opposite side and the arm is pulled down gently to depress the shoulder. Exaggerated positioning makes the landmarks more difficult to feel.

Landmarks

The interscalene groove is located using the method described for interscalene block (Fig. 12.7). Once the groove is found it is followed downwards as far as the subclavian artery. A finger is then placed over the artery to mark the site of injection. If the artery cannot be palpated, some anaesthetists remove the patient's pillow or even

get him to sit up. The technique can be used in the absence of a palpable pulse, but the inexperienced practitioner is advised to consider an alternative method because the failure rate is high and the risk of pneumothorax increased in this situation.

Technique

With the finger palpating the artery or in the groove, the needle is inserted immediately above the finger and advanced slowly in a caudal direction between the scalene muscles (Fig. 12.9) until paraesthesiae are elicited. A 'click' is sometimes felt as the needle penetrates the sheath and this is a helpful sign of correct positioning. If the first rib is contacted and no paraesthesiae are elicited, the needle is withdrawn and redirected more anteriorly or more posteriorly. It is important that the needle is not angled at all medially as this increases the risk of pneumothorax. If the subclavian artery is inadvertently punctured, the

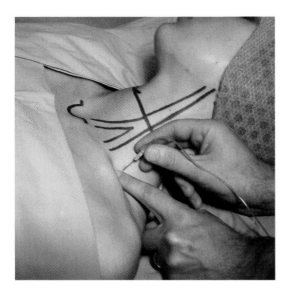

Fig. 12.9 Needle insertion for subclavian perivascular block. The left index finger lies on the artery.

pneumothorax. If the subclavian artery is inadvertently punctured, the needle should be withdrawn and directed a little more posteriorly.

To obtain successful blocks it is necessary to elicit paraesthesiae radiating to the arm or hand. Paraesthesiae in any other distribution indicate that the suprascapular, supraclavicular or long thoracic nerves have been stimulated and it is likely that the needle lies outside the sheath. Success with the subclavian approach is dependent on eliciting paraesthesiae or a response to nerve stimulation, so, if neither can be evoked after several attempts, an alternative method should be considered. When the appropriate paraesthesiae have been obtained an aspiration test is performed and the solution injected slowly with repeated aspiration.

Complications

Pneumothorax. As with the other supraclavicular techniques, pneumothorax is the principal complication of the subclavian perivascular block. Pneumothorax usually develops slowly and may take up to 24 hours to become clinically apparent. Cough, chest pain and dyspnoea are all symptoms which should alert the anaesthetist, and erect chest radiography should be performed. A film taken soon after injection may not show any

evidence of pneumothorax and should be repeated if doubt remains.

Block of adjacent nerves. Phrenic, recurrent laryngeal and stellate ganglion block can all occur. They are discussed in the section on interscalene block.

Axillary block

This offers a safe, relatively simple method of blocking the brachial plexus. Even when a large volume is used and directed proximally, the circumflex humeral and musculocutaneous nerves, which leave the sheath high in the axilla, may still remain unblocked. The radial nerve, which lies behind the axillary artery, is sometimes missed because septa separate the nerves in the axillary compartment.

Clinical application

The axillary approach consistently blocks the medial aspects of arm, forearm and those parts of the hand supplied by the ulnar and median nerves (Fig. 12.10). The lateral aspects of forearm and hand, supplied by the radial and musculocutaneous nerves, are blocked in 75% of cases. The circumflex humeral nerve, supplying the upper arm, is not reliably blocked. The main indication for axillary block is surgery to the hand and forearm although supplementary blocks of the radial nerve and the lateral cutaneous nerve of the forearm may be required.

Position

The patient lies supine with the arm abducted almost to 90° and with the elbow flexed so that the dorsum of the hand rests on the pillow (Fig. 12.11). If the arm is abducted further, the arterial pulse may be more difficult to palpate. In every patient it is wise to vary the degree of abduction and obtain maximum pulsation. In a patient with a fracture, pain may limit his ability to cooperate.

Technique

Although a needle can be used for axillary block, it is much easier and more reliable to use a catheter

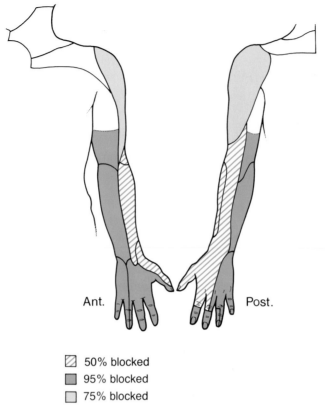

Ant.   Post.

▨ 50% blocked

■ 95% blocked

□ 75% blocked

Fig. 12.10 Distribution of axillary block.

technique. A 20 g or 22 g intravenous cannula is recommended.

The axillary artery is located and traced medially until it passes behind the anterior wall of the axilla. The index finger is placed over the artery and the cannula is inserted immediately above the finger at an angle of about 30° to the skin and directed parallel to, and just above, the artery (Fig. 12.12). The cannula is advanced slowly until a 'give' is felt as it pierces the sheath. The sheath lies quite superficially and once it has been penetrated the catheter is advanced from the needle just as if a vein were being cannulated (Fig. 12.13). The catheter will advance easily if it is in the sheath and if there is undue resistance it should be withdrawn and reinserted. If the artery or a vein is penetrated, the cannula and needle are withdrawn until blood can no longer be aspirated. The needle is then fixed and the catheter advanced again.

Once the catheter is in position it is connected to the syringe by an extension set. A finger is placed firmly over the artery distal to the injection site to ensure proximal spread of the solution. An aspiration test is performed and injection carried out slowly with repeated aspiration. Paraesthesiae are not sought deliberately, but if they are elicited they give additional confirmation that the cannula is correctly placed. If a vessel has been punctured it should be compressed for 5 minutes once the injection is complete to minimize haematoma formation.

Complications

The axillary technique is associated with fewer serious complications than any other. Intravascular injection is the principal risk.

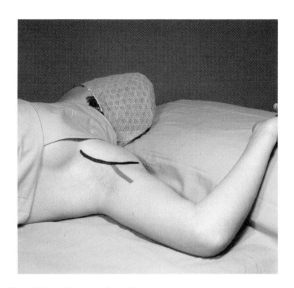

Fig. 12.11 Position for axillary block.

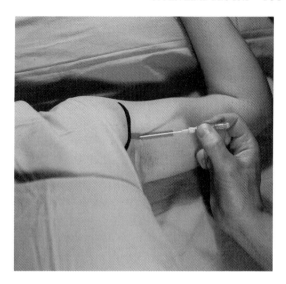

Fig. 12.12 Alignment of cannula for axillary block. During insertion the fingers of the left hand palpate and fix the artery.

Variations in technique

The risk of complications with axilliary block is low because injection does not take place in the root of the neck. In the last few years there has been a considerable amount of research aimed at improving the success rate of axillary block to take advantage of its inherent safety. This research has been reviewed (Brockway & Wildsmith 1990) and has confirmed the advice given above about volume and concentration of local anaesthetic to be used. Vester-Andersen and colleagues (1986) found that hyperabduction of the shoulder joint pulls the neurovascular bundle into the lateral wall of the axilla, where the head of the humerus may prevent circumferential spread of solution, especially to the radial, musculocutaneous and axillary nerves. Therefore, it is particularly important to ensure that the axillary pulse is readily palpable and that the arm is positioned by the patient's side soon after injection. It may also be helpful to ensure that the arm remains anterior to the coronal plane.

In 1987, Cockings and colleagues described a new technique – the transarterial axillary plexus block – to overcome the problem of inadequate spread of solution. In this method the needle is deliberately inserted into the axillary artery, and then advanced further until the tip is just beyond the vessel wall. In addition to this technical modification, the authors used a relatively large dose of drug, 50 ml of 1.5% mepivacaine. They reported extremely good results and attributed their success to several factors: the volume and concentration of drug used; injection deep to the

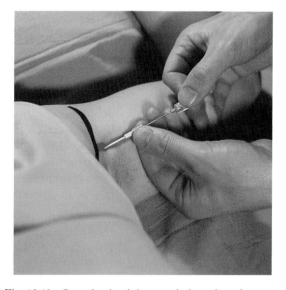

Fig. 12.13 Once the sheath is entered, the catheter is advanced from the needle.

axillary artery (and therefore close to the radial nerve); and precise landmark identification – injection very close to the artery.

However, when Youssef & Desgrand (1988) compared a transarterial technique with a 'conventional' method they were unable to demonstrate any significant differences between the two. They used a standard amount of drug so it may not have been arterial puncture per se that was responsible for the success rate claimed by Cockings and colleagues (1987). Deliberate puncture of a major artery cannot be advocated unless a very clear advantage can be shown for the patient.

An alternative approach to obtaining complete block of the upper limb is to accept the fact that no single technique will guarantee complete anaesthesia and to use a combined technique. Half the total dose of drug is injected by the axillary route and should ensure a block of the medial part of the arm. The other half of the dose is injected by either the interscalene or subclavian perivascular route to block the lateral half of the arm.

PERIPHERAL NERVE BLOCKS

With the careful application of brachial plexus techniques the role of individual nerve blocks in the arm is limited. Due to variations in anatomical course and wide cutaneous sensory overlap, multiple injections with supplementary infiltrations would be required for most surgical procedures. This is a particularly uncomfortable prospect for the patient.

Some blocks are of value for supplementing plexus anaesthesia or for providing analgesia during short procedures on the hand or fingers. Clinically, there is little difference between the effect of nerve block at the elbow or at the wrist, and only the simpler methods will be described. These are (with their preferred sites of performance):

1. Intercostobrachial nerve
2. Lateral cutaneous nerve of forearm (elbow)
3. Ulnar nerve (elbow)
4. Median nerve (wrist)
5. Radial nerve (wrist)
6. Digital nerve.

General remarks

For all these blocks 25 g needles are recommended as they minimize the risk of nerve trauma. The standard disposable 2 cm (1 inch) hypodermic needle is quite suitable. It is important to prevent intraneural injection which can be extremely painful and may produce a neuritis. It is wise to avoid these peripheral blocks when neuritis or nerve compression (e.g. carpal tunnel syndrome) are present.

The longer duration of bupivacaine makes this the drug of choice, although lignocaine and prilocaine may be used. The abundance of blood vessels in close proximity to nerves at the elbow and wrist means that intravascular injection and haematoma formation are potential complications. Even when blocking small nerves the action of a local anaesthetic is seldom instantaneous and up to 15 minutes should be allowed for its onset.

Techniques

Intercostobrachial nerve

The intercostobrachial nerve and the medial cutaneous nerve of the arm supply the skin of the axilla and the medial part of the upper arm (Fig. 12.2). None of the brachial plexus techniques is likely to block these nerves and the area they innervate may be a source of tourniquet discomfort. Both nerves may be blocked by injecting 5–10 ml of local anaesthetic solution subcutaneously across the axilla at right angles to the line of the artery. During axillary block this can be done simply by redirecting the needle prior to withdrawing it.

Lateral cutaneous nerve of forearm

The musculocutaneous nerve leaves the brachial plexus high in the axilla (Fig. 12.5). The lateral cutaneous nerve of the forearm is the sensory continuation of this nerve and may be blocked at the elbow to supplement axillary block. It perforates the deep fascia on the lateral side of the biceps muscle just proximal to the elbow joint, and supplies the skin on the lateral side of the forearm (Fig. 12.2). The needle is inserted at the point

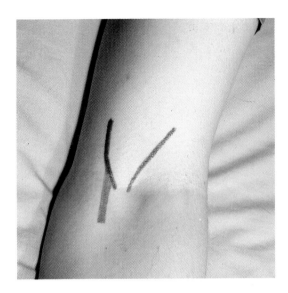

Fig. 12.14 Major landmarks at the left elbow. To block the lateral cutaneous nerve of the arm a needle is inserted in the line of the skin crease just lateral to the biceps tendon (outlined in black).

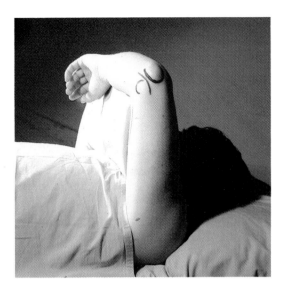

Fig. 12.15 Line of the ulnar nerve between the medial epicondyle of the humerus and the olecranon.

where the intercondylar line crosses the lateral border of the biceps tendon (Fig. 12.14), and 3–5 ml local anaesthetic is injected superficial to the fascia. Failure results if the needle is inserted too deeply.

Ulnar nerve

Ulnar nerve block is a useful supplement to interscalene block. It forms part of the triad of blocks required for anaesthesia of the hand and may be used in isolation for procedures on the little finger and ulnar aspect of the hand. As it approaches the elbow, the nerve crosses the medial head of triceps and lies in a groove behind the medial epicondyle (Fig. 12.15) where it is tightly bound in fibrous tissue. Injections made directly into the groove have been reported to produce neuritis so it is preferable to inject proximal to this point. With the elbow flexed, and the arm across the chest of the supine patient, the nerve is palpated 2–3 cm proximal to the medial epicondyle. The needle is inserted alongside the nerve and about 5 ml anaesthetic is injected. Paraesthesiae should not be sought because of the risk of neuritis.

The approach to this nerve at the wrist involves two needle insertions and is more difficult to perform.

Median nerve

Median nerve block affects the radial two-thirds of the palmar aspect of the hand (Fig. 12.2) and is usually combined with radial and ulnar nerve block. At the wrist the nerve lies quite superficially just under, and radial to, the palmaris longus tendon. Should this be absent, it lies between the tendon of flexor carpi radialis and the other flexor muscles. The tendons of palmaris longus and flexor carpi radialis become prominent when the wrist is flexed against resistance (Fig. 12.16). At the level of the proximal skin crease, the needle is inserted just radial to palmaris longus or, if it is absent, 1 cm medial to the flexor carpi radialis. The nerve is about 1 cm deep at this point, but fanwise needle movement in an ulnar direction may be required to obtain paraesthesiae. A 5 ml volume of local anaesthetic is adequate, but 1 ml should be injected subcutaneously on needle withdrawal to include the cutaneous branch to the palm of the hand.

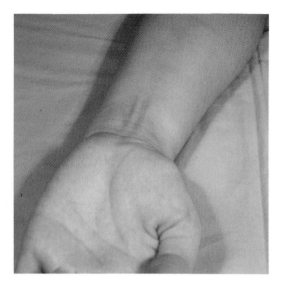

Fig. 12.16   The groove between the tendons of palmaris longus and flexor carpi radialis marks the position of the median nerve at the wrist.

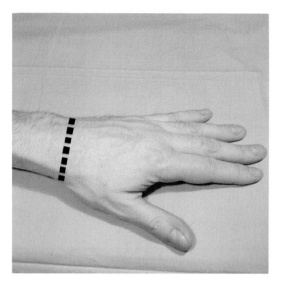

Fig. 12.17   A subcutaneous infiltration in the line marked will block the terminal branches of the radial nerve.

Radial nerve

About 7 cm proximal to the wrist the radial nerve passes underneath the tendon of brachioradialis to lie subcutaneously on the extensor aspect of the wrist. It divides into several terminal branches which supply the radial side of the dorsum of the hand (Fig. 12.2). The subcutaneous infiltration of 5–10 ml of solution across the radial and dorsal aspects of the wrist joint (Fig. 12.17) will block all of these terminal branches.

Digital nerves

Digital nerve block is very effective for outpatient procedures on the finger. *Under no cirumstances should solutions containing vasoconstrictor* be used because of the very real risk of ischaemia and subsequent gangrene. Each digit is supplied by four nerve branches (two dorsal and two palmar) which accompany the digital vessels. The needle is inserted into the dorsolateral aspect of the base of the finger. Subcutaneous injection of 1–2 ml of solution is made as the needle is advanced until pressure is felt on the anaesthetist's finger which is

placed under the patients finger (Fig. 12.18). The procedure is repeated on the other side of the finger to complete a subcutaneous ring infiltration.

INTRAVENOUS REGIONAL ANAESTHESIA (IVRA)

Injection of local anaesthetic into an exsanguinated limb was originally described by Bier in 1908, but only gained widespread acceptance following its reintroduction in the 1960s (Holmes 1963). Since then IVRA or 'Bier's block' has been used extensively, particularly in busy accident and emergency departments where its technical simplicity and reliability have enabled it to be successfully applied for many procedures on the upper limb. Unfortunately, this inherent simplicity is the source of potential danger. Inexperienced clinicians have used IVRA without understanding the technique or the need for reliable equipment, and without being able to cope with possible complications. As a result, fatalities have occurred with what should be a very safe technique (Heath 1982).

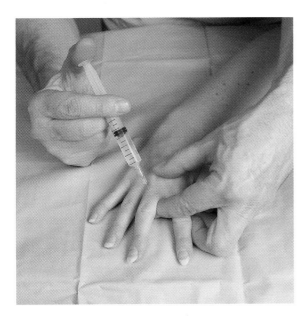

Fig. 12.18 Digital nerve block.

Clinical application

IVRA can be expected to provide satisfactory analgesia and muscle relaxation of the hand and forearm in up to 98% of cases. It is therefore suitable for most open or closed procedures performed below the elbow if these can be completed within 1 hour. Time limitation is related to tourniquet discomfort which cannot be easily avoided even with the use of double cuff systems. The reliability and rapid onset of analgesia with this method make it particularly useful for reduction of forearm fractures and other minor operations in the accident and emergency department. It can be considered for any patient over the age of 10 years and has been used in even younger patients. Unsatisfactory relaxation may occur in large, muscular arms, but poor distal analgesia is more likely to be associated with the use of proximal forearm veins or inadequate exsanguination.

Contraindications

Tourniquets should be avoided in patients carrying the sickle cell gene and those with Raynaud's disease. It is emphasized that the use of a method causing ischaemia in a limb which has suffered a crush injury may lead to necrosis of viable tissue.

The tourniquet

We recommend a single-cuff orthopaedic tourniquet with a 'bicycle-type' pump and high pressure tubing. This equipment should be regularly maintained. Double cuffs do not always reduce discomfort, and are potentially hazardous as there is a risk of confusion and accidental release of the wrong cuff. Sphygmomanometers are inappropriate. Automatic systems utilizing air reservoirs or a pressurized gas source are very useful, but can encourage a false sense of security, and may be confusing to use.

Drugs and dosage

Prilocaine is the drug of choice because of its low systemic toxicity. It is available specifically for IVRA in 50 ml single-dose vials, free of any preservative (Citanest 0.5% SDV, Astra Pharmaceuticals). The usual adult dose is 40 ml of this solution, but this should be reduced in frail elderly patients with thin forearms. Up to 50 ml may be used in well-built subjects with muscular forearms.

Precautions

IVRA should be approached with a level of caution which may appear to be disproportionate to its technical simplicity.

1. The patient should be starved for 4 hours preoperatively (Steedman et al 1991)
2. The procedure should be performed on a tipping trolley or operating table
3. There should be close supervision by a clinician experienced in the technique
4. Venous access should be established in the opposite arm
5. The full range of resuscitation equipment and drugs should be immediately available
6. The tourniquet should be checked for leaks prior to use and should be observed constantly during use.

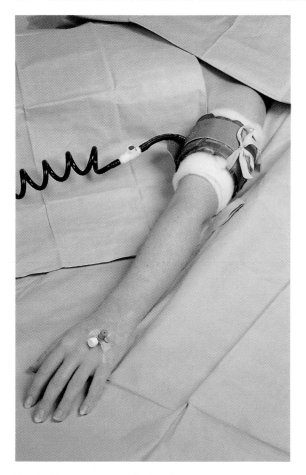

Fig. 12.19   Arrangement for IVRA.

Technique (Fig. 12.19)

With the patient supine the blood pressure is noted. An intravenous cannula is securely placed in a vein on the dorsum of the hand or distal forearm of the limb to be blocked. Antecubital veins should be avoided. The tourniquet is applied midway between axilla and elbow over a cushioning layer of orthopaedic padding.

The arm is exsanguinated by applying an Esmarch bandage from the finger tips to the tourniquet, or alternatively by elevating the limb for 2 minutes with compression applied to the brachial artery. The latter approach is more suitable in the presence of a fracture. The cuff is inflated to 100 mmHg above the systolic blood pressure. If there is any evidence of continuing arterial flow such as a palpable pulse or venous congestion, the tourniquet is released and the procedure restarted. When satisfactory ischaemic conditions are obtained the solution of 0.5% prilocaine is injected over 1–2 minutes. If the surgical procedure is to be performed on the hand or fingers it may be helpful to apply a venous tourniquet just proximal to the cannula to help direct the solution distally.

Within seconds of the end of the injection the patient may feel paraesthesiae and the skin may appear mottled. Sensory block is usually complete within 10 minutes, but muscle relaxation may take twice that time. Throughout the procedure the anaesthetist should monitor the pressure of the tourniquet cuff which should not be released for at least 20 minutes after injection. The patient should be closely observed and left supine for at least half an hour after the procedure.

Complications

Systemic toxicity. This is the major potential problem with this technique and it is usually associated with inadvertent, premature tourniquet deflation due to failure of equipment or technique. Strict attention to detail should avoid the problem.

There have been reports of convulsions (all with drugs other than prilocaine) which can only be explained by significant leakage of anaesthetic under adequately applied tourniquets. Simulated IVRA studies by El-Hassan and colleagues (1984) have shown that venous injection pressures in excess of tourniquet occlusion pressure can be achieved, with a risk of systemic leakage, particularly if antecubital veins are used. Rapid injection, poor exsanguination and manipulation of forearm fractures (Quinton et al 1988) may also contribute to this leakage.

The incidence of toxicity when the tourniquet is released after 20 minutes or more is variable. Minor symptoms (drowsiness, tinnitus, or tingling of lips) and signs (bradycardia or hypotension) can be observed even with prilocaine so there is no room for complacency. Neither major systemic toxicity nor methaemoglobinaemia have ever been described after IVRA with prilocaine at the doses recommended here.

Tourniquet problems. Reversible nerve damage due to tourniquet pressure has occasionally been reported (Fletcher & Healey 1983), but never in association with IVRA. It may be more likely when excessive tourniquet times (>90 minutes) are used, or when the cuff is applied too close to the elbow joint where the nerves are poorly cushioned by muscle.

Limb swelling after the procedure should be minimal and certainly no greater than if it had been performed under a tourniquet and general anaesthesia.

FURTHER READING

Winnie A P 1984 Perivascular techniques of brachial plexus block. Plexus anaesthesia, vol I. Churchill Livingstone, Edinburgh

REFERENCES

Brockway M S, Wildsmith J A W 1990 Axillary brachial plexus: method of choice. British Journal of Anaesthesia 64: 224–231

Brockway M S, Winter A W, Wildsmith J A W 1989 Prolonged brachial plexus block with 0.42% bupivacaine. British Journal of Anaesthesia 63: 604–605

Clarke A, Simpson K, Ellis F 1990 Continuous brachial plexus block in the management of intractable cancer pain in the arm. Palliative Medicine 4: 123–125

Cockings E, Moore P, Lewis 1987 Transarterial brachial plexus blockade using high doses of 1.5% mepivacaine. Regional Anesthesia 12: 159–164

de Jong R 1961 Axillary block of the brachial plexus. Anesthesiology 22: 215–225

El Hassan K, Hutton P, Black A 1984 Venous pressure and the arm volume changes during simulated Bier's block. Anaesthesia 39: 229–235

Farrar M, Scheybani, Nolte H 1981 Upper extremity block. Effectiveness and complications. Regional Anesthesia 6: 133–134

Fletcher I, Healy T 1983 The arterial tourniquet. Annals of the Royal College of Surgeons 65: 409–417

Gauman D M, Lennon R L, Wedel D 1988 Continuous axillary block for post operative pain management. Regional Anesthesia 13: 77–82

Heath M 1982 Deaths after intravenous regional anaesthesia. British Medical Journal 288: 913–914

Holmes C M 1963 Intravenous regional anaesthesia. Lancet i: 245–246

Lanz E, Theiss D, Janovic D 1983 The extent of blockade following various techniques of brachial plexus block. Anesthesia and Analgesia (Current Researches) 62: 58–58

Macintosh R, Mushin W 1967 Local anaesthesia; brachial plexus, 4th edn. Blackwell, Oxford

Partridge B, Katz J, Benirschke K 1987 Functional anatomy of the brachial plexus: implications for anesthesia. Anesthesiology 66: 743–747

Plevak D, Linstromberg J, Danielson D 1982 Paresthesiae vs nonparesthesiae: the axillary block. Anesthesiology 59: A216

Quinton D, Hughes J, Mace P, Aitkenhead A 1988 Prilocaine leakage during tourniquet inflation in intravenous regional anaesthesia – the influence of fracture manipulation. Injury 19: 333–335

Raj R, Montgomery S, Nettles D, Jenkins M 1973 Infraclavicular brachial plexus block: a new approach. Anesthesia and Analgesia (Current Researches) 52: 897–904

Selander D, Dhuner K, Lunberg F 1977 Peripheral nerve injury due to injection needles used for regional analgesia. Acta Anaesthesiologica Scandinavica 21: 27–33

Selander D, Edshage S, Wolff T 1979 Paraesthesia or no paraesthesia. Acta Anaesthesiologica Scandinavica 23: 27–33

Smith B E 1990 The role of electrical nerve stimulation in regional anaesthesia. Current Anaesthesia and Critical Care 1: 234–238

Steedman D J, Payne M R, McClure J M, Prescott L F 1991 Gastric emptying following Colles' fracture. Archives of Emergency Medicine 8: 165–168

Thompson G, Rorie D 1983 Functional anatomy of the brachial plexus sheath. Anesthesiology 59: 117–122

Urmey W, McDonald M 1990 Reductions in pulmonary function resulting from interscalene brachial plexus block. Regional Anesthesia 15(supplement): 15

Vester-Andersen T, Broby Johansen U, Bro-Rasmussen F 1986 Perivascular axillary block VI: the distribution of gelatine solution injected into the axillary neurovascular sheath of cadavers. Acta Anaesthesiologica Scandinavica 30: 18–22

Vongvises P, Panijayanond T 1979 A parascalene technique of brachial plexus anesthesia. Anesthesia and Analgesia 58: 267–273

Wildsmith J A W, Tucker G T, Cooper S, Scott D B, Covino B G 1977 Plasma concentrations of local anaesthetics after interscalene brachial plexus block. British Journal of Anaesthesia 49: 461–466

Winnie A 1969 An "immobile needle" for nerve block. Anesthesiology 31: 577–578

Winnie A 1970 Interscalene brachial plexus block. Anesthesia and Analgesia (Current Researches) 49: 455–466

Winnie A, Collins V 1964 The subclavian perivascular technique of brachial plexus anesthesia. Anesthesiology 25: 353–363

Yasuda I, Hirano T, Oijima T, Ohhira N, Kaneko T, Yamamuro M 1980. Supraclavicular brachial plexus block using an insulated needle. British Journal of Anaesthesia 52: 409–411

Youssef M S, Desgrand D A 1988 Comparison of two methods of axillary brachial plexus anaesthesia. British Journal of Anaesthesia 60: 841–844

13. Lower limb blocks

W. A. Macrae

While regional anaesthesia has become more widely used in recent years, lower limb blocks have not enjoyed the same popularity. Many anaesthetists feel that the techniques are complicated, difficult and unreliable and that much detailed anatomy has to be learnt before the blocks can be attempted. Spinal and epidural methods offer straightforward single-needle techniques for anaesthesia of the lower limb, whereas multiple injections are required to block the nerves more peripherally. However, the view that all nerve blocks of the lower limb are difficult and unreliable is incorrect. The aim of this chapter is to present simple techniques which give consistent results and may be used routinely. It is hoped that this approach will persuade the reader to include lower limb nerve blocks in his repertoire. Only brief reference will be made to nerve blocks which have not been found useful in daily clinical practice.

Anatomy

Some knowledge of anatomy is essential for the performance of nerve blocks in the lower limb, but no attempt will be made to describe the complete course of each nerve or to describe its anatomical relations since only comparatively small areas need to be understood in detail. The anatomy described is sufficient to permit the reliable identification of each nerve.

Lumbosacral plexus (Fig. 13.1)

The nerve supply of the lower limb is from the lumbosacral plexus which is formed from the anterior primary rami of the second lumbar to the third sacral roots. Each root divides into an anterior and posterior division, and these divisions then join and branch to form the individual nerves.

Cutaneous innervation

Whereas a knowledge of *dermatomal* distribution in the lower limb is needed for the proper use of spinal and epidural blocks, it is the *cutaneous* distribution of the various nerves (Fig. 13.2) which determines the practical application of peripheral nerve block. This cutaneous distribution varies. For example, the junction between the areas supplied by the saphenous (femoral) and the superficial peroneal (sciatic) nerves can be anywhere between the upper edge of the medial malleolus and the big toe. Such variation must be borne in mind if an operation is to be performed near the edge of the distribution of a nerve. It is essential to test carefully and block the neighbouring nerve if necessary.

Innervation of deep structures

The sensory nerve supply to deep tissues has not been as well elucidated as that of the skin. It is generally safe to assume that muscle and bones are supplied by the same nerves as the skin overlying them, but joints generally have a more complex nerve supply and receive innervation from all the nerves supplying structures around them. For example, the hip and knee joints are supplied by femoral, sciatic and obturator nerves and the ankle is supplied by both femoral and sciatic nerves. As in the upper limb, the *dermatomal innervation of deep structures* is quite different from that of the

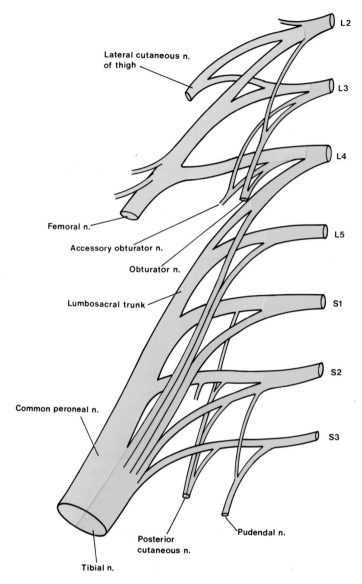

Fig. 13.1   The lumbosacral plexus.

skin. The foot is supplied by the lower roots (S_3–S_4) and the upper parts of the limb by the upper roots.

Choice of technique

The art of anaesthesia lies in giving each patient the most suitable anaesthetic for each operation. The choice of technique depends on the variables considered in the first section of this book, but a few points apply particularly to the use of local anaesthesia in the lower limb.

The patient. Peripheral nerve blocks have advantages in patients with cardiovascular disease since the extensive sympathetic block which may be associated with spinal or epidural anaesthesia is avoided. Spinal and epidural anaesthesia may also be contraindicated by spinal disease associated with the lower limb condition requiring surgery, or by the position of the patient who may, for

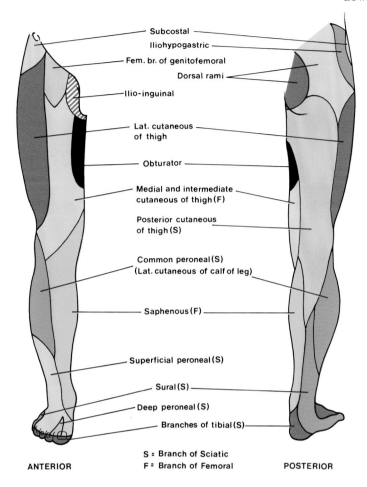

Subcostal
Iliohypogastric
Fem. br. of genitofemoral
Dorsal rami
Ilio-inguinal
Lat. cutaneous
of thigh
Obturator
Medial and intermediate
cutaneous of thigh (F)
Posterior cutaneous
of thigh (S)
Common peroneal (S)
(Lat. cutaneous of calf of leg)
Saphenous (F)
Superficial peroneal (S)
Sural (S)
Deep peroneal (S)
Branches of tibial (S)

S = Branch of Sciatic
F = Branch of Femoral

ANTERIOR   POSTERIOR

Fig. 13.2 Distribution of cutaneous nerves in the lower limb. See Figure 3.6 for corresponding dermatomes.

example, be in fixed traction and cannot be moved until anaesthesia has been induced. Conversely, a peripheral nerve block will be impossible if a plaster covers the injection site. Many lower limb nerves are blocked at points where they lie close to arteries. If the latter are affected by peripheral vascular disease it is important to avoid needle trauma to them.

A large volume of local anaesthetic is required for bilateral lower limb blocks. In the case of bilateral femoral and sciatic nerve blocks at the hip, this could amount to 80 ml which, in standard concentrations, is potentially toxic. It must be stressed that systemic concentrations after these blocks tend to be low (Misra et al 1991, Robison et al 1991) and toxicity is not a common problem,

but if factors are present which make such large doses particularly undesirable a technique requiring a smaller dose of drug, such as a spinal, may be preferable.

The patient's wishes must be taken into account. Most patients will accept regional anaesthesia if it is properly explained to them and if it is accepted practice in the unit. However, patients who are disturbed by injections or who are to undergo bilateral procedures are far more likely to accept the single injection required for a spinal or epidural than a technique involving multiple injections. On the other hand spinal and epidural anaesthesia are not entirely appropriate for outpatients for whom nerve blocks should be used wherever possible.

The operation. Obviously, the operation dictates what sort of block is appropriate. For most orthopaedic operations on the leg, a tourniquet is used and the block must eliminate pain from the tourniquet as well as from the operative site. If tourniquet discomfort does develop it must be dealt with promptly and well before the patient's response disrupts the operation. Sedation, even with an opioid analgesic, may not be adequate and recourse to a light general anaesthetic may well be necessary, although many of the benefits of a nerve block for a peripheral procedure are then lost.

The time factor. Sciatic and femoral nerve blocks take a relatively long time because the patient has to be positioned twice and two separate injections are required. The blocks take between 15 and 30 minutes to become effective so if speed is important, a spinal anaesthetic is a better choice. When lower limb blocks are being performed it is particularly important to organize the operating list to take this time factor into account, otherwise delay will occur and the anaesthetist will find himself becoming unpopular. Having the support and cooperation of colleagues is as important as knowing where to put the needle!

General recommendations

Choice of block for operations on the lower limb in the average patient is not difficult. The most useful blocks are undoubtedly epidurals and spinals. They are adaptable to almost all operations on the lower limb and are so easy to perform and so reliable that they are an essential part of every anaesthetist's repertoire. They are the methods of choice for hip and knee surgery and operations involving the femoral shaft, and are also useful for bilateral operations below the knee.

Nerve blocks do have their place. For skin grafts from the thigh, block of the lateral cutaneous nerve of the thigh and the femoral nerve are useful. For unilateral varicose veins, femoral nerve block, together with local infiltration to the groin, is often adequate. For unilateral operations below the knee, femoral and sciatic nerve blocks are, in the opinion of many, the methods of choice.

Individual nerve blocks are also useful in the diagnosis and treatment of chronic pain and every anaesthetist involved in this work should be familiar with the common lower limb nerve blocks.

General aspects of technique

The general principles of technique for blocks of the major nerves of the lower limb (factors such as choice of equipment, aseptic technique and the dosage, latency and duration of drugs) are much the same as for the brachial plexus (see Ch. 12). Lignocaine 1–2% and bupivacaine 0.25–0.5%, with or without adrenaline, are suitable for most lower limb blocks, but prilocaine 1–2% has much to commend it in many situations. Nerve stimulators are widely used for location of the sciatic because it is so deeply situated, but the author does not find the use of stimulators helpful.

The choice of tourniquet site should be discussed. For operations on the knee, it must be applied to the thigh, but, for operations on the ankle and foot, it may be applied to the calf. This position is widely used in some Scandinavian countries and has been used by the author for many years without any problems, although the precise siting is important. If it is placed too high, there may be pressure on the common peroneal nerve as it winds around the neck of the fibula or on the saphenous nerve where it lies on the anteromedial surface of the tibia just below the knee. If the tourniquet is too low, it will be in the surgeon's way. The advantage of placing the tourniquet on the middle of the calf (Fig. 13.12) for operations on the ankle and foot is that nerve block at the knee will provide anaesthesia for both the tourniquet and the operation (Fig. 13.2)

NERVE BLOCK AT THE HIP

Femoral nerve block

Anatomy (Fig. 13.3)

The femoral nerve (L_2–L_4) runs down the postero-lateral wall of the pelvis behind the fascia iliaca, lying on the psoas and iliacus muscles. The femoral artery and vein lie anterior to the fascia iliaca which sweeps downwards and forwards from the posterior and lateral walls of the pelvis and blends with the inguinal ligament. When the

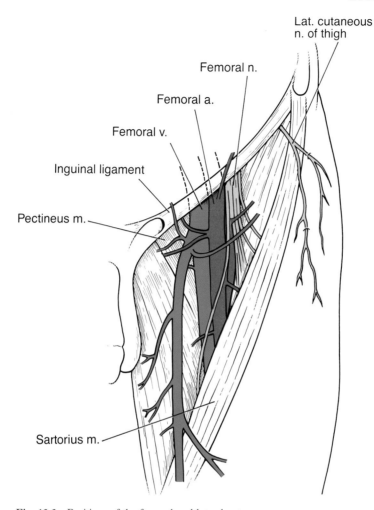

Fig. 13.3 Positions of the femoral and lateral cutaneous nerves.

vessels pass behind the inguinal ligament they draw a fascial sheath down around them. The femoral nerve lies *behind and lateral to* this sheath and, unlike the vessels, is not within it. All three are deep to the fascia lata, but unfortunately the exact position of the nerve in relation to the artery is inconstant. It may be close to the sheath or several centimetres lateral to it, as well as being more deeply placed. Just below the inguinal ligament the nerve divides into several branches. Because of these factors, femoral nerve block is not as easy as may be thought. Moore (1965a) states that when sciatic and femoral nerve blocks are

combined, and found to be inadequate, it is usually the femoral nerve which has been missed.

Clinical application

It is important to stress that, although femoral nerve block is not always easy, it is a useful technique, and well worth mastering. The majority of incisions for varicose vein surgery are made within its distribution and it may be used alone or in combination with block of the lateral cutaneous nerve for the taking of skin grafts from the thigh. It is suitable for many orthopaedic operations on

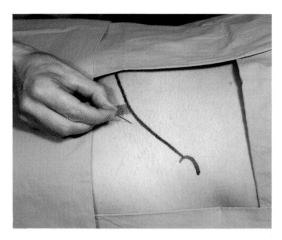

Fig. 13.4 Femoral nerve block.

the leg and foot and can provide analgesia of a fracture of the upper part of the femoral shaft. Serpell and colleagues (1991) have shown that continuous femoral nerve block is useful for controlling pain after knee surgery.

Technique (Fig. 13.4)

A line drawn between the anterior superior iliac spine and the pubic tubercle marks the position of the inguinal ligament. The femoral artery is palpated as it passes behind the midpoint of the ligament. The needle is inserted just below the ligament, 1 cm lateral to the artery, parallel with the course of the nerve, but inclined superiorly at an angle of about 45°. A 'click' is felt as the needle passes through the fascia lata and it should be advanced with a gentle probing motion until paraesthesiae are elicited. In many patients, particularly those with a little subcutaneous fat, a second 'click' can be felt as the needle penetrates the fascia iliaca. If the needle has been inserted to a depth of 3 or 4 cm and paraesthesiae have not been obtained it is withdrawn and the direction changed slightly, either medial or lateral. Once paraesthesiae are obtained, the needle is immobilized and an aspiration test performed before 10–15 ml of local anaesthetic solution is injected. If paraesthesiae are not obtained, despite a careful search, 20 ml of local anaesthetic should be injected fanwise from the artery to a point about

3 cm lateral to it. This usually produces an effective block, although it cannot be guaranteed to do so.

Lateral cutaneous nerve of thigh

Anatomy

The lateral cutaneous nerve of the thigh (lateral femoral cutaneous nerve) (L_2–L_3) runs forward in a curve on the iliacus muscle outside the pelvic viscera and fascia iliaca. Anteriorly it passes behind the inguinal ligament to enter the thigh deep to the fascia lata, 1–2 cm medial to the anterior superior iliac spine (Fig. 13.3). In the thigh, it divides into two branches, anterior and posterior, which pierce the fascia lata about 10 cm below the anterior superior iliac spine and supply the skin of the lateral aspect of the thigh.

Technique

The nerve is blocked where it emerges below the inguinal ligament. The patient lies supine and the anterior superior iliac spine is palpated and marked. The needle is introduced perpendicularly through the skin 1 cm medial to, and 2 cm below, the anterior superior iliac spine. After passing through skin and subcutaneous tissue, slight resistance to needle advancement is felt and then a 'click' as the needle passes through the fascia lata. After aspiration, 2 ml local anaesthetic solution is injected. The needle tip is then withdrawn into the subcutaneous tissues, redirected laterally and advanced deep to the fascia lata. A further 2 ml of local anaesthetic is injected 1 cm from the original injection point. This process is repeated medial to the original injection point.

This is a fairly easy block with a high success rate, although, like many blocks, it can be difficult in obese patients since the key to success is to insert the needle into the correct tissue plane. In these patients the following procedure may aid correct needle placement. Once the needle tip is in the subcutaneous tissues, a finger is placed on the skin either side of the needle shaft. When these two fingers are moved from side to side the needle will move with the subcutaneous tissues, but once it has penetrated the fascia lata it will be anchored in place.

Obturator nerve block

The obturator nerve (L_2–L_4) slants down the side wall of the pelvis to the upper part of the obturator foramen, through which it passes into the thigh. In the foramen, it divides into anterior and posterior branches. The obturator nerve sends branches to the hip and knee joints and supplies a variable area of skin on the inside of the thigh. It also supplies the adductor muscles.

Block of the obturator nerve is both difficult and uncomfortable, sometimes painful, for the patient. The success rate even in experienced hands is poor (Moore 1965b) and the block is of little value on its own. It is used occasionally to complement sciatic and femoral nerve blocks for knee operations or to prevent tourniquet pain, but a spinal, an epidural or a 'there-in-one' block are more useful.

The 'three-in-one' block

The sheath concept

This interesting and useful block was first described by Winnie and his colleagues (1973). The aim is to block the femoral, the lateral cutaneous and the obturator nerves with a single injection. The principle upon which the block is based is that all three nerves are branches of the lumbar plexus and lie sandwiched between the same muscles and fascia. If a large volume of local anaesthetic is injected into this musculofascial plane, it will spread centrally to affect all three nerves. In order to make the drug spread in the right direction, pressure is applied distal to the site of injection. The original description (Winnie et al 1973) showed that spread to all three nerves could be demonstrated radiographically after femoral injection and confirmation of the concept came from Sharrock (1980), who reported inadvertent 'three-in-one' block after injection around the lateral cutaneous nerve of the thigh.

Technique (Fig. 13.5)

'Three-in-one' block is essentially a modification of femoral nerve block. Paraesthesiae must be elicited, after which the needle should be held firmly to prevent it moving. Firm pressure is applied distal to the needle with the thumb, and the local anaesthetic is injected. It is best if an assistant holds the syringe and injects the drug while the anaesthetist holds the needle with one hand and presses below it with the other.

In the original paper a 20 ml volume of local anaesthetic was said to be adequate to block all three nerves, but many anaesthetists now find that 30 ml gives better results. This is a most useful block, but it only works well when paraesthesiae are elicited and, as mentioned in the section on femoral nerve block, this may not be easy. If, despite a long and thorough search, paraesthesiae are not obtained, it is wiser to use a spinal or epidural block.

Sciatic nerve block

Anatomy

The sciatic nerve is the largest nerve in the body. It starts in the pelvis as the continuation of the sacral plexus (Fig. 13.1) and passes from the pelvis into the buttock through the greater sciatic foramen. At this point, it is accompanied by the

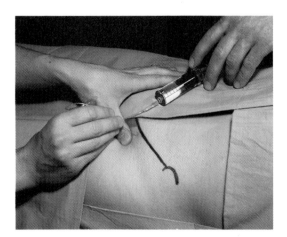

Fig. 13.5 'Three-in-one' block.

posterior cutaneous nerve of the thigh which can be thought of as a branch of the sciatic.

After emerging from the greater sciatic foramen, the nerve is just posterior to the acetabulum and the head of the femur. It lies on the muscles around the hip joint and is covered by gluteus maximus. It then runs vertically downwards in the hamstring compartment of the thigh to reach the popliteal fossa, where it divides into common peroneal and tibial branches (Fig. 13.9). Occasionally this division occurs much higher in the thigh. The tibial nerve passes vertically downwards through the calf to supply the heel and sole of the foot. The common peroneal nerve winds diagonally across the popliteal fossa to the lateral part of the calf before descending to the foot where its branches innervate the dorsal structures. The sural nerve is formed from components of both tibial and common peroneal branches and supplies the lateral border of the foot (Fig. 13.9).

Clinical application

Block of the nerve in the buttock is easy and reliable. It produces anaesthesia of the back of the thigh because the posterior cutaneous nerve lies close to the sciatic and is blocked by the same injection. It also provides anaesthesia of the anterolateral part of the leg and most of the foot. In combination with femoral or saphenous nerve block, it provides anaesthesia for the whole of the leg below the knee. It causes motor block of the hamstrings as well as of the muscles of the leg.

Techniques

Four methods have been described for blocking the sciatic nerve at the level of the hip joint:

1. Posterior approach (of Labat)
2. Anterior approach
3. Supine block (Raj et al 1975)
4. Lateral approach (Ichiyangi 1959).

The easiest block with the highest success rate is undoubtedly the posterior approach. However, the anterior approach can be useful if the patient is in pain and cannot be moved. The supine and the lateral approaches will not be described.

Posterior approach (Fig. 13.6). Positioning is vital if this block is to be carried out effectively. The patient lies with the side to be blocked uppermost. The lower leg is straight and the upper leg is flexed at the hip and knee so that the thigh is at right angles to the body. The greater trochanter is palpated and its upper border marked. The iliac crest is traced posteriorly and the posterior superior iliac spine is marked. Between these two points a line is drawn and from its midpoint a perpendicular is dropped. The point for needle insertion is about 5 cm along this perpendicular and its position can be checked by drawing a line between the coccyx and the top of the greater trochanter. The needle is inserted where the two lines intersect.

After skin cleansing, local anaesthetic is infiltrated into the skin and muscle. A 9 cm ($3\frac{1}{2}$ inch), 22 g spinal needle is inserted at right angles to the skin and advanced until either paraesthesiae are obtained or bone is encountered. If bone is encountered, the needle is withdrawn and redirected medially or laterally until paraesthesiae are obtained. While inserting the needle, the anaesthetist should try to imagine the anatomy of the pelvis underneath (Fig. 13.7). The sciatic nerve is emerging through the greater sciatic foramen, which forms a bony arch, and if this arch can be visualized, block of the nerve will become easier. Once paraesthesiae, which must radiate to the foot rather than to the knee joint, have been obtained,

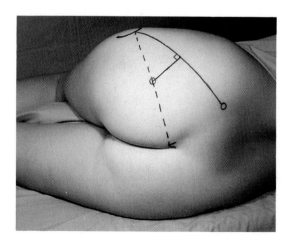

Fig. 13.6   Posterior approach to the sciatic nerve.

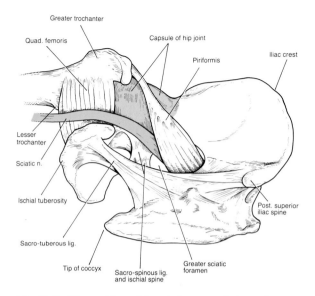

Quad. femoris
Greater trochanter
Capsule of hip joint
Piriformis
Iliac crest
Lesser trochanter
Sciatic n.
Ischial tuberosity
Post. superior iliac spine
Sacro-tuberous lig.
Tip of coccyx
Sacro-spinous lig. and ischial spine
Greater sciatic foramen

Fig. 13.7 The position of the sciatic nerve relative to the major structures near the hip joint.

the needle is held firmly and 20 ml of local anaesthetic is injected.

Anterior approach (Fig. 13.8). For this the patient lies supine. The anterior superior iliac spine and the pubic tubercle are palpated and marked, and a line is drawn between them to represent the inguinal ligament. This line is divided into three equal parts and a perpendicular dropped from the junction of the medial and middle thirds. A line is then drawn from the top of the greater trochanter parallel to the line of the inguinal ligament and the point where it meets the perpendicular is the point of needle insertion. This overlies the lesser trochanter on the inner aspect of the femur and at this level the sciatic nerve lies close behind the acetabulum and the head of the femur. The anterior approach requires a fairly long needle. A 9 cm ($3\frac{1}{2}$ inch) spinal needle is often not long enough and the author uses a 125 mm (5 inch) 20 g needle which was originally designed for chemical sympathectomy.

After skin cleansing, a wheal of local anaesthetic is raised, the needle is inserted and directed slightly laterally so that it strikes the medial surface of the femur. It is then withdrawn and 'walked off' the femur so that it passes medial to the femoral head.

Some anaesthetists believe that if the needle is inserted 5 cm deeper than its point of contact with the femur it will lie very close to the nerve and that if the local anaesthetic can be injected easily and without resistance, a good block will result. However, this is not always the case and it is better to seek paraesthesiae which radiate to the foot. Computerized tomography (Charlton, personal communication) has shown that the sciatic nerve often lies more laterally behind the femur than was previously appreciated. When using the classical landmarks described above, it may be impossible to bring the tip of the needle close enough to the nerve. Use of a more medial insertion point with more lateral direction of the needle may lead to a higher success rate. After careful aspiration, 20 ml of local anaesthetic is injected.

NERVE BLOCK AT THE KNEE JOINT

Sciatic nerve (popliteal fossa) block

Block of the sciatic nerve in the popliteal fossa is relatively easy and anaesthetizes the foot and most of the leg. Its advantage is that widespread motor block is avoided. In the author's opinion, sciatic nerve block in the popliteal fossa, combined with saphenous nerve block, is the method of choice for unilateral operations on the ankle or foot.

Technique (Fig. 13.9)

The patient lies prone and the leg is gently lifted to flex the knee joint so that the tendons of the biceps femoris (laterally) and semimembranosus with semitendinosus (medially) stand out. A line is drawn in the flexion crease between these tendons and from the middle of this line a perpendicular is drawn upwards for 10–15 cm to the apex of the fossa. The point of needle insertion is 1 cm lateral to the top of this perpendicular, since the sciatic nerve does not lie in the middle of the popliteal fossa, but slightly to the lateral side. The needle is inserted parallel to the perpendicular, pointing slightly upwards and is gently advanced until paraesthesiae to the foot are elicited. The nerve normally lies 3–5 cm deep to the skin. If paraesthesiae are not obtained the needle is

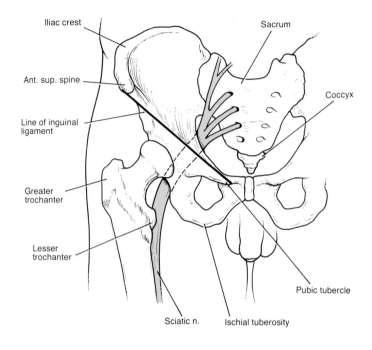

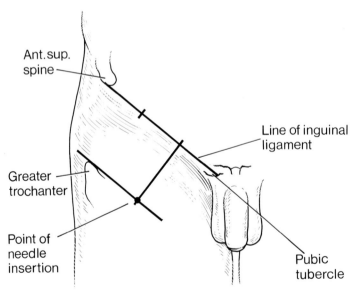

Fig. 13.8   Landmarks for the anterior approach to the sciatic nerve.

withdrawn almost to skin, and redirected slightly laterally or medially. It is important to make only small changes in direction as the nerve may otherwise be missed. Once paraesthesiae have been elicited, 15–20 ml of local anaesthetic is injected.

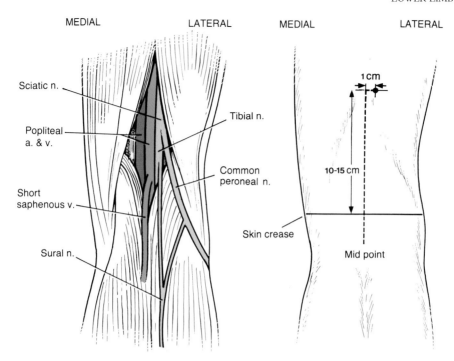

Fig. 13.9 Sciatic nerve block in the popliteal fossa. The perpendicular from the skin crease is extended to overlie the apex of the fossa.

Saphenous nerve block

The saphenous nerve (Fig. 13.10) is the terminal branch of the femoral nerve and supplies the skin of the anteromedial aspect of the leg. The lower border of the area supplied by this nerve is variable. Since most operations on the ankle and foot require a tourniquet, saphenous nerve block is needed for a mid-calf tourniquet even if the operation is carried out in the sciatic nerve territory.

The nerve runs down through the thigh in the adductor canal under the sartorius muscle. It pierces the fascia lata between the tendons of sartorius and gracilis on the inner aspect of the knee joint and becomes subcutaneous. In thin subjects, the nerve can often be rolled under the fingers where it lies on the medial aspect of the head of the tibia about 2 cm below the lower border of the patella. The long saphenous vein is a close relation here and is a useful landmark. The nerve is blocked by infiltrating 10 ml of local anaesthetic in the subcutaneous tissue at this point. Paraesthesiae are not sought. The proximity of the vein makes aspiration particularly important.

DISTAL BLOCKS OF THE LOWER LIMB

Ankle block

In order to anaesthetize the foot by injecting at the level of the ankle, it is necessary to block five nerves. They are the saphenous nerve (the terminal branch of the femoral nerve) and four nerves derived from the sciatic, the tibial, sural, superficial peroneal and deep peroneal nerves. Ankle block, although technically straightforward, has very limited use. It is uncomfortable for the patient because multiple injections are required and incomplete blocks occur with depressing regularity. It is seldom adequate for surgery to the foot because it does not provide anaesthesia for a tourniquet. It will be described only briefly.

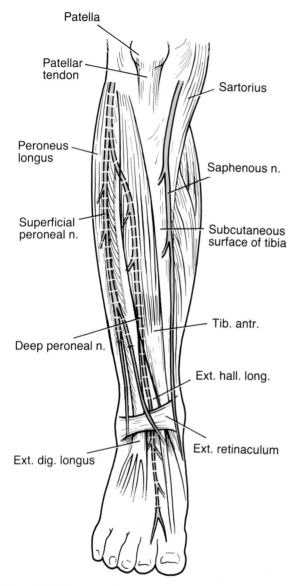

Fig. 13.10 Nerves on the anterior aspect of the leg and foot.

The saphenous nerve is blocked just above and slightly anterior to the medial malleolus (Fig. 13.10); the tibial nerve immediately behind the medial malleolus and deep to the posterior tibial artery (Fig. 13.11); the sural behind the lateral malleolus (Fig. 13.11); the deep peroneal between the tendons of tibialis anterior and extensor digitorum longus on the anterior aspect of the ankle (Fig. 13.10); and the superficial peroneal nerve by infiltrating subcutaneously across the anterior aspect of the ankle joint (Fig. 13.10).

Ring (digital nerve) block

Ring block is a simple, safe, effective and extremely useful technique and is probably underused, especially as a means of postoperative analgesia. After operations on the toes in which periosteum is damaged (e.g. osteotomy or nail bed ablation) postoperative pain can be severe and out of all proportion to the scale of the procedure. Even if a general anaesthetic is used for the operation itself, a ring block with 0.5% *plain* bupivacaine can provide analgesia for more than 12 hours. The technique is essentially the same as that described for the upper limb (see Ch.12).

Bier's block

Bier's block (Fig. 13.12) is not as widely used for lower limb procedures as it is for those in the upper limb. Although this may be because conditions for which it is suited are seen less often in the lower limb, it is more probably because the technique is not considered to be practical. The large dose of local anaesthetic required when the tourniquet is placed on the thigh can result in a significant incidence of problems due to systemic toxicity, yet operative and tourniquet pain are very frequent (Valli et al 1987). If the tourniquet is placed at mid-calf level the dose of drug used is the same as in the upper limb and the technique is identical in every respect (see Ch.12). However, tourniquet discomfort can still be a problem and some workers find that anaesthesia is not as reliable as in the upper limb technique (Fagg 1987, Valli & Rosenberg 1986). This suggests that case selection is very important for the use of this technique.

Local anaesthesia for knee arthroscopy

Spinal and epidural blocks are the most convenient techniques for operations on the knee. 'Three-in-one' block combined with sciatic block at the hip is an alternative, but tourniquet pain is often a

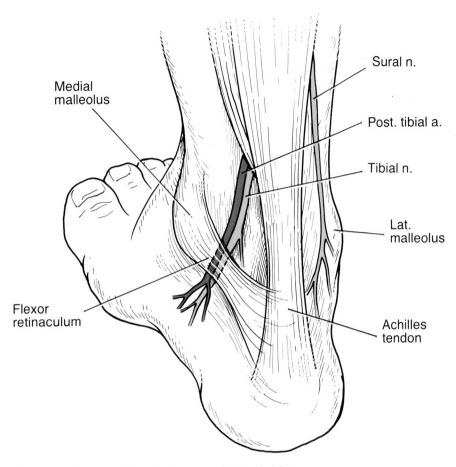

Fig. 13.11   Nerves on the posterior aspect of the ankle joint.

problem. Femoral nerve block on its own is insufficient.

For arthroscopy alone, or for operations carried out through the arthroscope, a simple infiltration technique can be used. This has the advantage that both general anaesthesia and central neural blocks are avoided, so it is particularly suitable for day patients. It is vital that the surgeon and anaesthetist work together for this technique to be effective. The anaesthetist must know where the surgeon intends to insert the flushing needles, the arthroscope and any other instrument.

The skin and deeper tissues are infiltrated with local anaesthetic (0.5% prilocaine with 1:200 000 adrenaline), and the area infiltrated is marked with an indelible pen. A 20 ml volume of solution is

normally sufficient. A 19 g needle is then inserted into the knee joint and 50 ml of the same local anaesthetic solution is injected. The knee is passively flexed and extended a few times to spread the local anaesthetic, and after 10 minutes the procedure can start. No tourniquet is used because the adrenaline provides excellent operating conditions. If the knee is flushed with standard solutions of local anaesthetic there is no loss of anaesthesia, but if an effusion is present it is wise to drain it prior to injection of any solution to avoid dilution and to improve the surgeon's view.

This technique can be used satisfactorily for the great majority of patients undergoing arthroscopy, but it is contraindicated in certain groups. Those with severe osteoarthritis of the hip will require

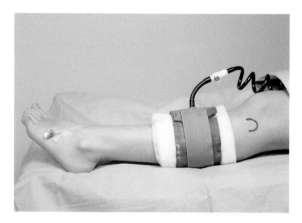

Fig. 13.12   Intravenous regional anaesthesia in the lower limb. The head of the fibula has been marked. Note that the tourniquet is well below that level.

spinal or epidural anaesthesia to allow the surgeon to manipulate both joints during the arthroscopy. It may be impossible to provide satisfactory analgesia in patients with widespread scarring of the knee due to injury or previous surgery. Finally, infiltration may be unsuitable for patients with an acutely painful knee. Spasm of the quadriceps muscles may make it difficult to perform the block and for the surgeon to do a proper arthroscopy. However, it may be possible to improve the situation by performing a femoral nerve block in addition to the local infiltration. If these limitations are borne in mind the block can be used successfully for a wide range of arthroscopic procedures (Buckley et al 1989).

REFERENCES

Buckley J R, Hood G M, Macrae W 1989 Arthroscopy under local anaesthesia. Journal of Bone and Joint Surgery 71B: 126–127

Fagg P 1987 Intravenous regional anaesthesia for lower limb orthopaedic surgery. Annals of the Royal College of Surgeons of England 69: 274–275

Ichiyangi K 1959 Sciatic nerve block: lateral approach with the patient supine. Anesthesiology 20: 601–604

Misra U, Priddie A K, McClymont C, Bower S 1991 Plasma concentrations of bupivacaine following combined sciatic and femoral 3-in-1 nerve block in open knee surgery. British Journal of Anaesthesia 66: 310–313

Moore D C 1965a Regional block, 4th edn, p 287. Thomas, Springfield

Moore D C 1965b Regional block, 4th edn, p 293. Thomas, Springfield

Raj P P, Parks R I, Watson T D, Jenkins M T 1975 New single position supine approach to sciatic–femoral nerve block. Anesthesia and Analgesia 54: 489

Robison C, Ray D C, McKeown D W, Buchan A S 1991 Effect of adrenaline on plasma concentrations of bupivacaine following lower limb nerve block. British Journal of Anaesthesia 66: 228–231

Serpell M G, Millar F A, Thomson M F 1991 Comparison of lumbar plexus block versus conventional opioid analgesia after total knee replacement. Anaesthesia 46: 275–277

Sharrock N E 1980 Inadvertent '3 in 1 block' following injection of the lateral cutaneous nerve of the thigh. Anesthesia and Analgesia 59: 887–888

Valli H, Rosenberg P H 1986 Intravenous regional anesthesia below the knee. Anaesthesia 41: 1196–1201

Valli H, Rosenberg P H, Hekali R 1987 Comparison of lidocaine and prilocaine for intravenous regional anesthesia of the whole lower extremity. Regional Anesthesia 12: 128–134

Winnie A P, Ramamurthy S, Durrani Z 1973 The inguinal paravascular technic of lumbar plexus anesthesia: the '3 in 1 block'. Anesthesia and Analgesia 52: 989–996

14. Head, neck and airway

R. S. Neill

Regional nerve blocks, performed by the dental, maxillofacial, ophthalmic, or ear, nose and throat surgeon, have an established place as sole anaesthetics for relatively minor operations on the head and neck. The size of the workload, particularly in dentistry, is such that there are insufficient trained anaesthetists to provide a service. In any case general anaesthesia would be quite inappropriate for such minor surgery.

Since specialist anaesthetists are involved only in the management of the more major procedures they have tended to limit themselves to the use of general anaesthesia. The relative complexity of the innervation of the head and neck is another reason why few anaesthetists have explored the possibilities of regional anaesthesia in this area, even though most have personally experienced its benefits during a visit to the dentist.

Innervation of the head and neck

The structures of the head and neck are supplied by a relatively large number of nerves – the 12 cranial and the upper four cervical. Much of this innervation subserves very specialized sensory or secretomotor function and is of no relevance to nerve block for surgery. The nerves which serve somatic functions contain, for all practical purposes, only sensory or motor fibres. Thus sensory block may be produced without motor paralysis. This is a distinct advantage with the intra-oral blocks because it means that the muscles controlling the airway are unaffected. In other situations it may be important to ensure that both sensory and motor nerves are blocked. For example, when a retrobulbar block is used for a procedure on the open eye, the orbital branch of the facial nerve must be blocked. This paralyses the orbicularis oculi muscle and reduces the risk of vitreous prolapse.

For the purposes of nerve block for surgery the most important nerves of the head and neck are those which provide somatic sensation to the skin (Fig. 14.1) and the mucous membranes of the airway. Some knowledge of the distribution of the motor nerves is also required.

Trigeminal nerve (Figs. 14.2 and 14.3)

The trigeminal (fifth) is the largest cranial nerve. It supplies sensation to the face, the greater part of the scalp, the teeth, mouth and nasal cavity, and controls the muscles of mastication. The trigeminal (semi-lunar) ganglion lies in the middle cranial fossa in a recess near the apex of the petrous temporal bone. On leaving the ganglion the sensory root divides into three divisions – ophthalmic, maxillary and mandibular. The smaller motor root lies inferior to the ganglion and joins the mandibular division.

The *ophthalmic nerve* enters the orbit through the superior orbital fissure and divides into frontal, nasociliary and lacrimal nerves. The terminal cutaneous branches of the frontal are the supraorbital and supratrochlear nerves. Those of the nasociliary are the infratrochlear and external nasal nerves. The lacrimal continues without major branches.

The *maxillary nerve* leaves the cranial cavity through the foramen rotundum and crosses the pterygopalatine fossa to enter the orbit through the inferior orbital fissure. It traverses the infra-orbital

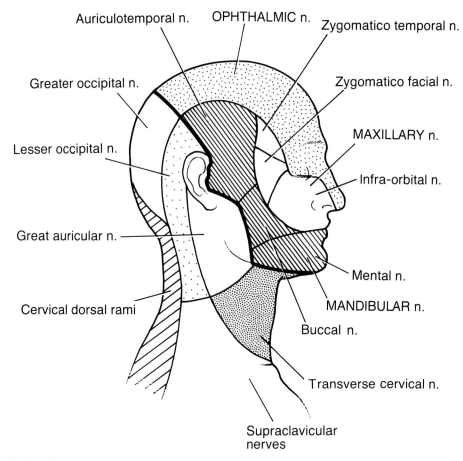

Fig. 14.1   Distribution of nerves supplying the superficial tissues of the head and neck.

canal to emerge as the infra-orbital nerve. In the infra-orbital fissure an inconstant branch may be given off to form the zygomaticotemporal nerve. A connection between the zygomaticotemporal and the lacrimal nerves may replace one or other of these two.

The *mandibular nerve* is the largest division of the trigeminal and it leaves the skull through the foramen ovale with the motor root. The two then unite before dividing into a small anterior and a large posterior trunk. At this point the nerve lies in the pterygopalatine fossa anterior to the neck of the mandible and posterior to the lateral pterygoid plate. The anterior trunk supplies most of the muscles of mastication and has one sensory

branch, the buccal nerve, which supplies the skin over, and the mucous membrane deep to, the buccinator muscle.

The posterior trunk is sensory (apart from a branch to mylohyoid) and has three main branches – the auriculotemporal, inferior dental and lingual nerves. The auriculotemporal emerges from behind the temporomandibular joint to lie close to the superficial temporal vessels and supply the skin of the temple. The inferior dental nerve enters the inferior dental foramen on the medial surface of the ramus of the mandible and runs through the bone to emerge as the mental nerve. The lingual nerve runs between the ramus of the mandible and the medial pterygoid muscle and supplies the

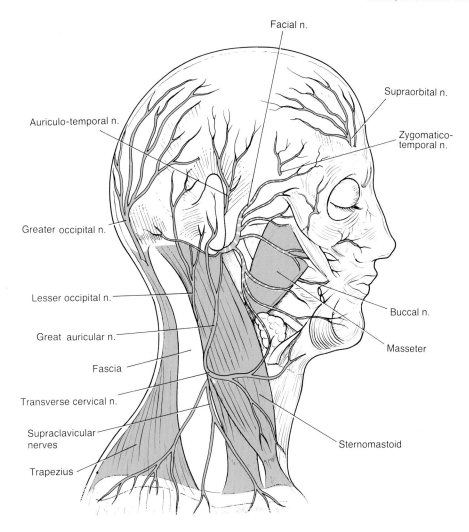

Fig. 14.2   Positions of the nerves supplying the side of the face and neck.

anterior two-thirds of the tongue. At the level of the third molar it is covered only by mucous membrane.

Facial nerve

As the facial (seventh) nerve traverses the parotid gland it divides into five main branches – temporal, zygomatic, buccal, mandibular and cervical – which radiate out to supply the muscles of expression in the respective parts of the face. The mandibular branch runs forward below the angle of the mandible before turning upwards and forwards to supply the angle of the mouth.

Glossopharyngeal nerve

The glossopharyngeal (ninth) nerve supplies sensory fibres to the posterior part of the tongue, to the pharynx and the tonsil, secretomotor fibres to the parotid and motor fibres to stylopharyngeus. It emerges from the skull through the jugular fora-

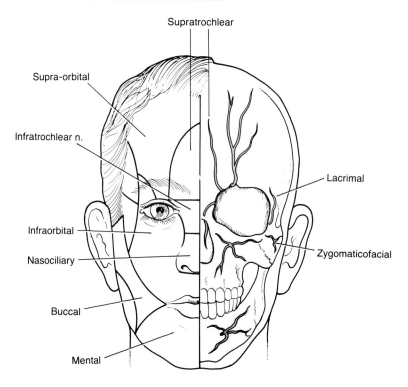

Fig. 14.3 Positions of the nerves supplying the face. Note the straight-line relationship between the supra-orbital notch, the infra-orbital foramen and the mental foramen.

men and passes forward between the internal jugular vein and internal carotid artery to pierce the superior constrictor muscle of the pharnyx.

Vagus nerve

In the head and neck the vagus (tenth) nerve, which lies within the carotid sheath, has two branches which are of interest here. The *superior laryngeal nerve* arises from the inferior ganglion of the vagus and runs downwards, forwards and medially to cross in front of the greater horn of the hyoid bone where it divides into two branches. The internal branch pierces the thyrohyoid membrane to supply the mucous membrane of the larnyx down to the level of the vocal cords. The external branch is the motor nerve to the cricothyroid muscle.

The *recurrent laryngeal nerve*, having looped under the aorta on the right and the subclavian artery on the left, ascends in the groove between the trachea and oesophagus. It enters the larynx posteriorly, behind the articulation between the cricoid cartilage and the inferior cornu of the thyroid cartilage. It supplies the mucous membrane of the larynx below the vocal cords and all the muscles of the larynx except cricothyroid.

Hypoglossal nerve

The hypoglossal (twelfth) nerve is the motor nerve to the tongue. From the base of the skull, where it is closely related to the glossopharyngeal and vagus nerves, it passes between the internal jugular vein and the internal carotid artery and curves downwards and forwards to the base of the tongue.

Cervical nerves

The dorsal rami of the upper cervical nerves (C_2–C_4) supply the skin of the back of the neck and, through the greater occipital nerve, a portion of the scalp (Fig. 14.2).

The first four ventral rami form the cervical plexus, which may be divided into two parts. The deep branches supply only muscles, including, of course, the diaphragm. The superficial branches all pierce the deep fascia at the middle of the posterior border of sternomastoid and run upwards (great auricular, lesser occipital), transversely (transverse cervical) and downwards (supraclavicular) to supply skin over a wide area (Fig. 14.2). The supraclavicular nerves supply sensation to the skin of the chest and shoulder down to the level of the second rib – the 'cape' area.

Possible blocks – problems and hazards

Techniques for blocking the main trunks of all the cranial nerves mentioned above have been described. These methods involve injection near the base of the skull, are often technically difficult and require very precise knowledge of anatomy. The main divisions of the trigeminal nerve lie in very vascular areas and the main trunks of other nerves are closely related to each other, the carotid artery and the jugular vein. There is significant risk of intravascular injection, haematoma formation or needle damage to other important structures. Both sensory and motor innervation to the airway may be affected with consequent risk of obstruction and aspiration.

Similar disadvantages apply to the classical technique of 'deep' cervical plexus block. This is performed by making separate injections on to the transverse processes of the second to fourth cervical vertebrae. Careful needle angulation should avoid complications such as injection into the vertebral artery, epidural or subarachnoid space, but it is not an easy method. A simpler, single-injection technique has been described (Murphy 1981), but both methods will paralyse the diaphragm. Cervical epidural block has been used for surgery of the neck, but the potential problems and the availability of alternative methods mean that it is rarely used.

Some individuals do obtain a comprehensive knowledge and experience of these techniques, but opportunities to learn and maintain such skills occur only in very specialized units and these complex methods offer little advantage over the more distal blocks. These are usually much easier technically and may be reliably employed, even by the occasional user, with advantage to patient and surgeon. The techniques which are described below meet these criteria and have much to offer, not only as sole anaesthetics, but also as adjuncts to general anaesthesia (Neill 1983).

Clinical applications

The use of nerve blocks in the head and neck may confer significant advantages in four situations:

1. *Out-patients*. Obviously the vast majority of dental work falls into this category. When blocks are used with general anaesthesia the residual action of the local anaesthetic provides analgesia without central depression, reduces the incidence of general systemic upset and allows early ambulation.
2. *Poor-risk patients*. Carefully selected nerve blocks can avoid the need for, or considerably reduce the dosage of, general anaesthesia if this carries a greater than normal risk.
3. *Postoperative airway problems*. The combination of the effects of narcotic analgesics with the anatomical derangements seen after maxillofacial surgery may imperil the airway. Nerve block with long-acting agents can provide high quality analgesia with less risk to the patient. Unfortunately, several of the more proximal blocks may be needed.
4. *Awake intubation*. In patients with airway abnormalities it may be safer to perform endotracheal intubation (or tracheostomy) under regional block before induction of general anaesthesia. It must be appreciated that the technique will abolish the protective reflexes so the patient is at risk from pulmonary aspiration until the local anaesthetic is absorbed.

Murphy (1980) divides patients for whom head and neck blocks should be considered into similar groups and adds a fifth – those undergoing carotid artery surgery. Consciousness is fully preserved to assess the adequacy of the cerebral circulation when the carotid artery is clamped. Few British patients will accept this technique, but a superficial cervical plexus block may be used to supplement general anaesthesia and provide analgesia into the postoperative period. The reduction in afferent input helps to reduce the incidence and severity of the hypertension seen after these operations.

A number of other situations may be mentioned to illustrate the usefulness of the more distal head and neck blocks. Skin tumours, particularly the basal cell carcinoma, occur frequently on the face and neck. Often these patients are elderly and frail, are dealt with as outpatients and have multiple or extensive lesions. Infiltration techniques may distend and distort the tissues so that accurate definition of the lesion and neat approximation of the wound edges may be difficult. Careful use of nerve blocks, supplemented by discrete infiltration if necessary can overcome these difficulties and requires a smaller dose of local anaesthetic. Similar cosmetic considerations apply to the repair of facial lacerations. Superficial cervical plexus block, with or without general anaesthesia, may be used for any procedure in the neck including lymph node biopsy, tracheostomy and thyroidectomy. Block of the great auricular nerve alone is sufficient to produce very good postoperative analgesia in children who have had prominent ears corrected. The reader can readily add to these by adapting to his own practice combinations of the methods described below.

SUGGESTED TECHNIQUES

As has been indicated proximal nerve blocks of the head and neck have little to offer outside specialist units. These techniques are described in the larger texts (e.g. Garber 1980, Boberg Ans & Barner 1980, Neill 1989) and only the more distal methods will be described here. Aspiration tests are vital with each of these blocks, even though only small doses of local anaesthetics are employed. Major toxic

reactions to injection in these areas have been described and have been attributed to retrograde spread along branches into the carotid artery.

Trigeminal branches

Figure 14.3 illustrates the areas of facial skin which are supplied by the terminal branches of the three divisions of the trigeminal nerve and shows the various foramina through which they emerge to lie in the superficial tissues of the face. Identification of the three main nerves is aided by the fact that the supra-orbital notch, the infra-orbital foramen and the mental foramen are in line. The nerves which supply the side of the face and the rest of the scalp are shown in Figures 14.1 and 14.2.

Supratrochlear and supra-orbital block

These nerves can be blocked, bilaterally if needed, from a single injection site on the nasal bridge. The needle is first directed downwards and laterally towards the medial canthus and then directly laterally under the supra-orbital rim. Solution should be deposited at least 1 cm either side of the notch and 1–2 ml is adequate for both blocks.

Auriculotemporal block

The superficial temporal artery is palpated just above the temporomandibular joint in front of the ear. The nerve will be blocked by 2–3 ml of local anaesthetic infiltrated around the vessels.

Infra-orbital block

The infra-orbital foramen can usually be palpated 1 cm below the orbital rim and 1 cm from the lateral wall of the nose. Injection of 1–2 ml of local anaesthetic at this point should produce a block. The needle may be inserted through the skin or through the upper buccal sulcus, just lateral to the lateral incisor tooth, but in either case the point must be kept below the orbital rim and well away from the eye. The needle should not be inserted into the foramen. This is unnecessary and potentially hazardous because the nerve, or the accompanying artery, may be damaged and it is quite easy to puncture the floor of the orbit.

Zygomaticofacial and lacrimal block

The zygomatic foramen can be palpated 1–2 cm from the lower lateral margin of the orbit. An injection should be made to encircle the foramen since the nerve's branches radiate in all directions.

The same injection point is used to block the lacrimal nerve. The needle is directed up towards the lateral margin of the orbit.

Inferior dental and lingual nerves

The inferior dental foramen lies in the centre of the medial aspect of the vertical ramus of the mandible. It may be located by palpating the concavity of the retromolar trigone with the index finger, the nail identifying the medial ridge. With the barrel of the syringe resting on the contralateral premolar, the needle is inserted parallel to the occlusal surface just beyond the midpoint of the palpating finger. As the injection (2 ml) is made, the syringe is swung across to allow the needle to be inserted a further 2 cm parallel to the horizontal ramus of the mandible. The injection will anaesthetize both nerves.

Buccal block

The needle is inserted into the mucous membrane of the cheek at the level of the occlusal surface of the first mandibular molar. It is then directed backwards and 2–3 ml of solution is infiltrated parallel to the lateral aspect of the mandibular ramus.

Mental block

The mental foramen is situated below the first premolar tooth, half-way between the gum margin and the lower border of the body of the mandible. Injection of 1–2 ml local anaesthetic solution close to the bone in that region should produce a block.

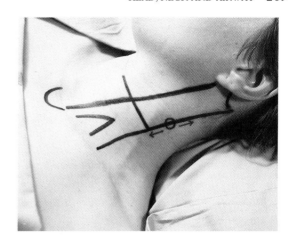

Fig. 14.4 Landmarks for superficial cervical plexus block. The circle marks the point of needle insertion and the arrows indicate the direction in which solution will be seen to spread in a thin individual.

Because the opening of the foramen is directed backwards, it is not readily palpable. Its position may be confirmed by using the straight-line relationship with the other foramina.

Cervical nerves

Superficial plexus block (Fig. 14.4)

The superficial branches of the plexus are blocked by an injection made at the midpoint of the posterior border of sternomastoid. To help identify this point the patient should turn the head slightly to the opposite side and lift it just clear of the pillow to contract the muscle. Usually the external jugular vein crosses the posterior border of the muscle 1–2 cm below this point. Solution is directed upwards and downwards from the injection point. If the injection is made into the correct tissue plane, solution will be seen to 'flow' along the border of the muscle in a thin subject. A solution of 5–10 ml of local anaesthetic will be sufficient and bilateral blocks may be performed safely.

Great auricular block

The branches of the plexus which form the great auricular nerve and supply the ear (Fig. 14.2) may be blocked by injecting 2–3 ml of local anaesthetic 2–3 cm anteriorly and posteriorly from the tip of the mastoid process.

Greater occipital block

The nerve penetrates the semispinalis capitis and trapezius muscles and enters the subcutaneous tissues of the scalp about 2.5 cm lateral to the occipital protuberance. Infiltration of 2–3 ml of solution just above this point should block the nerve.

Awake intubation

Oral intubation

The upper airway is innervated by branches of the trigeminal, glossopharyngeal and vagus nerves. Nerve block is not a practical proposition and a technique which is essentially topical is recommended. The quality of local anaesthesia required for awake intubation will depend on the general condition of the patient and the technique employed will have to take this into account. Local anaesthetic drugs are absorbed very rapidly from mucous membranes and care should be taken to ensure that dosage is limited to 200 mg of lignocaine or its equivalent. A pressurized aerosol containing 10% lignocaine is available for topical application and it delivers metered doses of 10 mg.

The patient lies in the standard position for intubation, with all the usual facilities to hand. Intravenous sedation is helpful, but is usually contraindicated by the very need for awake intubation. The most effective way of anaesthetizing the mucous membrane of the mouth and pharnyx is to give the patient a benzocaine lozenge to suck. If atropine is to be used to dry secretions it should not be given until after this stage. The alternative to the lozenge is to spray the mouth and pharnyx with 10% lignocaine, using a laryngoscope smeared with a little lignocaine gel to aid access. Each spray of local anaesthetic should be allowed about 30 seconds to act before the laryngoscope is advanced further. In many patients it is possible to complete the procedure by spraying on to and through the vocal cords, but a

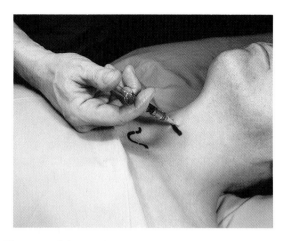

Fig. 14.5 Cricothyroid puncture.

robust subject will require a more specific approach.

Cricothyroid injection (Fig. 14.5). This is the simplest and most effective way of applying local anesthetic to the larynx itself. With the patient's head absolutely straight, the cricoid cartilage is palpated. A 25 g needle, attached to a syringe containing 2–4 ml of 4% lignocaine, is inserted in the midline, just above the cricoid and advanced gently through the cricothyroid membrane. The inpiration of a little air will confirm the position of the needle tip. The patient is instructed to take a deep breath and then to cough. As inspiration becomes maximal the lignocaine is injected rapidly and the needle withdrawn. The cough will ensure that the local anaesthetic spreads to the area above the cords supplied by the internal laryngeal nerve. This branch of the superior laryngeal nerve can be blocked where it crosses the hyoid bone and pierces the thyrohyoid membrane (Raj 1983). However, the cricothyroid puncture will still be needed to anaesthetize the mucosa below the cords supplied by the recurrent laryngeal nerve. The above technique makes the separate nerve block unnecessary.

Nasal intubation

Essentially the same technique may be used for nasal intubation or fibreoptic bronchoscopy. A pack soaked in 4% cocaine or 4% lignocaine with adrenaline 1:100 000 is inserted for 30 minutes to anaesthetize the nasal airway and shrink the mucosa. The tube should be well lubricated with lignocaine gel.

Tracheostomy

A tracheostomy may be performed under simple infiltration, but this may cause some distortion of

the anatomy. A bilateral cervical plexus block will avoid this and a cricothyroid injection may be performed before the trachea is opened.

REFERENCES

Boberg Ans J, Barner S S 1980 Neural blockade for ophthalmologic surgery. In: Cousins M J, Bridenbaugh P O (eds) Neural blockade, p 443. Lippincott, Philadelphia
Garber J 1980 Neural blockade for dental, oral and adjoining areas. In: Cousins M J, Bridenbaugh P O (eds) Neural blockade, p 426. Lippincott, Philadelphia
Murphy T M 1980 Somatic blockade. In: Cousins M J, Bridenbaugh P O (eds) Neural blockade, p 423. Lippincott, Philadelphia
Murphy T M 1981 Nerve blocks in anesthesia. In: Miller

R D (ed) Anesthesia, p 624. Churchill Livingstone, New York
Neill R S 1983 Head and neck surgery. In: Henderson J J, Nimmo W S (eds) Practical regional anaesthesia, p 165. Blackwell, Oxford
Neill R S 1989 Head and neck. In: Nimmo W S, Smith G (eds) Anaesthesia, p 1134. Blackwell, Oxford
Raj P P 1983 Bronchoscopy and tracheal intubation. In: Henderson J J, Nimmo W S (eds) Practical regional anaesthesia, p 165 Blackwell, Oxford

15. Regional techniques in ophthalmology

A. P. Rubin

Many minor operations on the lids or conjunctiva may be performed with simple infiltration or topical (conjunctival) application of local anaesthetic. As well as sensory block, more complex ophthalmic surgery requires akinesia (immobility) of the globe and *often* a reduction in intra-ocular pressure. To produce these requirements, local anaesthetic must be injected to produce not only sensory block within the orbit, but also block of the motor supply to the extra-ocular muscles (the four recti and two obliques), the levator palpebrae superioris and the orbicularis oculi. The traditional method of producing these aims, the retrobulbar block, has been in use for over 100 years (Knapp 1884) and involves injection within the cone formed by the extra-ocular muscles. It must be combined with a facial nerve block to ensure paralysis of the orbicularis oculi muscle. The peribulbar block is more recent (Davis & Mandel 1986) and does not normally require this supplementation because the injections are performed outside the muscle cone and the solution spreads directly to the orbicularis oculi muscle.

ANATOMY OF THE ORBIT (Figs 15.1, 15.2 and 15.3)

The globe lies within the orbit (Fig. 15.1) and is between 2 and 2.5 cm long (the axial length). Knowledge of this important measurement (which is usually obtained as part of the work-up for lens implant surgery) is needed to reduce the risk of globe perforation during retrobulbar block, particularly in myopic eyes, which are longer. The equator of the globe is at half the axial length.

The orbit itself is a cone-shaped cavity with its apex placed posteriorly and its base formed by the orbital margin (Fig. 15.2). It is important to appreciate that the medial wall runs backwards parallel to the saggital plane, but that the lateral wall is angled towards the midline.

The four rectus muscles arise from the annulus of Zinn (Fig. 15.3) at the back of the orbit and are inserted close to the equator of the globe (Fig. 15.1). The muscle cone forms the boundary between two compartments: the central or retrobulbar space and the peripheral or peribulbar space (Fig. 15.1). Within the cone lie the optic nerve, ophthalmic artery, ciliary ganglion and the nerves to the muscles. All of these structures are vulnerable to damage secondary to trauma, vasoconstriction or pressure. The peribulbar compartment is similar to the epidural space or brachial plexus sheath, containing fat, connective tissue septa and small blood vessels. The least vascular parts of the peribulbar space are the inferotemporal, nasal and superotemporal sections and it is usual to make injections there (Hamilton 1990).

The sensory supply of the orbit is provided by the lacrimal, frontal and nasociliary branches of the ophthalmic division of the trigeminal nerve (V), each of which enters the orbit through the superior orbital fissure (Fig. 15.3). Autonomic fibres run from the ciliary ganglion, which is situated within the cone near to the orbital apex. The oculomotor nerve (III) supplies the superior, inferior and medial rectus muscles as well as the levator palpebrae superioris; the trochlear nerve (IV) supplies the superior oblique; the abducent nerve (VI) supplies the lateral rectus; and the facial nerve

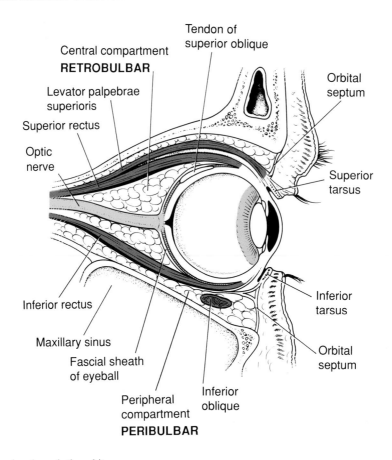

Fig. 15.1 Vertical section through the orbit.

(VII) the orbicularis oculi. After traversing the stylohyoid foramen the facial nerve passes through the parotid gland, posterior to the vertical ramus of the mandible. The orbicularis oculi is usually supplied by the temporal and zygomatic branches.

GENERAL MANAGEMENT

Indications

In adults virtually all ophthalmic operations may be performed under local anaesthesia, the limiting factor being the ability of the patient to lie still for long enough. Its advantages include less need for inpatient management, earlier discharge, fewer emetic or other side-effects and improved post-operative analgesia.

Contraindications

These methods should not be used when surgery is expected to be prolonged and they are not appropriate in children, patients who cannot lie reasonably flat or those who suffer from pathological anxiety, claustrophobia, dementia or involuntary movements, including uncontrolled coughing or sneezing.

Preparation of the patient

The use of regional anaesthesia should not be an excuse for inadequate preoperative assessment. A complete history should be taken and physical examination and relevant investigations performed well in advance of surgery so that the late

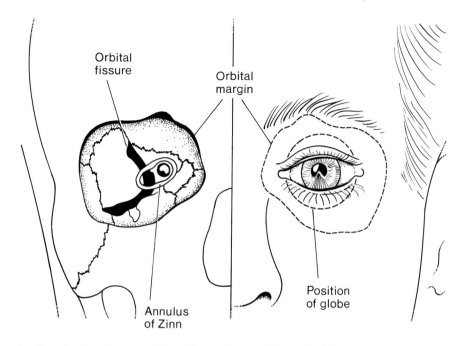

Fig. 15.2 Anterior view of orbit and contents. Dotted lines indicate positions of orbital margin and globe.

cancellation rate is minimized. Full discussion of the proposed technique should allay the patient's anxiety and most will accept it once they are reassured that they will feel no pain during the block or the operation, and that they will not see frightening things. Patients should be fasted as for a general anaesthetic because of the small, but real, risk of unconsciousness due to intravascular injection or intracranial spread of local anaesthetic. The bladder must be empty, but premedication is rarely required in this predominantly elderly population.

General principles

The patient must be kept comfortable at all times with pillows and padding as required. A pillow under the knees helps to alleviate back strain and it is particularly important to ensure that the neck is in a comfortable position in the elderly patient. Sedation is very rarely required, but a few patients benefit from small (1 mg) doses of midazolam, usually prior to performance of the block.

Every care should be taken to ensure that the local anaesthetic technique is painless. This may be achieved by the use of very fine needles, the preliminary application of warmed local anaesthetic solution diluted in ten times its volume of balanced salt solution (Bloom et al 1984, Korbon et al 1987), very slow injections, gentle technique, and constant explanation and reassurance. Injections through the conjunctiva, which may be anaesthetized first with 1% topical amethocaine, are less painful than those through the skin of the eyelid. Great care should be taken to choose relatively avascular areas, to withdraw the needle very carefully and to apply gentle pressure immediately to control any potential haemorrhage. Great care must be taken at all times to avoid damage to the anaesthetized cornea.

A pressure device such as the Buys mercury bag (Buys 1980) or Honan balloon (Davidson et al 1979) should be applied over the closed padded eye after injection to aid dissipation of the solution and ensure a low intra-ocular pressure.

Monitoring

A pulse oximeter, electrocardiograph and blood pressure recorder should be used. Intravenous

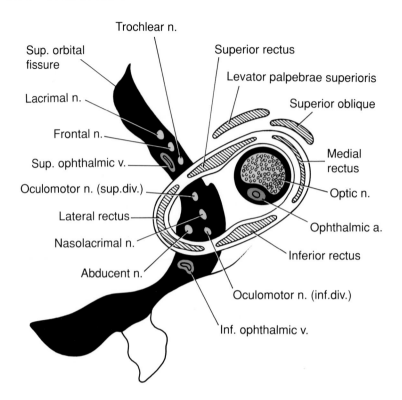

Fig. 15.3 Structures at the apex of the orbit.

access should be ensured and full resuscitation equipment available.

LOCAL ANAESTHETIC SOLUTIONS

Topical. Amethocaine 1% is usually used to anaesthetize the conjunctiva, but it stings on application. The preliminary application of this solution diluted in ten times its volume of balanced salt solution is painless, but allows subsequent application of the full strength solution without discomfort.

Injection. High concentrations of local anaesthetic are required to produce motor, as well as sensory block, and the most commonly used solution is a mixture of equal parts of 2% lignocaine and 0.75% bupivacaine (Feibel 1985, Hamilton et al 1988). It is usual to add hyaluronidase 7.5 IU ml^{-1} (Thomson 1988) to improve diffusion of the solution through the fat-filled spaces of the orbit. Adrenaline 5 μg ml^{-1} is also

added to improve the quality and duration of block, but may be omitted if contraindicated (House et al 1991).

TECHNIQUES

Retrobulbar block (Fig. 15.4)

Topical anaesthesia of the conjunctiva is produced with amethocaine as described above. The patient is then asked to look straight ahead and the lower eyelid pulled down. A 31 mm (1.25 inch) 23 g needle, with a syringe containing 3 ml of anaesthetic solution attached, is inserted through the inferior conjunctival cul de sac level with the lateral border of the iris (Fig. 15.5) The bevel of the needle should face the globe to reduce the risk of perforation and the needle is initially directed parallel to the floor of the orbit. Once the needle tip has passed the equator of the globe, the needle is redirected upwards and inwards towards the lower part of the superior orbital fissure (Feitl &

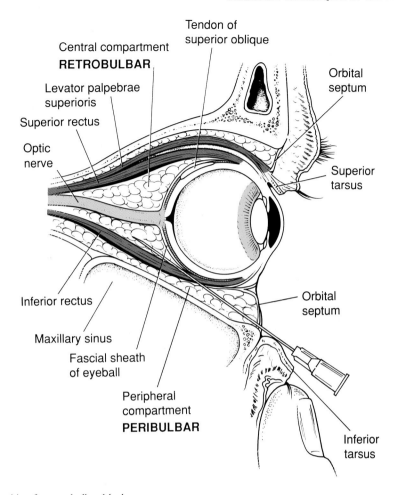

Fig. 15.4 Needle position for retrobulbar block.

Krupin 1990). It should not cross the mid-sagittal plane of the orbit. A 'give' may be felt as the needle perforates the muscle cone, but this is less likely with sharp needles than with the traditional short-bevel Atkinson needle (Atkinson 1961). After a careful aspiration test, solution should be injected slowly while the patient is watched closely. The needle is withdrawn carefully and firm digital pressure applied to the eye for 5 minutes.

Complications

The most common complication is *retrobulbar haemorrhage*, which occurs in 1–2% of patients (Morgan et al 1988). This causes proptosis, chemosis (subconjunctival oedema), subconjunctival haemorrhage and a dramatic increase in intra-orbital pressure, which usually necessitates postponement of the operation. *Retinal artery compression* may follow and require urgent decompressive surgery.

Globe perforation is especially likely with long myopic eyes (Ramsay & Knobloch 1978; Feibel 1985) and must be discussed immediately with the ophthalmic surgeon. *Optic atrophy* and *retinal vessel occlusion* may occur even in the absence of obvious haemorrhage. These may be due to injection into the optic nerve sheath, direct damage to the optic nerve or central retinal artery, or haemorrhage within the nerve sheath.

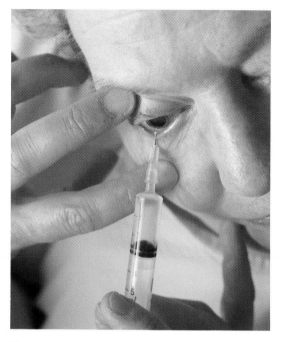

Fig. 15.5   Needle insertion point for retrobulbar block.

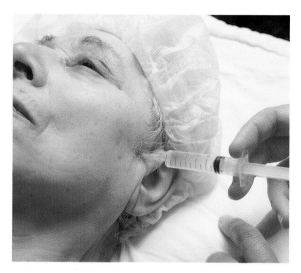

Fig. 15.6   O'Brien method of facial nerve block.

Systemic complications include confusion, convulsions, loss of consciousness and respiratory or cardiac arrest (Feitl & Krupin 1990). These may be due to systemic drug toxicity, intra-arterial injection with retrograde flow of anaesthetic solution, injection into cerebrospinal fluid within a cuff of dura around the optic nerve, or allergic or vasovagal reactions.

Facial nerve block

Retrobulbar block must be supplemented by this block to ensure paralysis of the orbicularis oculi muscle. A number of techniques – Nadbath-Rehman, O'Brien, Atkinson and Van Lint – have been described (Zahl 1990) but only two will be considered here.

O'Brien (1929) method

The patient is asked to open and close his mouth to allow palpation of the condyle of the mandible in front of the ear. The needle is inserted perpendicularly until it strikes the periosteum, where 2 ml of solution is injected (Fig. 15.6). A further 1 ml is injected as the needle is withdrawn and the area is then massaged. This method has the disadvantages that it is painful to perform and a complete facial nerve block ensues, producing drooping of the mouth which is very disfiguring.

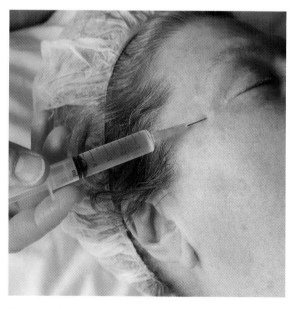

Fig. 15.7   Van Lint method of facial nerve block.

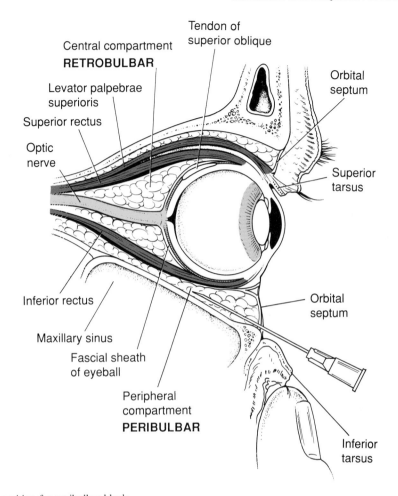

Fig. 15.8   Needle position for peribulbar block.

Van Lint (1914) method

The needle is inserted 1 cm lateral to the lateral canthus (Fig. 15.7). Up to 4 ml of solution is injected in a 'V' towards the upper and lower lids. This limits the block to the relevant terminal branches of the nerve, but the technique has the disadvantage of frequently producing bruising of the lids, which may be enough to produce pressure on the eye.

Peribulbar block (Fig. 15.8)

Topical anaesthesia of the conjunctiva is produced with amethocaine as outlined above. All needles are initially inserted tangentially to the globe to reduce the risk of perforation. A preliminary injection of 1.5 ml of 0.2% lignocaine (2% lignocaine mixed with ten times its volume of balanced salt solution) is made with a 1 cm 27 g needle through the inferotemporal area of the conjunctival cul de sac, level with the lateral border of the iris.

After 2 minutes, 5 ml of the standard drug mixture is injected through a 2.5 cm 25 g needle inserted at the same inferotemporal site (Fig. 15.9). If the needle strikes the orbital floor, its direction is changed to a more horizontal one. At a depth of 2.5 cm, and after careful aspiration, the solution is injected very slowly (Davis & Mandel 1986, Hamilton 1990). During the injection, the lower lid may fill with solution and there may be

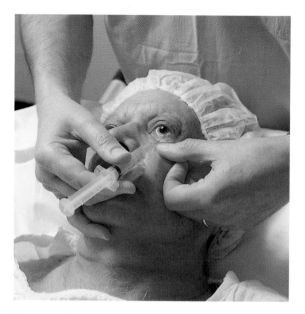

Fig. 15.9   Initial injection for peribulbar block.

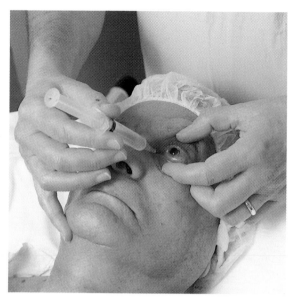

Fig. 15.10   Second injection for peribulbar block.

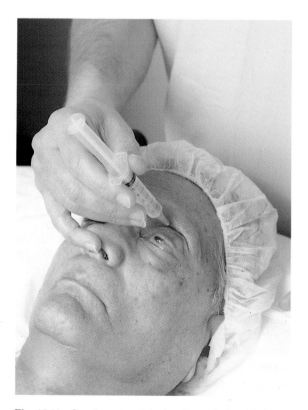

Fig. 15.11   Supplementary injection for peribulbar block.

some conjunctival oedema. However, if there is evidence of a significant increase in orbital or globe pressure the injection must be stopped. Normally the globe should feel soft and move freely within the orbit and there should be no proptosis. If these criteria are met, a full volume should be injected, the needle withdrawn carefully and pressure applied with a swab on the closed eye.

Within 5 minutes of this one injection, 20% of patients will develop adequate anaesthesia and akinesia, but the majority will require another injection. The same needle is inserted through the conjunctiva on the nasal side, medial to the caruncle and directed straight back parallel to the medial orbital wall (Fig. 15.10). A further 5 ml of solution is injected at a depth of about 1.5–2 cm. However, 20% of patients will require further injections to achieve complete akinesia. These injections are performed at sites appropriate to the clinical deficiencies of the block. Common sites for such supplementary injections are superonasal and superotemporal through the upper lid level with either the medial or lateral margins of the iris (Fig. 15.11).

These subsequent injections are usually painless because the initial one produces adequate anaes-thesia of the orbit. Each injection should be followed by a period of firm digital pressure and a pressure device should be applied for at least 20 minutes after the last injection to ensure a low intra-ocular pressure. Before surgery commences, complete paralysis of all the relevant muscles must be confirmed by careful testing and the orbital pressure should be sufficiently low for surgery to proceed.

Peribulbar block is the author's preferred technique. It has the great advantage that all injections are performed outside the muscle cone so that the complication rate is very low. Significant haemorrhage is unusual, but if it should occur the operation can usually still proceed. The block is less painful to perform, a separate facial nerve block is not required and the patient rarely loses complete light perception during the block. However, the technique is more time-consuming and requires larger volumes of local anaesthetic solution.

Complications of peribulbar block

Minor haemorrhage or *conjunctival oedema* may occur, but are usually controlled easily by firm pressure.

Perforation of the globe is the most serious complication and should be avoided by inserting the needles tangentially to the globe so that they are directed towards the orbital margin. Pain or resistance to either needle advancement or solution injection are warning signs.

Systemic toxicity might result from the larger doses of local anaesthetic required and the patient must be monitored carefully.

Myotoxicity due to the direct injection of high concentrations of local anaesthetic into the muscle has been described (Rainin & Carlson 1985). This causes muscle palsy, the commonest sign of which is prolonged ptosis.

REFERENCES

Atkinson W S 1961 The development of ophthalmic anesthesia. American Journal of Ophthalmology 51: 1–14

Buys N S 1980 Mercury balloon reducer for vitreous and orbital volume control. In: Emery J (ed) Current concepts in cataract surgery, pp 258–259. C V Mosby, St Louis

Bloom L H, Scheie H G, Yanoff M 1984 The warming of local anesthetic agents to decrease discomfort. Ophthalmic Surgery 15: 603

Davidson B, Kratz R, Mazzocco T 1979 An evaluation of the Honan intraocular pressure reducer. American Intraocular Implant Society Journal 5: 237

Davis D B II, Mandel M R 1986 Posterior peribulbar anesthesia; an alternative to retrobulbar anesthesia. Journal of Cataract and Refractive Surgery 12: 182–185

Feibel R M 1985 Current concepts in retrobulbar anesthesia. Survey of Ophthalmology 30: 102–110

Feitl M E, Krupin T 1990 Retrobulbar anesthesia. In: Zahl K, Meltzer M A (eds) Ophthalmology clinics of North America. Regional anesthesia for intraocular surgery, pp 83–91. W B Saunders, Philadelphia

Hamilton R C 1990 The complications of regional anesthesia. In: Zahl K, Meltzer M A (eds) Ophthalmology clinics of North America. Regional anesthesia for intraocular surgery, pp 111–125. W B Saunders, Philadelphia

Hamilton R C, Gimbel H V, Strunin L 1988 Regional anaesthesia for 12 000 cataract extraction and intraocular lens implantation procedures. Canadian Journal of Anaesthesia 35: 615–623

House P H, Hollands R H, Schulzer M 1991 Choice of anesthetic agents for peribulbar anesthesia. Journal of Cataract and Refractive Surgery 17: 80–83

Knapp H 1884 On cocaine and its use in ophthalmic and general surgery. Archives of Ophthalmology 13: 402–448

Korbon G A, Hurley D P, Williams G S 1987 pH-adjusted lidocaine does not "sting". Anesthesiology 66: 855–856

Morgan C M, Schatz H, Vine A K et al 1988 Ocular complications associated with retrobulbar injections. Ophthalmology 95: 660–665

O'Brien C S 1929 Akinesis during cataract extraction. Archives of Ophthalmology 1: 447–449

Rainin E A, Carlson B M 1985 Postoperative diplopia and ptosis: a clinical hypothesis based on the myotoxicity of local anesthetics. Archives of Ophthalmology 103: 1337–1339

Ramsay R C, Knobloch W H 1978 Ocular perforation following retrobulbar anesthesia for retinal detachment surgery. American Journal of Ophthalmology 86: 61–64

Thomson I 1988 Addition of hyaluronidase to lignocaine with adrenaline for retrobulbar anaesthesia in the surgery of senile cataract. British Journal of Ophthalmology 72: 700–702

Van Lint M 1914 Paralysie palpebrale temporaire provoquee dans l'operation de la cataracte. Annales D'Oculistique 151: 420–424

Zahl K 1990 Blockade of the orbicularis oculi. In: Zahl K, Meltzer M A (eds) Ophthalmology clinics of North America. Regional anesthesia for intraocular surgery, pp 93–100. W B Saunders, Philadelphia

16. Regional anaesthesia in children

E. N. Armitage

It is only in recent years that the use of local anaesthesia has gained a secure place in paediatric anaesthetic practice. There are several reasons for this:

1. Major medical contraindications to general anaesthesia are relatively rare in children.
2. Most children require a general anaesthetic if a nerve block is to be performed easily and safely, and it can then be argued that the patient has been subjected to hazards of two anaesthetic procedures instead of one.
3. There has been no general agreement as to which blocks are appropriate, which operations are most suitable for blocks, what dose of local anaesthetic is required or which parameters should be used for calculating the dose. Although some information on the pharmacokinetics of local anaesthetics in children is now available, many anaesthetists, in their anxiety to avoid systemic toxicity, tend to employ inadequate doses.
4. Since technical procedures such as venepuncture and intubation can be more difficult than in adults, it has been assumed (incorrectly) that this is also true of regional blocks.
5. There has been a tendency to underestimate the analgesic requirements of children and they have probably suffered even more than adults from conservative attitudes towards postoperative pain control. Systemic analgesia has not always been considered essential after procedures such as circumcision and herniotomy, so it is

hardly surprising that local analgesia has also been thought unnecessary.
6. Until the advent of long-acting local anaesthetic drugs, postoperative analgesia – the area in which blocks have most to offer children – has been impractical. Lignocaine is too short-acting to provide useful postoperative analgesia and it is far from ideal for continuous techniques.

Recent developments in pharmacology, changes in clinical practice and alterations in attitudes towards surgical pain in children have rendered some of these traditional objections invalid. General anaesthesia remains desirable if a major block is to be performed, but it can be maintained at a light plane once the block has become effective. Recovery is much faster and the combination of light general with local anaesthesia is particularly suitable for out-patient and day stay surgery – an increasingly popular form of care for children. The benefits far outweigh the potential hazards.

In district general hospital practice, paediatric surgery consists predominantly of straightforward procedures (circumcision, herniotomy, orchidopexy, etc.) which take less than an hour. The long duration of bupivacaine contributes much to the early postoperative period in these cases since the child wakes free of pain and the administration of analgesia can be timed so that it is effective before the block wears off. If oral analgesics are inappropriate or might be inadequate, the first dose of an intramuscular drug may be given painlessly within the area of the block. If subsequent analgesia is given at regular intervals, rather than 'as needed', postoperative pain is minimized. Many children are too young to understand the need for surgery and are naturally upset and perplexed when they experience pain. The period of analgesia after a block provides an excellent psychological environment for the child in the early recovery phase.

Some of the factors to be considered before a block is performed are the same as in adults. The technique should be safe, effective and have a high success rate if patient, anaesthetist and other staff are not to be disappointed. It should be easy to perform and require no cooperation from the patient. If analgesia is produced over a wide area the technique will be suitable for a variety of operations. The anaesthetist then acquires regular practice and the block becomes an accepted part of his routine. Techniques which are widely used in adults are not always ideal for children. Fortunately the converse is also true – some techniques which are of limited value or are difficult to perform in adults are very suitable for children.

Caudal block

This fulfils most of the above requirements and its use in children differs from that in adults in two ways. Firstly, it is easy to perform. Bony irregularities, asymmetry of the cornua and overlying pads of fat, all of which can make identification of the sacrococcygeal ligament difficult in adults, rarely become obvious until the second decade of life. Secondly, the block may extend over a much wider anatomical area than in the adult so it can be used for surgery at levels up to and including the umbilicus. Indeed, it is possible to produce blocks which extend considerably higher, although use of a caudal injection to provide analgesia of the upper trunk is neither elegant nor logical, and large, potentially toxic doses of local anaesthetic are required (McGown 1982). In practice, therefore, the umbilicus acts as a very convenient upper limit since much paediatric surgery is performed below that level. The more extensive spread of a caudal injection in children is attributed to the lower density of their epidural fat (Schulte-Steinberg & Rahlfs 1977).

Technique

No special equipment is needed. The block is applicable to children of all ages and the dose depends on the level of block required as well as on the child's size. Therefore, a wide range of volumes will be injected for which different size syringes are required. However, it is best to standardize on the 21 g needle for all but the smallest infants because this gives a more consistent 'feel'.

The sacral hiatus is near to the anus in a child so the overlying skin, which must be *clean, healthy and dry* if a caudal block is to be used, is more likely to be contaminated than in an adult. The antiseptic solution must be allowed to dry after application so that it is fully effective and not carried through to deeper tissues by the needle. Some anaesthetists believe that a full 'scrub-up' and a formal skin preparation are necessary, while others feel that a simple, but meticulously performed, 'no-touch' technique suffices for a single injection.

General anaesthesia is administered and the child turned into the left lateral position (for a right-handed anaesthetist) with the trunk rotated 45° towards the prone (Fig. 16.1). This position is obtained by lifting the buttocks on to a small sandbag or other support and allows the anaesthetist to perform the block without having to bend

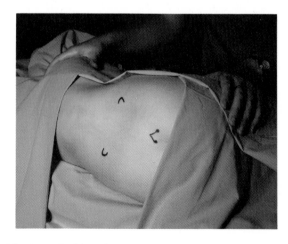

Fig. 16.1 Position of a child for caudal block.

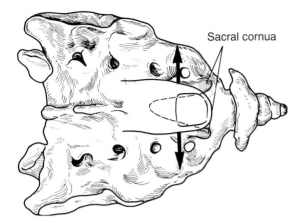

Fig. 16.2 Identification of the sacral cornua using sideways movement of the thumb.

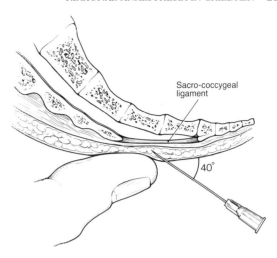

or stoop. An assistant continues the inhalational anaesthetic and maintains the airway.

Accurate location of the sacral cornua is the first step in the procedure and is essential for success. It is important to realize that these bony excrescences, representing the unfused laminae of the fifth sacral segment, appear to be more cephalad in the child than in the adult. They are best palpated by moving the left thumb up and down across the base of the sacrum (Fig. 16.2) and they may be thought of as forming the base of an isosceles triangle whose apex points cephalad. The apex is formed by the fusion of the sacral bones in the midline and the area of the triangle is filled by the sacrococcygeal ligament (Fig. 16.3).

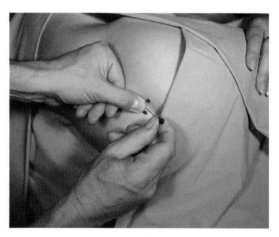

Fig. 16.4 Needle insertion for caudal block in a child.

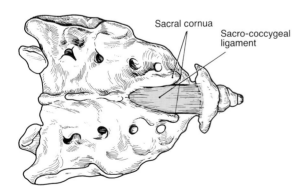

Fig. 16.3 Sacrococcygeal ligament.

In cases where the cornua are difficult to palpate, reassurance is needed to confirm their position. The child's hip are flexed to exactly 90° and a line is drawn along the long axis of the femur. When projected posteriorly, this will cross the midline at the level of the sacral cornua. This surface marking will discourage insertion of the needle too caudad – the commonest mistake of the 'adult' anaesthetist using the technique in children. Use of the tip of the coccyx as a landmark may be misleading as it also encourages needle insertion to be too caudad.

Once the cornua have been identified, the thumb is moved cephalad so that it lies over the apex of the isosceles triangle. The needle is inserted immediately caudad to the thumb and at an angle of about 40° (Fig. 16.4). After the needle has penetrated the skin and subcutaneous fat, it meets the resistance of the sacrococcygeal ligament. As the tip passes through the ligament and into the sacral canal a distinct loss of resistance is felt. The needle should be inserted close to the apex of the triangle because the sacral cavity is comparatively deep at that point and, once it has been entered, the anaesthetist is aware that the needle has 'dropped' into the sacrum.

If the needle is too caudad it will immediately strike the posterior surface of the anterior table of sacral bone (Fig. 16.5) and there will be no feeling that the needle is properly within the canal. If bone is encountered before ligament, the needle should be withdrawn and the landmarks checked before a second attempt is made. Occasionally a loss of resistance may follow too cephalad a needle insertion because one of the ligaments bridging the vestigial sacral spines has been penetrated. However, any attempt to advance the needle is prevented by bone, and attempts at injection meet increasing resistance.

When the needle has entered the sacrum it should be advanced 2–3 mm (no more) to ensure that it lies freely within the cavity. It is inappropriate in children to flatten the angle of the needle and advance it along the canal as is sometimes

recommended in adults, because blood vessels will be damaged and, in babies and small children, the theca may be penetrated.

If blood appears at the hub, the needle is withdrawn until the flow ceases, and the lumen is cleared with saline. Aspiration may then produce blood-stained saline, but as long as frank blood does not appear the local anaesthetic may be injected. Usually, blood is obtained only when the needle has been inserted too far, but occasionally it appears as soon as the ligament has been penetrated. In such a case the needle may be advanced a little in the hope that it will emerge from the vessel to lie freely in the sacral canal. Aspiration tests for blood sometimes give false negative results because the vessel wall is sucked on to the needle bevel. This risk can be minimized by the prior injection of 1 ml of solution to distend the vein and by gentle aspiration. The appearance of blood is not an indication for abandoning the block as long as the needle can be repositioned satisfactorily, although the author has some data to suggest that higher plasma concentrations of local anaesthetic result when a blood vessel has been damaged.

If the needle is inserted correctly, a dural tap is rare (approximately 1 in 800 cases) even in small babies. When it does occur, attempts to produce a spinal block are usually unsuccessful and it is best to abandon the procedure.

Drugs and dosage

Since the usual intention is to produce prolonged analgesia without profound block, 0.25% bupivacaine is the agent of choice. Motor block should be avoided because children become very upset if they cannot move freely. They are also very intolerant of paraesthesiae and these seem to be more prevalent when large volumes of 0.25% bupivacaine are used. A warning about such effects at the preoperative visit is helpful, but avoidance is better. Dilution of the bupivacaine to 0.19% (3 parts 0.25% solution to 1 part saline) minimizes these unpleasant symptoms when volumes in excess of 20 ml are needed.

Several dose regimes have been described (Kay 1974, Schulte-Steinberg & Rahlfs 1977, Armitage 1979), some of them based on the amount of drug

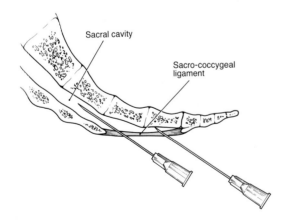

Sacral cavity

Sacro-coccygeal ligament

Fig. 16.5 Position of the needle within the sacral canal. If the point of insertion is too inferior it will immediately strike bone (the right-hand needle shows this).

Table 16.1 Dose schedule for caudal block with bupivacaine in children. Use 0.25% solution if the volume is <20 ml, 0.19% if >20 ml

Block required	Volume (ml kg^{-1})
Lumbosacral	0.5
Thoracolumbar	1.0
Mid-thoracic	1.25

per dermatome. Complicated arithmetic is sometimes involved and in practice a three-tier scale (Table 16.1) is simple and effective. For short cases producing brief pain, such as anal dilatation and separation of labial adhesions, 1% lignocaine may be used instead of 0.25% bupivacaine. The required volume is calculated using exactly the same regime. Schulte-Steinberg & Rahlfs (1970) have shown that age is a slightly better index for calculating dose than either weight or height. However, because of improvements in obstetric and neonatal care, many very premature infants now present for surgery. Since the 'ages' of these children are obstetrically determined, weight is the more appropriate index.

The regime shown in Table 16.1 produces satisfactory blocks in virtually every case and will provide analgesia lasting for 6–8 hours after circumcision and perineal procedures. The duration of analgesia after operations in the thoracolumbar region is shorter, but it is rarely less than 3 hours. The doses of drug are high and comparable with those given to adults by the lumbar epidural route. For example, a 20 kg, 5-year-old child would require 20 ml of 0.25% bupivacaine for inguinal herniotomy. Eyres and colleagues (1978) administered 2 mg kg^{-1} of 0.5% bupivacaine (equivalent to 0.8 ml kg^{-1} of 0.25% bupivacaine) caudally and found that plasma concentrations were well within safe limits. Later, the same group (Eyres et al 1983) used 0.25% bupivacaine in a dose of 3 mg kg^{-1} (that is 1.2 ml kg^{-1} – virtually the same as the mid-thoracic dose in Table 16.1). The greatest plasma concentration found was 2 µg ml^{-1}, and this was in only two of a total of 45 patients.

Complications

The need to avoid motor block and paraesthesiae has been stressed. *Retention of urine* is virtually unknown in children as long as the concentration of bupivacaine does not exceed 0.25%, but a watch must be kept to ensure that it does not occur. Persistent questioning of the child about this should be avoided because it will cause anxiety which itself predisposes to retention. *Hypotension* is rarely seen in children – an observation made repeatedly by those employing regional anaesthesia in children. Very occasionally a child is troubled by *severe itching* in the area between the normal and analgesic skin, and scratching may be aggressive enough to draw blood.

Caudal opioids

Children have not escaped the recent enthusiasm for epidural opioids. Caudal morphine in a dose of 0.05 mg kg^{-1} produces analgesia for 10–36 hours after circumcision and other genital operations (Jensen 1981). Epidural opioids have become popular in adults because it is claimed they provide prolonged analgesia without sympathetic block. However, the effects of sympathetic block are minimal in children, so opioids offer no advantage and it is unnecessary to use such long-acting agents when simpler regimes are so effective.

Caudal catheters

In the past, anaesthetists have been unwilling to insert a catheter so near the anus because it is difficult to ensure that the area remains clean. Like any other foreign body, a catheter increases the risk of infection. Busoni & Sarti (1987) have minimized this risk by taking advantage of the fact that the sacral vertebrae do not fuse until early adult life. They insert the needle, and then the catheter, at the second sacral interspace.

Epidural block

Although a caudal is suitable for many paediatric operations, it will be inadequate for major surgery. The need for effective analgesia extends over days rather than hours, oral analgesia is likely to be ineffective and is also inappropriate if oral fluids are forbidden. An epidural, established before surgery and continued into the postoperative period, can provide very effective analgesia, but it is a major undertaking and the anaesthetist must be experienced in both paediatric and regional anaesthesia. Special equipment is required and the expected benefits must be considerable for the technique to be justified. Operations such as the removal of large abdominal tumours, transthoracic repair of hiatus hernia and major renal reconstructions are suitable and if a tranverse incision (much favoured by paediatric surgeons) is used, an accurately placed block can easily cover the few dermatomes involved.

The nature of the surgery is not the only criterion for selection. It is possible to perform an epidural on very small children, but it is rarely satisfactory if they are unable to communicate and cooperate with those looking after them. Pain-free young children are active so they require additional sedation if intravenous infusions, nasogastric tubes, urinary catheters and wound drains are to remain unmolested. Because of this an epidural is not really practical in children younger than 4 years of age.

The attitude of the parents to an epidural should be taken into account and its use should be discussed with them. Preconceived ideas abound and it is unwise to embark on an epidural if the parents remain anxious about its safety or benefits. On the other hand, a mother who has had a successful obstetric epidural is a valuable ally. The attitude of the nurses is also important. They cannot be expected to embrace a technique with enthusiasm unless it has been fully explained to them and their role in its management has been clearly defined.

Technique

It is usual to induce general anaesthesia before performing the block. The epidural space is narrower in the child than in the adult and this fact influences the approach to the space, the design of the needle and the method of its insertion. With the midline approach the needle takes the shortest route across the epidural space, but with the paramedian it crosses the space obliquely so there is less risk of dural puncture. There is also a better chance that the catheter will advance easily rather than impinge upon, and perhaps puncture, the dura.

A special needle is required because the standard Touhy is too big. The needle manufactured by Steriseal (Fig. 16.6) is 5 cm (2 inches) long and graduated in centimetres. It is 18 g, but is thin walled so that it accepts a standard 18 g Portex catheter. The point has a conventional short bevel since a Huber type is unnecessary when the paramedian approach is used. When this needle enters the epidural space it should be rotated so that the bevel faces anteriorly (away from the anaesthetist and parallel to the dura). Portex also market a 19 g paediatric epidural needle for use with a 23 g nylon catheter. The shaft is 5 cm long, is graduated every 0.5 cm and has a Huber bevel (Desparmet 1986).

With the above exceptions, the technique (Fig. 16.7) is the same as is used for an adult (see Ch. 8).

Drugs and dosage

Ecoffey and colleagues (1986) give 0.75 ml kg^{-1} of 0.5% bupivacaine with adrenaline. Murat and colleagues (1987) use 0.25% bupivacaine with adrenaline for children less than 8 years of age, and 0.375% or 0.5% solution for older children when abdominal relaxation is required. They give an

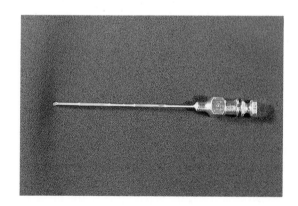

Fig. 16.6 Paediatric epidural needle.

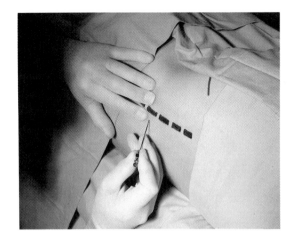

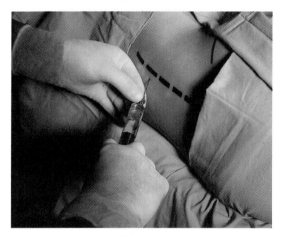

Fig. 16.7 Epidural needle insertion using the paramedian approach in a child.

initial dose of 0.75 ml kg^{-1} to children weighing less than 20 kg, and 1 ml per 10 cm of height to children taller than 100 cm. The dose is halved for top-up injections, which may be required hourly during major surgery.

Postoperative management

Ideally the last incremental dose should be given about 20 minutes before the end of surgery so that the child wakes free of pain and remains so while an epidural infusion of 0.1% bupivacaine is established. This is delivered through a paediatric infusion set which delivers 60 drops ml^{-1} so that the number of drops per minute is equal to the number of millilitres per hour. The initial infusion

rate is 0.1–0.2 ml kg^{-1} h^{-1}. This is usually insufficient in the long term, but allows the anaesthetist to observe the rate at which the block is regressing. If the infusion rate needs to be increased a bolus dose of 0.2 ml kg^{-1} should be given first.

Epidural infusions in children are more difficult and time-consuming to manage than in adults and require review every 4–6 hours if they are to be continuously effective. Even with a good block, additional parenteral sedation is almost always required and a small dose of an opioid does much to reduce activity and relieve anxiety and distress. This combined technique produces a relaxed pain-free child who cooperates with the physiotherapist and is easy to nurse. Also, there is the advantage that it is unnecessary to add opioid to the epidural infusion of local anaesthetic when it is already being given for its systemic effect. All injections can be given painlessly and if the block extends into the lower limbs intravenous infusions can be sited in (and blood samples taken from) warm, analgesic feet. The epidural infusion is usually continued for 48 hours.

Complications

Difficulties arise more commonly in the management of the block than in its performance. The author has yet to puncture the dura with either needle or catheter, and accidental venous cannulation does not seem to occur any more often than in adults. Most of these children require bladder catheterization on surgical grounds, so retention of urine is not a problem. Persistent motor block, on the other hand, is potentially serious in children since pressure due to prolonged immobility can easily damage a child's soft skin.

Subarachnoid block

Until recently, spinal anaesthesia has had little place in paediatric practice. It does not provide long-term analgesia, yet it requires the same meticulous aseptic precautions as an epidural. For the simpler surgical procedures, caudal block is more versatile and quicker to perform.

However, advances in neonatology have produced a new challenge for the paediatric anaesthetist who is now being asked to provide anaesthesia for surgery such as inguinal herniotomy in infants who were born prematurely. These children, some delivered as early as 12 weeks before term, have usually been treated for the respiratory distress syndrome and, although they may no longer require mechanical ventilation, they still suffer from bronchopulmonary dysplasia. Intubation and general anaesthesia are tolerated badly. Even when they have grown up to or past normal birth weight, these children show an increased incidence of postoperative complications such as apnoeic attacks (Steward 1982). Alternatives to general anaesthesia have been sought which do not affect the respiratory system. Spinal anaesthesia has the advantages of rapid onset, profound block and minimal systemic effects because of the low dose of local anaesthetic required. Abajian and colleagues (1984) and Harnik (1984) have both shown the technique to be feasible using 0.5% amethocaine in 5% dextrose in doses between 0.05 and 0.13 ml kg^{-1}. The larger dose gives more consistent results for inguinal herniotomy. Heavy bupivacaine (0.5% in 8% glucose) is also satisfactory.

Lumbar puncture is performed caudad to the third lumbar vertebra to avoid damage to the spinal cord. A 22 g 3.5 cm ($1\frac{1}{2}$ inch) needle is introduced after infiltration of the skin and deeper tissues with 1% lignocaine. The dead space of the needle is 0.04 ml and this should be allowed for in drawing the solution into a 1 ml syringe. Abajian and colleagues (1984) recommend that the needle and syringe are left in place for about 5 seconds after injection.

Spinal anaesthesia in small babies is a relatively new technique and its place in their management has yet to be established. It is possible that it will prove to be a real advance in this small group of patients although they are unlikely to present for surgery outside specialist units.

Peripheral blocks

As the advantages of combining light general anaesthesia with regional block have become more widely recognized, further refinements have been sought. In an attempt to limit the area of block to the operative field, peripheral blocks have been tried as they cause minimal paraesthesiae and motor weakness. They may also be applicable where central blocks are contraindicated. However, there are disadvantages:

1. There is a slightly increased risk of needle damage to nerves when blocks are performed under general anaesthesia.
2. Unless the anaesthetist has plenty of opportunity to practise the various techniques he is unlikely to attain the necessary level of competence.
3. Peripheral blocks in children do not have the same high success rate as caudals.

Inguinal field block

A 23 g needle is inserted just medial and caudad to the anterior superior iliac spine and advanced until there is a loss of resistance as it penetrates the external oblique aponeurosis. Solution is injected in two directions: laterally towards the iliac crest and mediocaudally towards the inguinal ligament.

Smith & Jones (1982), using 0.25% bupivacaine in a dose of 0.5 ml for each year of age, found that 56 out of 58 children were free of pain 4 hours after inguinal herniotomy, although five had required paracetamol before assessment. In the control group 35 out of 49 were free of pain, but ten had required paracetamol.

Penile block

The technique is essentially the same as for adults (see Ch. 11). White and colleagues (1983), using 0.2 ml kg^{-1} of 0.5% *plain* bupivacaine, found that the mean duration of analgesia was 12 hours. In that series of 27 patients, two small haematomas were produced. Yeoman and colleagues (1983) also used 0.5% plain bupivacaine, but in a dose of 1 ml in boys under 3 years of age and 0.3 ml year^{-1} thereafter. Over 40% were free of pain for at least 6 hours after operation.

Upper limb blocks

An axilliary brachial plexus block is useful for operations on the hand, such as correction of syndactyly. The artery is immobilized between two fingers of the left hand and a 25 g, 1.5 cm ($\frac{5}{8}$ inch) needle is advanced until it is judged to lie in the axillary sheath. A 'give' as the needle enters the sheath is not always noted in children, but if the needle moves with arterial pulsation, a successful block usually results. A dose of 0.3 ml kg^{-1} of 0.25% bupivacaine with adrenaline produces blocks which may last up to 22 hours.

More peripheral limb blocks, particularly digital nerve block, are useful for minor procedures on fingers and toes. It is essential that *plain* solutions of local anaesthetic are used.

Lower limb blocks

McNicol (1985) has described block of the sciatic nerve by the anterior approach in children. In this, great reliance is placed on the loss of resistance felt as the needle passes through the adductor muscles and enters the neurovascular compartment. Bupivacaine 0.5% in a dose of 0.5–1.0 ml kg^{-1} was used

and 78 of the 82 blocks in his series were successful. There were no complications. The same author has described combined blocks of the femoral and lateral cutaneous nerve of the thigh for surgery on the femur and thigh (McNicol 1986). He had two failures in 50 patients.

Although such nerve blocks are anatomically specific, it is at least arguable that caudal block is more reliable and less invasive.

Infiltration

Simple infiltration provides excellent analgesia after the removal of the superficial lesions (moles, naevi and cysts) which form a significant part of paediatric surgery. The solution should surround the lesion, but must be placed some distance from it to avoid obliterating it or distorting the operative field. If the surgeon wishes to apply skin markings it may be better to delay infiltration until the operation has been completed.

FURTHER READING

Arthur D S, McNicol L R 1986 Local anaesthetic techniques in paediatric surgery. British Journal of Anaesthesia 58: 760–778

Saint-Maurice C, Schulte-Steinberg O 1990 Regional anaesthesia in children. Mediglobe SA, Fribourg, Switzerland

REFERENCES

Abajian J C, Mellish R W P, Browne A F, Perkins F M et al 1984 Spinal anesthesia for surgery in the high-risk infant. Anesthesia and Analgesia 63: 359–362

Armitage E N 1979 Caudal block in children. Anaesthesia 34: 396

Busoni P, Sarti A 1987 Sacral intervertebral epidural block. Anesthesiology 67: 993–995

Desparmet J 1986 Equipment for paediatric epidurals. Anaesthesia 41: 337–338

Ecoffey C, Dubousset A-M, Samii K 1986 Lumbar and thoracic epidural anesthesia for urologic and upper abdominal surgery in infants and children. Anesthesiology 65: 87–90

Eyres R L, Kidd J, Oppenheim R C, Brown T C K 1978 Local anaesthetic plasma levels in children. Anaesthesia and Intensive Care 6: 243–247

Eyres R L, Bishop W, Oppenheim R C, Brown T C K 1983 Plasma bupivacaine concentrations in children during caudal epidural analgesia. Anaesthesia and Intensive Care 11: 20–22

Harnik E 1984 Spinal anaesthesia for inguinal hernia repair

in the premature infant. Poster presentation: Centennial Meeting of Regional Anaesthesia, Vienna

Jensen B H 1981 Caudal block for postoperative pain relief in children after genital operations. A comparison between bupivacaine and morphine. Acta Anaesthesiologica Scandinavica 25: 373–375

Kay B 1974 Caudal block for postoperative pain relief in children. Anaesthesia 29: 610–611

McGown R G 1982 Caudal analgesia in children. Five hundred cases for procedures below the diaphragm. Anaesthesia 37: 806–818

McNicol L R 1985 Sciatic nerve block for children. Sciatic nerve block by the anterior approach for postoperative pain relief. Anaesthesia 40: 410–414

Mc Nicol L R 1986 Lower limb blocks for children. Lateral cutaneous and femoral nerve blocks for postoperative pain relief in paediatric practice. Anaesthesia 41: 27–31

Murat I, Delleur M M, Esteve C, Egu J F, Raynaud P, Saint-Maurice C 1987 Continuous extradural infusion in children. Clinical and haemodynamic implications. British Journal of Anaesthesia 69: 1441–1450

Schulte-Steinberg O, Rahlfs V W 1970 Caudal anaesthesia in children and spread of 1% lignocaine. British Journal of Anaesthesia 42: 1093–1099

Schulte-Steinberg O, Rahlfs V W 1977 Spread of extradural analgesia following caudal injection in children. A statistical study. British Journal of Anaesthesia 49: 1027–1034

Smith B A C, Jones S E F 1982 Analgesia after herniotomy in a paediatric day unit. British Medical Journal 285: 1466

Steward D J 1982 Preterm infants are more prone to complications following minor surgery than term infants. Anesthesiology 56: 304–306

White J, Harrison B, Richmond P, Procter A, Curran J 1983 Postoperative analgesia for circumcision. British Medical Journal 286: 1934

Yeoman P M, Cooke R, Hain W R 1983 Penile block for circumcision? A comparison with caudal blockade. Anaesthesia 38: 862–866

17. Pain and autonomic blocks

D. M. Justins, A. P. Rubin

The sympathetic nervous system has been the target of pain-relieving techniques since the early part of the 20th century, but because the pathophysiology of many chronic pains remains poorly understood, it is difficult to suggest why or how sympathetic nerve block helps some of these conditions. The mechanism may simply involve the interruption of afferent nociceptive fibres which run in the autonomic nerves, or it may be more complex and be linked to the interruption of sympathetic efferent fibres and the disruption of reflex control systems so that peripheral somatosensory processing is altered. Sympathetic blocks distal to the site of injury may produce relief of pain even when sympathetic abnormality is not evident (Loh & Nathan 1978).

Sympathetic blocks should never be used as the sole therapy in the management of chronic pain conditions. A multidisciplinary approach is usually indicated and may utilize other treatments such as systemic drugs, physiotherapy, transcutaneous electrical nerve stimulation (TENS) and psychological techniques. In some cases, such as peripheral vascular disease, the anaesthetist may just provide a nerve block service without being involved in other aspects of patient management, but the performance of the block still requires a full understanding of the anatomy and pathophysiology involved, as well as experience and skill in dealing with chronic pain problems. The complications of sympathetic blocks can be very serious. The patient must have a full understanding of what is planned and what the block aims to achieve. These techniques are palliative, not curative. An image intensifier is mandatory for coeliac and lumbar sympathetic blocks, and for

any neurolytic procedure. It allows a faster, safer procedure, overcomes the problem of variable anatomical landmarks, allows precise needle placement, demonstrates the spread of injected solution and reveals inadvertent intravascular injection even when aspiration tests have been negative. Finally, it allows injection of minimal volumes of neurolytic solution.

Indications

Peripheral vascular disease

Autonomic blocks may be of value in:

1. *Acute vascular disorders*: post-traumatic vasospasm; acute arterial or venous occlusion; cold injury; inadvertent intra-arterial thiopentone
2. *Chronic vasospastic conditions*: Raynaud's syndrome; acrocyanosis; livedo reticularis; sequelae of spinal cord injury or disease (e.g. polio)
3. *Chronic obliterative diseases*: thromboangiitis obliterans (Buerger's disease); atherosclerosis (Reid et al 1970)
4. *Perioperative*: microvascular surgery; fistula formation for dialysis

Neurolytic lumbar sympathetic blocks will relieve rest pain and improve healing of skin ulcers in about 65–75% of patients with atherosclerosis, but the procedure is of little benefit for claudication. The successful block may last for 6–9 months and during this time the patient may develop collateral circulation. The results are comparable to surgical sympathectomy whilst producing much less morbidity and mortality. If amputation is necessary then preoperative sympathetic blocks may aid in defining the level of tissue viability and also encourage healing of the stump. There is some evidence to suggest that preoperative blocks might also diminish the incidence of postamputation stump or phantom pain. Established postamputation pain is occasionally helped by sympathetic block, but treatment is generally difficult.

Visceral pain

Nociceptive afferent pathways from the viscera accompany sympathetic nerves. Sympathetic block interrupts these pathways and also the efferent viscerovisceral reflexes so that ischaemia and spasm are relieved. Situations in which the blocks may be considered are :

Abdominal cancer. Neurolytic coeliac plexus block produces good pain relief which lasts for the remainder of life in about 80% of patients with pain from carcinoma of the pancreas, stomach, gall bladder or liver (Brown et al 1987). The pain of other abdominal malignancies and rectal tenesmus can also be helped (Bristow & Foster 1988).

Chronic non-malignant abdominal pain does not respond as well and the results of coeliac plexus block for chronic pancreatitis are disappointing. Unilateral L_1 sympathetic blocks are sometimes helpful in the loin pain haematuria syndrome. Some chronic perineal pain syndromes respond to bilateral lumbar sympathetic block (Foster 1990).

Acute abdominal pain due to acute pancreatitis and ureteric colic.

Cardiac pain. The pain of acute myocardial infarction and intractable angina is eased by upper thoracic sympathetic or stellate ganglion block.

Perioperative. Anaesthesia for upper abdominal surgery may be achieved using a combination of coeliac and intercostal blocks.

Hyperhydrosis

Sympathetic blocks produce anhydrosis, but the effect is rarely sustained and totally unacceptable

side-effects such as Horner's syndrome are common if neurolytic procedures are attempted.

Nerve damage

The sympathetic nervous system may be involved in a number of chronic pain states, especially when there is nerve damage.

Major nerve injury. Major nerve injury is classically associated with causalgia and this term is still widely used. *Causalgia* is defined as burning pain, allodynia and hyperpathia, usually in the hand or foot, after partial injury of a nerve or one of its major branches (International Association for the Study of Pain 1986). The nerves most commonly involved are the median, ulnar, sciatic and tibial. The limb has cold, discoloured, clammy skin and increased sweating. Eventually atrophic changes develop. Sympathetic block may produce relief early in the course of the disease, but this is not inevitable. Resolution becomes less likely once atrophic changes are established and the condition can follow an unremitting course of ever increasing pain, distress and disability.

Acute herpes zoster. There is convincing evidence to suggest that sympathetic blocks reduce pain and promote healing during the acute phase, but claims that the incidence of postherpetic neuralgia can be reduced remain unproven. Sympathetic blocks are of doubtful value in established postherpetic neuralgia.

Carcinomatous neuropathy. Invasion by carcinoma, particularly of the brachial or lumbar plexus, and carcinoma of head and neck may produce a neuropathic, burning pain which is partially responsive to sympathetic block.

Reflex sympathetic dystrophy (RSD). In the English language alone there are over 30 descriptive labels for painful conditions in which sympathetic activity is claimed to be abnormal. RSD is one of the most commonly used terms and is defined as continuous pain in a portion of an extremity after trauma (not involving a major nerve), associated with sympathetic hyperactivity (International Association for the Study of Pain 1986). The clinical spectrum ranges from cases in which pain is the sole manifestation, to those in which the predominant findings are devastating trophic changes with virtually no pain (Schwartzman & McLellan 1987).

Attempts have been made to explain this group of conditions as a purely peripheral phenomenon caused by abnormal sympathetic activity or, alternatively, as a central phenomenon in which heightened spinal activity enhances reflex sympathetic outflow. This in turn stimulates the chemosensitive peripheral receptors and increases afferent input to the spinal cord (Roberts 1986). Janig (1988) attempts to channel the various possible causes and consequences through a central link that he describes as distorted information processing in the spinal cord. The role of the sympathetic nervous system in many chronic pain states may have been overemphasized and sympathetic overactivity is certainly not the common denominator (Schott 1986).

One way out of the difficulties in the classification of these conditions is simply to describe pain as being either *sympathetically maintained* or *sympathetically independent*, based solely on the results of diagnostic sympathetic nerve blocks. False positive or false negative responses to the blocks cause confusion and many patients will have 'mixed' pains which do not fit into either category (Campbell et at 1988).

Sympathetically maintained pain (SMP) has been described in a wide range of situations and even spontaneous onset is possible. Minor trauma such as a fracture is a frequent precipitant. A number of neurological conditions are associated with SMP, including cerebrovascular accidents, multiple sclerosis and spinal cord and peripheral nerve injury. Cerebrovascular accidents are the main cause of the central pain syndromes which are often called thalamic pain. Peripheral sympathetic blocks will relieve pain in some of these patients even though the primary lesion is intracranial (Loh et al 1981).

Recent research fails to support the idea that nerve damage is a prerequisite to involvement of the sympathetic nervous system in a chronic pain state, or that abnormal sympathetic activity is diagnostic of underlying nerve damage (Frost et al 1988). Sympathetic involvement should be suspected when the patient reports a continuous burning pain which may be accompanied by swelling, changes in temperature, sweating and colour, and eventually trophic changes in skin, nails, joints and bones. Hyperalgesia to cold stimuli is a sensitive, but not specific, sign of SMP (Frost et at 1988).

When sympathetic involvement is proven or suspected, aggressive therapy initiated as soon as possible would seem to provide the best outcome for these patients. Even when a sympathetically dependent pain is identified a successful result is not inevitable and some cases remain intractable despite every therapeutic endeavour. Sympathetic nerve blocks and vigorous physiotherapy form the cornerstone of most treatment programmes (Schutzer et al 1984). TENS may be helpful. High-dose corticosteroids and numerous other drugs have also been suggested (Charlton 1990).

Clinical application of sympathetic blocks

Sympathetic blocks can be used for both diagnosis and therapy.

Diagnostic blocks can be used to differentiate between somatic and visceral pain, to identify a sympathetic component, to see if blood flow increases, or sweating decreases. If an attempt is being made to define the sympathetic contribution to any particular pain syndrome the diagnostic block must be a pure sympathetic block without any accompanying somatic block. This can only be achieved with precise interruption of the sympathetic chain. Epidural injections and intravenous regional techniques with local anaesthetic or guanethidine are not selective and do not aid in the diagnosis of the sympathetic component of a pain syndrome. An image intensifier is mandatory to confirm precise needle position and the spread of injected solution. Objective signs of sympathetic block must be identified using changes in skin temperature or conductivity, or tests of sweat production with ninhydrin, cobalt blue or starch iodine. When a limb has been blocked, dilated veins become visible and the increase in blood flow can be measured using a Doppler flow probe or venous plethysmography (Lofstrom & Cousins 1988).

False positive results may be due to spread of solution on to adjacent somatic nerves, systemic effects of absorbed local anaesthetic taken up from the injection site, or the placebo response. False negative results may follow an incomplete or inappropriate block and inadequate assessment before or after the block. A complete sympathetic block is difficult to achieve (Malmqvist et al 1987). Many patients will have both sympathetic and somatic components to their pain. There is no clear correlation between the degree or duration of pain relief and the actual period of sympathetic block and the same patient may show variable responses on different occasions. Some patients demonstrate unexpected or unusual responses, such as contralateral or delayed blocks, and some pain is made worse (Purcell-Jones & Justins 1988).

A *prognostic block* can be used to demonstrate to the patient its effect on pain, blood flow or sweating, but there is sometimes poor correlation between the result of the prognostic block and the outcome of any subsequent surgical or neuro-ablative procedure. The local anaesthetic block produces widespread disruption of nerve function. If neuro-ablation is to be based upon the results of prognostic blocks, more than one should be performed and a consistent response demonstrated. Sometimes the prognostic block will produce an increase in pain or an uncomfortable increase in limb temperature which the patient finds unacceptable.

Therapeutic blocks may be performed with local anaesthetics, neurolytics such as phenol or alcohol, and (for intravenous regional techniques) drugs such as guanethidine. Neurolytic blocks are primarily indicated for painful abdominal cancer and peripheral vascular disease, and should be used with great caution and reluctance in all other conditions. Local anaesthetic sympathetic blocks have been shown to be superior to conservative therapy in a series of RSD patients (Wang et al 1985). Intravenous guanethidine blocks may be superior to ganglion blocks (Bonelli et at 1983, Eriksen 1981). Axillary brachial plexus block produced better results than stellate ganglion block in a series of patients with upper limb RSD (Defalque 1984). Sometimes a single block produces long-term relief, but most patients require more than one. Continuous upper limb sympathetic block can be established using an infusion into a brachial plexus catheter. This technique has been used in the treatment of RSD and after reconstructive microvascular surgery (Manriquez & Pallares 1978). There are no clear guidelines as to the indications for different techniques and the optimal frequency and duration of treatment have not been established. Many questions about the pathology and treatment of RSD remain to be answered.

Contraindications

Anticoagulants or haemorrhagic disorders

There is constant risk of damage to blood vessels with these techniques and the nerves are deeply placed. Thus, a large haematoma may be produced if there is *any* coagulation disorder.

Local infection or neoplasm

Needles should not be inserted through infected or neoplastic tissue as there is a risk of spread to deeper structures.

Local anatomical or vascular anomalies

Anatomical distortion makes the block more difficult and reduces the success rate. Anomalous vessels increase the risk of accidental needle puncture and of haematoma formation.

Inadequate facilities

The use of neurolytic solutions without full evaluation of the patient, or in the absence of proper safeguards such as radiographic control, may have disastrous consequences.

Neurolytic solutions used for sympathetic blocks

A number of different solutions will destroy nerves, but phenol and alcohol are the most often used.

Phenol destroys all nerve fibre types by protein denaturation. It is not selective and will destroy motor and sensory nerves, but the fibres can regenerate so the blocks should not be regarded as permanent. The strongest aqueous solution is 6.6%, but higher concentrations can be obtained using an oily base such as a radiographic contrast medium. Contact with somatic nerves may cause neuritis. Toxic reactions may occur if a dose of 600 mg is exceeded in a 70 kg man.

Alcohol has a similar non-selective destructive action on nerves, but it produces a very high incidence of neuritis and is usually reserved for coeliac plexus block where the large injection volumes preclude the safe use of phenol.

SYMPATHETIC BLOCKS

Stellate ganglion block

Anatomy

The stellate (cervicothoracic) ganglion is formed by the fusion of the seventh and eighth cervical and first thoracic sympathetic ganglia. It lies anterior to the transverse process of the seventh cervical and first thoracic vertebrae and the neck (and possibly the head) of the first rib (Fig. 17.1). It is anterior to the paravertebral fascia, may be covered in its lower parts by the dome of the pleura and lies posterior to the carotid sheath.

Technique

Many approaches to the stellate ganglion have been described, but the simplest and most satisfactory is the anterior paratracheal. In the supine position the head is extended and a point is marked 3 cm above and 2 cm lateral to the suprasternal notch. Pressure is applied with two fingers in the groove between the trachea and the carotid sheath (Fig. 17.2). In a very thin patient it may be possible to feel the transverse process of C_6, which lies at

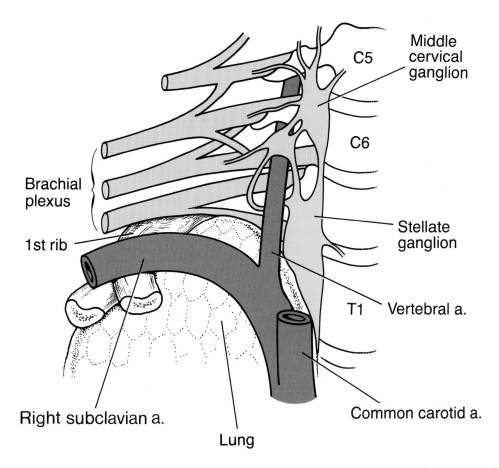

Fig. 17.1   Position of the stellate ganglion. Note that, at the level of injection (C_6), the vertebral artery is a posterior relation.

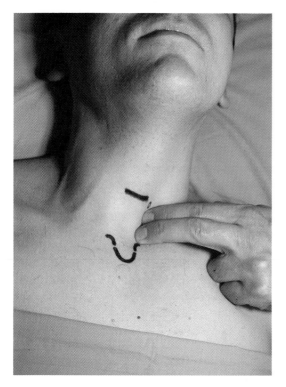

Fig. 17.2   Landmarks for stellate ganglion block. The cricoid cartilage and the tip of the transverse process of C$_6$ have been marked.

the level of the cricoid cartilage. A 23 g 30 mm needle is inserted directly backwards to pass between the trachea and the carotid sheath until it strikes the transverse process of C$_6$ some 2.5–3 cm from the skin. The needle should then be withdrawn 2–3 mm so that it lies anterior to the prevertebral fascia. The needle is fixed in this position with one hand, whilst an aspiration test is performed. Thereafter, 10–15 ml of solution is injected slowly, with aspiration after every 2 ml. The use of a short catheter between the needle and syringe allows an assistant to perform the injection whilst the needle is kept immobile. The patient must not talk or swallow during the injection. If the needle is in the correct fascial plane there should be no resistance to injection and no swelling should be apparent. For full sympathetic block of the upper limb the solution should extend to the T$_3$ ganglion and larger volumes are necessary. There is little advantage in sitting the patient to aid spread (Hardy & Wells 1987).

Other approaches (Atkinson et al 1982). Lateral and posterior approaches should only be used when the anterior approach is difficult because of anatomical distortion. These approaches have a much higher incidence of complications, including epidural and intrathecal injection.

Choice of solution

Lignocaine 1% is suitable for a diagnostic block, but bupivacaine 0.25% or 0.5% is preferred for other blocks. Neurolytic stellate ganglion block is potentially very hazardous and should be performed only by an experienced practitioner. If the technique is used, very small volumes (less than 1 ml) containing radio-opaque medium can be injected under radiographic control to ensure that surrounding structures are not damaged. Surgical techniques may be preferable.

Complications

Systemic toxicity. The stellate ganglion is closely related to several major blood vessels, particularly the vertebral artery. Intra-arterial injection of a minute dose of local anaesthetic will produce immediate and startling signs of central toxicity as the drug is delivered directly to the brain stem.

Vasovagal reactions. These are readily triggered from the neck and should be distinguished from local anaesthetic toxicity. The patient becomes anxious, pale, sweaty and nauseated, with bradycardia and hypotension. Withdrawal of the needle and elevation of the legs is usually sufficient treatment.

Horner's syndrome. Horner's syndrome (unilateral meiosis, ptosis and enophthalmos) is an inevitable result of successful stellate ganglion block and the patient must be warned of this beforehand. Conjunctival vasodilatation and unilateral nasal congestion will also occur. No special treatment is required although the meiosis may be reversed with 10% phenylephrine drops.

Brachial plexus block. If the injection is in the wrong tissue plane, the local anaesthetic may affect the roots of the brachial plexus. No treatment is required, but it may lead to diagnostic and prognostic confusion.

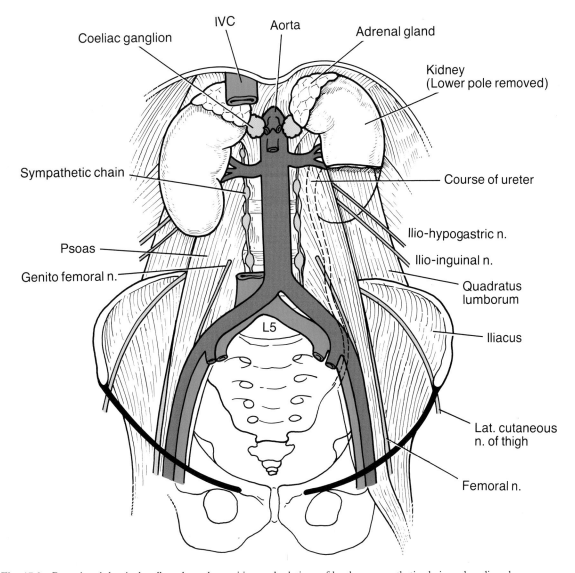

Fig. 17.3 Posterior abdominal wall to show the position and relations of lumbar sympathetic chain and coeliac plexus.

Recurrent laryngeal nerve palsy. Local anaesthetic may spread to the recurrent laryngeal nerve and cause hoarseness.

Phrenic nerve block. This will occur if the solution is injected too far anteriorly, but rarely causes any problems.

Pneumothorax. The dome of the pleura rises above the first rib and is closely related to the ganglion. It becomes vulnerable if the needle is inserted in a caudad direction.

Because of the risk of the last three complications, bilateral stellate blocks should never be performed.

Lumbar sympathetic block

Anatomy (Figs 17.3 and 17.4)

The lumbar sympathetic trunk is situated in the retroperitoneal connective tissue anterior to the vertebral bodies and the medial margin of psoas muscle. The genitofemoral nerve lies laterally on

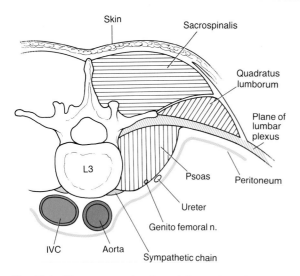

Fig. 17.4   Transverse section through L₃, to show the position and relations of the lumbar sympathetic chain.

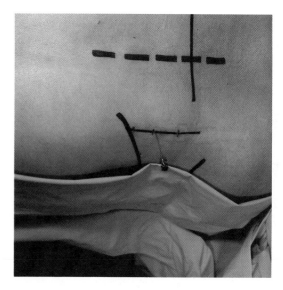

Fig. 17.5   Landmarks and angle of needle insertion for lumbar sympathectomy at the level of L₃.

psoas. The aorta and the inferior vena cava are anterior relations; the kidney and ureter are posterolateral. All the sympathetic fibres pass through or synapse at the L_2 ganglion. Therefore, a block at the upper level of L_3 should abolish all sympathetic supply to the lower limb. However, opinions differ over the number of levels which need to be injected to produce optimal lower limb sympathectomy. Boas (1983) examined 500 cases and was unable to demonstrate any difference between single-level injection (L_2 or L_3), double-level injection (L_2L_3 or L_3L_4) or triple-level injections ($L_2L_3L_4$). Walsh and colleagues (1984) reported over 400 cases and claimed that triple-level injection produced the best results. Umeda and colleagues (1987) studied 19 cadavers and concluded that the optimal site was either the lower third of the second lumbar vertebral body or the upper part of the third. A single-level injection is certainly safer and faster to perform and the spread of solution can be observed with the image intensifier. If it is insufficient, the injection can be repeated at an adjacent level.

Technique

The injection can be performed with the patient prone, or in a lateral position. The patient and the various anatomical landmarks are more stable in the prone position, and bilateral blocks can be performed easily. The prone approach is thus essentially the same for splanchnic nerve block, coeliac plexus block and lumbar sympathetic block at any level, the lateral approach being reserved for the patient who cannot lie prone.

An intravenous cannula is required for all patients, and facilities for the treatment of hypotension must be available, particularly if bilateral blocks are to be performed. Sedation with drugs such as alfentanil and midazolam is sufficient for most cases.

In 1926 Mandl described the classical approach, which depended upon needle contact with the transverse process to gauge depth (Mandl 1926, 1947). A more lateral approach, which was developed to avoid the transverse process altogether, was described by Reid and colleagues (1970). The transverse process can be visualized with an image intensifier and the needle inserted so as to miss this obstacle.

Prone position. With the image intensifier the spine of L₃ is identified and a point is marked 7–10 cm lateral to this, but midway between the transverse processes of L₃ and L₄ (Fig. 17.5). The skin and deeper tissues are infiltrated, a 15 cm

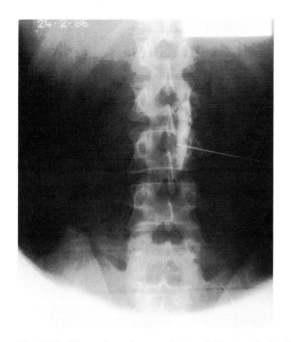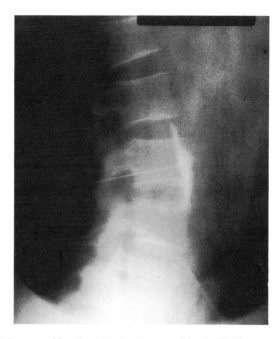

Fig. 17.6 Films taken after completion of injection for lumbar sympathectomy. Note how the dye has spread longitudinally from the single injection point.

20 g needle is inserted at this point and directed towards the side of the body of L3. The direction is at approximately 60° to the coronal plane. Once contact is made with the vertebral body, a lateral radiograph should be used to help manoeuvre the needle anteriorly. The needle tip should remain close to the vertebra and its final position should be level with the anterior edge of the vertebral body (Fig. 17.6). A characteristic click is often felt as the needle passes through the psoas fascia. An anteroposterior radiograph at this stage should show the needle point midway between the lateral edge of the vertebral body and its spine. Injection of contrast solution should demonstrate spread in the longitudinal axis alone without any lateral or posterior extension (Fig. 17.6). Injection into the psoas produces a characteristic pattern which radiates inferolaterally away from the vertebral body. Occasionally the solution will be 'whisked' away in a small vessel, even though aspiration tests were negative.

If the pattern of spread from the initial level of injection is satisfactory, then all the solution is injected. If the spread is unsatisfactory the same procedure is repeated one vertebral level above or below.

Lateral position. A major problem with this approach is ensuring that the patient's back is absolutely vertical so that the radiographs are truly anteroposterior and lateral. Once the patient is accurately positioned the procedure is basically as above.

Continuous block

An epidural catheter can be inserted into the prevertebral area and a continuous sympathetic block maintained by an infusion of local anaesthetic (Betcher et al 1953). Some authors recommend this prognostic block for up to 5 days as a prerequisite to neurolytic block (Lofstrom & Cousins 1988).

Choice of solution

A diagnostic block requires a small volume which has been precisely placed: 2–5 ml of

0.5% bupivacaine at each level should suffice. Therapeutic local anaesthetic injections may use 5–10 ml of 0.5% bupivacaine at a single level. Neurolytic injections should be made with 6.6% aqueous phenol or a stronger solution mixed with radiographic contrast medium. A volume of about 2–5 ml is usually satisfactory, but recommendations range from 0.1 to 10 ml (Boas 1983, Walsh et al 1984). The needle should be flushed with local anaesthetic before withdrawal to avoid leaving a track of phenol through more superficial tissues.

Complications

Major complications such as *inadvertent injection* of phenol into the *vertebral canal*, the *peritoneal cavity* or a *blood vessel* should not occur with a correct technique performed under radiographic control. Similarly, *needle or phenol damage* to the *kidney, renal pelvis, ureter* and *intervertebral discs* should also be avoidable. Injury to blood vessels in the posterior abdominal wall is not uncommon, but a significant retroperitoneal haematoma is unlikely in a patient with normal coagulation. However, phenol damage to blood vessels may explain some otherwise unaccountable neurological complications (Clarke 1984).

Mild backache is common and is likely to be more severe if neurolytic solution is deposited inadvertently in the posterior abdominal wall. Destruction of sympathetic fibres may cause a characteristic cramp-like burning pain and dysaesthesia in the anterior thigh – so-called 'sympathalgia' (Boas 1983) – which may also follow surgical sympathectomy (Tracy & Cockett 1957). A more definitive *neuritis* may be caused by spread of phenol to the genitofemoral nerve where it lies on the psoas. Occasionally other somatic nerves may be damaged by the needle or phenol. Treatment of both sympathalgia and neuritis may include carbamazepine or amitriptyline and TENS, but these are not always immediately effective and the patient will need to be reassured that remission should occur over a period of several weeks.

The vasodilatation that is produced by sympathectomy may result in *hypotension* especially in the elderly or after bilateral blocks. The blood pressure should be monitored for at least 2 hours after the procedure and the patient supervised during mobilization in case there is postural hypotension. Hypotension usually responds quickly to elevation of the legs so that vasopressors or intravenous fluids are rarely required. *Intravascular 'steal'* may occur after sympathectomy in arteriosclerotic patients and result in diversion of blood from compromised distal vessels into the more proximal cutaneous circulation.

Failure of ejaculation is a real risk after bilateral block and this must be explained to male patients (Baxter & O'Kafo 1984).

Coeliac plexus block

Anatomy (Figs 17.3 and 17.7)

The coeliac plexus , the largest of the prevertebral plexuses, is formed by the union of the greater $(T_5–T_{10})$, lesser $(T_{10}–T_{11})$ and least (T_{12}) splanchnic nerves, with the coeliac branch of the right vagus. It therefore contains both sympathetic and parasympathetic fibres. There are usually two semilunar ganglia at the level of the lower part of the 12th thoracic and the upper part of the first lumbar vertebra. The ganglia lie in the retroperitoneal tissue between the suprarenal glands, posterior to the stomach, pancreas and the left renal vein, anterior to the crura of the diaphragm, and mainly anterolateral to the aorta. The ganglia surround the origin of the coeliac and superior mesenteric arteries and bilateral injection is necessary to ensure a complete block.

Technique

The patient should lie prone on the radiography table as for lumbar sympathetic block. Using the image intensifier the spine and transverse processes of the first lumbar vertebra are identified and a point is marked 6–7 cm lateral to the spine, making sure that it is just inferior to the transverse processes and the 12th rib (Fig. 17.8). The skin and deeper tissues are infiltrated with local anaesthetic, a 15 cm 20 g needle is inserted at the marked point and directed towards the side of the

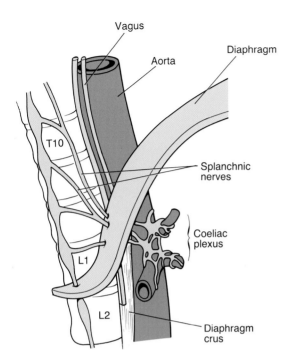

Fig. 17.7 Position of the coeliac plexus. Note that it lies more anterior than the sympathetic chain.

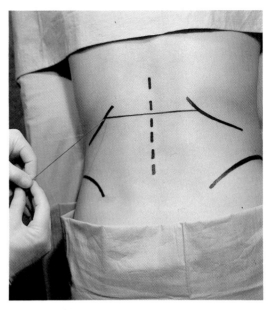

Fig. 17.8 Landmarks and needle alignment (patient supine, pictured from above) for coeliac plexus block. The posterior spines of T_{12}–T_5 have been marked.

body of L_1 (Fig. 17.9). The needle is likely to damage the kidney if the insertion point is more than 7 cm lateral to the spine (Moore et al 1981). The needle is advanced slightly cephalad and at 60° to the coronal plane. Once contact has been made with the vertebral body a lateral radiograph should be used to help manoeuvre the needle anteriorly. Its tip should be kept close to the vertebral body until it lies at the anterior edge of the body. A second needle is inserted on the opposite side.

The coeliac plexus lies more anterior than the sympathetic chain so the right needle should be advanced to lie about 1–2 cm anterior to the vertebral body, the left a little less because of the presence of the aorta. An anteroposterior radiograph at this stage should show the needle points situated medial to the lateral edge of the vertebra (Fig. 17.10). Injection of contrast solution should demonstrate spread in the longitudinal axis, without any lateral or posterior extension. Careful aspiration tests should precede the injection, which should be very easy – any resistance suggests that

the needle tip is in the wrong place. A small volume of local anaesthetic should be injected before the alcohol because the latter can be extremely uncomfortable. Sedation, or even general anaesthesia, is always necessary. Computerized tomography has been used during coeliac plexus block with great success (Filshie et al 1983).

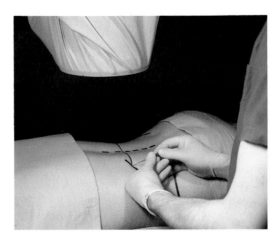

Fig. 17.9 Needle inserted for coeliac plexus block.

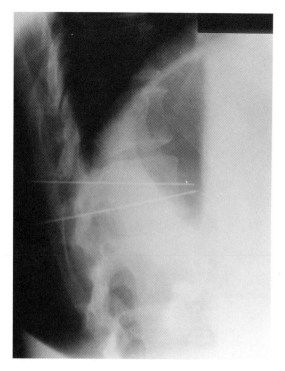 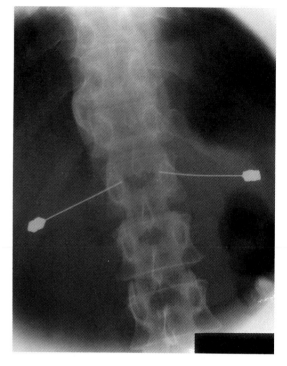

Fig. 17.10   Correct needle position for bilateral coeliac plexus block.

Choice of solution

Diagnostic and therapeutic local anaesthetic injections are performed with 20 ml of 0.25% plain bupivacaine on each side. Depot preparations of steroid can be added for chronic pancreatitis, although the value of this remains unproven (Kennedy 1983). For a neurolytic block up to 20 ml of 50% alcohol is injected on each side. Absolute alcohol can be diluted with 0.25% bupivacaine. Repeated aspirations tests must be performed and the dispersion of the contrast solution observed.

Complications

In general, the complications of coeliac plexus block are similar to those lumbar sympathectomy.

Hypotension is an almost inevitable consequence and it can persist for many days after neurolytic block. Intravenous fluids, support stockings, and bed rest are the first lines of treatment.

Blood vessel damage can be caused to the aorta and the coeliac or superior mesenteric arteries by the needle or alcohol.

Failure of ejaculation is a significant risk so neurolytic blocks must be avoided in young males or any man unwilling to accept this side-effect.

Splanchnic nerve block

Anatomy (Fig. 17.7)

The greater, lesser and least splanchnic nerves cross the lateral side of the body of T_{12} as they sweep forward to penetrate the diaphragm and form the coeliac plexus. The pleura lies lateral, and the crura of the diaphragm anterior to the nerves. The pleura attaches posteriorly to the vertebral bodies and creates a well-defined compartment (Boas 1983).

Technique

The patient should lie prone. Using the image intensifier the lateral end of the transverse process of L_1 is identified. The needle is inserted just lateral to it and is directed to pass beneath the 12th rib on to the side of the body of T_{12}. Using a lateral view the needle is manoeuvred until the tip is just posterior to the anterior edge of the vertebra. Injection of contrast will show that spread of dye is limited anteriorly and inferiorly by the crus of the diaphragm, and posteriorly by the attachment of the pleura to the vertebrae.

Choice of solution

Up to 15 ml of either bupivacaine or phenol can be injected using constant radiographic monitoring.

Complications

Pneumothorax may occur if the needle is not kept close to the side of the body of T_{12}.

Intravenous regional sympathetic blocks

Intravenous regional sympathetic block is a development of intravenous regional anaesthesia. It involves the injection of a drug into an exsanguinated limb isolated from the circulation by a tourniquet. Guanethidine (Hannington-Kiff 1974) is the drug most frequently used, but others include ketanserin (Davies et al 1987), bretylium (Ford et at 1988), reserpine (Lief et al 1987), labetalol (Parris et al 1987), hydralazine, methyldopa and droperidol. Guanethidine causes depletion of noradrenaline stores in sympathetic nerve endings. Complete repletion of these stores takes up to 10 days, but the effect of the block may persist for much longer.

The mode of action of the so-called intravenous regional sympathetic blocks is not well understood and the effects are not confined to the sympathetic nervous system (Loh et al 1980). The solution in which the active drug is dissolved, the tourniquet pressure and the ischaemic period may influence the final result (Glynn et al 1981, McKain et al 1983). When used to treat RSD a series of intravenous blocks may produce relief of longer duration than repeated sympathetic chain block (Bonelli et al 1983, Eriksen 1981). None of these treatments has been subjected to rigorous double-blind trial (Charlton 1990).

The blocks are easy to perform and may be used in the presence of anticoagulants. Pain arising from central lesions may be helped even though only the distal portion of the limb is blocked.

Technique

Firm scientific guidelines do not exist so there is wide variation in recommendations from different centres and choice is made on a purely empirical basis. The procedure involves essentially the same technique as for intravenous regional anaesthesia with local anaesthetic. Sedation may be necessary before the tourniquet is inflated and, if the limb is particularly sensitive, exsanguination with an Esmarch bandage may not be possible. It would seem reasonable to keep the tourniquet inflated for about 15 minutes. Reactive hyperaemia follows release of the tourniquet and the blood pressure should be carefully monitored. Prolonged hypotension (Sharpe et al 1987) may require active treatment.

It is impossible to give firm guidelines on the optimal frequency or the total number of blocks if a series is planned, but an interval of 1 week is often convenient. It may seem pointless continuing beyond 3–4 blocks if no benefit is apparent, although some authorities would disagree.

Choice of solution

For an arm, guanethidine 10–20 mg in up to 40 ml of 0.5% preservative-free prilocaine is used, and for a leg, guanethidine 20–30 mg in up to 50 ml of prilocaine.

Complications

Pain on injection may occur despite the use of the prilocaine. The onset may be immediate or it may develop during the period that the tourniquet is inflated.

Worsening of the presenting condition occurs occasionally and the patient returns next day with a painful, red, swollen hand or foot. In this case the block should not be repeated.

REFERENCES

Atkinson R S, Bushman G B, Lee J A 1982 A synopsis of anaesthesia, p 674. Wright, Bristol

Baxter A D, O'Kafo B A 1984 Ejaculatory failure after chemical sympathectomy. Anesthesia and Analgesia 63: 770–771

Betcher A M, Bean G, Casten D F 1953 Continuous procaine block of paravertebral sympathetic ganglions: observations on one hundred patients. Journal of the American Medical Association 151: 288–292

Boas R A 1983 The sympathetic nervous system and pain. In: Swerdlow M (ed) Relief of intractable pain, p 215–237. Elsevier, Amsterdam

Bonelli S, Conoscente F, Movilia P G, Rostelli L, Francucci B, Grossi E 1983 Regional intravenous guanethidine verses stellate ganglion blocks in reflex sympathetic dystrophy: a randomised trial. Pain 16: 297–307

Bristow A, Foster J M G 1988 Lumbar sympathectomy in the management of rectal tenesmoid pain. Annals of the Royal College of Surgeons of England 70: 38–39

Brown D L, Bulley C K, Quiel E L 1987 Neurolytic celiac plexus block for pancreatic cancer pain. Anesthesia and Analgesia 66: 869–873

Campbell J N, Raja S N, Meter R A 1988 Painful sequelae of nerve injury. In: Dubner R, Gebhart G F, Bond M R (eds) Proceedings of the Vth World Congress on Pain, pp 135–143. Elsevier, Amsterdam

Charlton J E 1990 Reflex sympathetic dystrophy: non-invasive methods of treatment. In: Stanton-Hicks M, Janig W, Boas R A (eds) Reflex Sympathetic Dystrophy, pp 151–164. Kluwer, Boston

Clarke I M C 1984 Nerve blocks. Clinics in Oncology 3: 181–193

Davies J A H, Beswick T, Dickson G 1987 Ketanserin and guanethidine in the treatment of causalgia. Anesthesia and Analgesia 66: 575–576

Defalque R J 1984 Axillary versus stellate ganglion blocks for reflex sympathetic dystrophy of the upper extremity. Regional Anesthesia 9: 35

Eriksen S 1981 Duration of sympathetic blockade. Stellate ganglion versus regional guanethidine block. Anaesthesia 36: 768–771

Filshie J, Golding S, Robbie D S, Husband J E 1983 Unilateral computerised tomography guided coeliac plexus block: a technique for pain relief. Anaesthesia 38: 498–503

Ford S R, Forrest W H, Eltherington L, 1988. The treatment of reflex sympathetic dystrophy with intravenous regional bretylium. Anesthesiology 68: 137–140

Foster J M G 1990 Personal communication.

Frost S A, Raja S N, Campbell J N, Meter R A, Khan A A 1988 Does hyperalgesia to cooling stimuli characterize patients with sympathetically maintained pain (reflex sympathetic dystrophy)? In: Dubner R, Gebhart G F,

Bond M R (eds) Proceedings of the Vth World Congress on Pain, pp 151–156. Elsevier, Amsterdam

Glynn C J, Basedow R W, Walsh J A 1981 Pain relief following postganglionic sympathetic blockade with iv guanethidine. British Journal of Anaesthesia 53: 1297–1302

Hannington-Kiff J G 1974 Intravenous regional sympathetic block with guanethidine. Lancet i: 1019–1020

Hardy P A J, Wells J C D 1987 Stellate ganglion blockade with bupivacaine: effect of volume on extent of sympathetic blockade. British Journal of Anaesthesia 59: 933P–934P

International Association for the Study of Pain 1986 Classification of chronic pain. Pain Supplement: 3

Janig W 1988 Pathophysiology of nerve following mechanical injury. In: Dubner R, Gebhart G F, Bond M R (eds) Proceedings of the Vth World Congress on Pain, pp 89–108. Elsevier, Amsterdam

Kennedy S F 1983 Celiac plexus steroids for acute pancreatitis. Regional Anesthesia 8: 39–40

Lief P A, Reisman R, Rocco A, McKay W, Kaul A, Benfell K 1987 IV regional guanethidine vs. reserpine for pain relief in reflex sympathetic dystrophy (RSD): a controlled, randomised, double-blind, crossover study. Pain Supplement 4: 398

Lofstrom B J, Cousins M J 1988 Sympathetic neural blockade of the upper and lower extremity. In: Cousins M J, Bridenbaugh P O (eds) Neural blockade, pp 461–500. Lippincott, Philadelphia

Loh L, Nathan W 1978 Painful peripheral states and sympathetic blocks. Journal of Neurology, Neurosurgery and Psychiatry 41: 664–671

Loh L, Nathan P W, Schott G D, Wilson P G 1980 Effects of regional guanethidine infusion in certain painful states. Journal of Neurology, Neurosurgery and Psychiatry 43: 446–451

Loh L, Nathan P W, Schott G D 1981 Pain due to lesions of central nervous system removed by sympathetic block. British Medical Journal 282: 1026–1028

McKain C W, Urban B J, Goldner J L 1983 The effects of intravenous regional guanethidine and reserpine. Journal of Bone and Joint Surgery (American) 65: 808–811

Malmqvist L-A, Bengtsson M, Bjornsson G, Jorfeldt L, Lofstrom J B 1987 Sympathetic activity and haemodynamic variables during spinal analgesia in man. Acta Anaesthesiologica Scandinavica 31: 467–473

Mandl F 1926 Die Paravertebrale Injektion. Springer Verlag, Vienna

Mandl F 1947 Paravertebral block. Heinemann, London

Manriquez R G, Pallares V 1978 Continuous brachial plexus block for prolonged sympathectomy and control of pain. Anesthesia and Analgesia 57: 128–130

Moore D C, Bash W H, Burnett L L 1981 Celiac plexus block: a roentgenographic, anatomic study of technique and spread of solution in patients and corpses. Anesthesia and Analgesia 60: 369–379

Parris W C V, Harris R, Lindsay K 1987 Use of intravenous regional labetalol in treating resistant sympathetic dystrophy. Pain Supplement 4: 399

Purcell-Jones G, Justins D M 1988 Delayed contralateral sympathetic blockade following chemical sympathectomy – a case history. Pain 34: 61–64

Reid W, Watt J K, Gray T G 1970 Phenol injection of the sympathetic chain. British Journal of Surgery 57: 45–50

Roberts W J 1986 A hypothesis on the physiological basis for causalgia and related pains. Pain 24: 297–311

Schott G D 1986 Mechanisms of causalgia and related clinical conditions. Brain 109: 717–738

Schwartzman R J, McLellan T L 1987 Reflex sympathetic dystrophy. A review. Archives of Neurology 44: 555–561

Schutzer S F, Gossling H R, Connecticut F 1984 The treatment of reflex sympathetic dystrophy syndrome. Journal of Bone and Joint Surgery 66 1(4): 625–629

Sharpe E, Milaszkiewicz R, Carli F 1987 A case of prolonged hypotension following intravenous guanethidine block. Anaesthesia 42: 1081–1084

Tracy G D, Cockett F B 1957 Pain in the lower limb after sympathectomy. Lancet i: 12–14

Umeda S, Arai T, Hatano Y 1987 Cadaver anatomic analysis of the best site for chemical lumbar sympathectomy. Anesthesia and Analgesia 66: 643–646

Walsh J A, Glynn C J, Cousins M J, Basedow R W 1984 Blood flow, sympathetic activity and pain relief following lumbar sympathetic blockade or surgical sympathectomy. Anaesthesia and Intensive Care 13: 18–24

Wang J K, Johnson K A, Tucker G T 1985 Sympathetic blocks for reflex sympathetic dystrophy. Pain 23: 13–17

Index

249